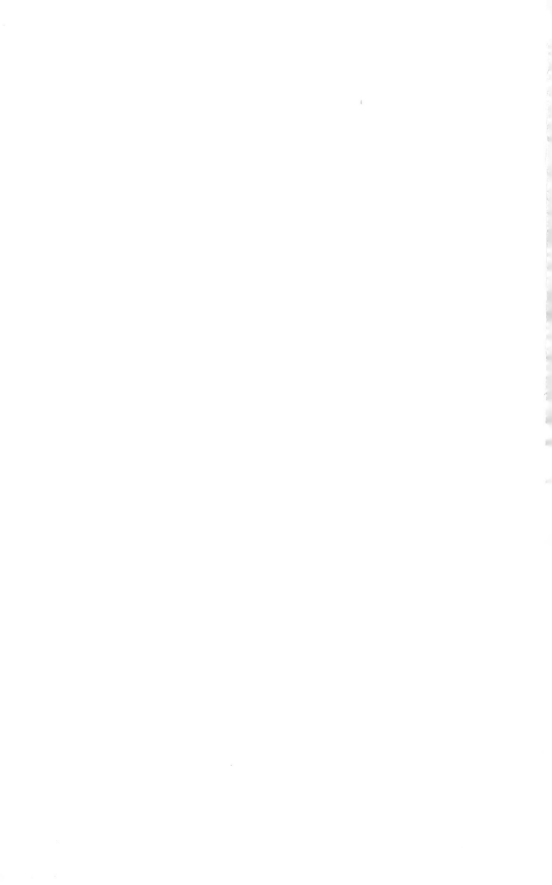

AIDS
CLINICAL REVIEW
2000/2001

AIDS CLINICAL REVIEW 2000/2001

edited by

Paul A. Volberding
Mark A. Jacobson

University of California, San Francisco, and
San Francisco General Hospital
San Francisco, California

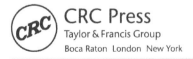

CRC Press
Taylor & Francis Group
Boca Raton London New York

CRC Press is an imprint of the
Taylor & Francis Group, an **informa** business

Preface

The HIV pandemic has stimulated a remarkable response from the biomedical scientific community. Basic science discoveries in the virology, immunology, and pharmacology of HIV disease have been made at an astonishing rate in the two decades since AIDS was first described. These biological insights have been quickly translated into new clinical management strategies that are being rapidly tested in prospective clinical trials and observational studies. The result is an exponentially growing mass of clinical research data that is being adapted by the physicians, nurses, microbiologists, therapists, pharmacists, and epidemiologists who deal directly with patients suffering from HIV disease. The HIV pandemic has generated a new subspecialty of medicine for these clinicians—one that combines elements of infectious diseases, virology, immunology, oncology, endocrinology, neurology, epidemiology, psychiatry, and the behavioral sciences. The need to disseminate the abundance of cutting-edge clinical research results to these practitioners in a timely and coherent manner is obvious.

Since 1989, the *AIDS Clinical Review* has attempted to meet the need for a single-volume update for HIV practitioners in which some of the most important and controversial clinical issues are discussed in depth. *AIDS Clinical Review 2000/2001* is the eighth in this series, focusing on specific areas in which important new advances have occurred in the diagnosis, therapy, and prevention of HIV infection and HIV-associated complications. Although less encyclopedic than a conventional textbook, the *Review* has the advantage of more rapid publication. All the chapters in this edition were written within one year of publication, an interval that compares favorably with that for a review article published in a major medical journal. However, unlike a series of review articles, the *Review* offers a broader perspective and a greater possibility of interdisciplinary insights. Thus, the editors seek in this volume to bridge the gap between journal review articles and book chapters.

Each *Review* author is an investigator directly involved in prospective clinical research relevant to his or her topic. Our authors have critically examined the results of the most recent clinical trials and observational studies, including results presented at scientific meetings but not yet published in peer review journals, as well as results of their own recent investigations. Finally, they have strived to identify important research questions for future investigators to ponder and answer. Hence, many of the most important issues surrounding recent HIV clinical research have been illuminated in this single-source reference for the worldwide clinical community that deals directly with HIV infection and disease.

The first chapter of the *2000/2001 Review*, by Tom Coates of the University of California, San Francisco, Anke Ehrhardt of Columbia University, and David Celentano of Johns Hopkins University, reviews the latest information concerning behavioral interventions to prevent HIV transmission. In the second chapter, Barbara Ensoli and Aurelio Cafaro of the Istituto Superiore di Sanità in Rome present an overview of the current status of HIV vaccine development, clarifying the substantive advancements that have been made and providing a realistic assessment of the potential efficacy and likely clinical limitations that vaccines will have. Ann Melvin and Lisa Frenkel of the University of Washington, Seattle, explore in Chapter 3 what is known about the mechanism of mother–child vertical HIV transmission and the striking results that short-term antiretroviral therapy has had in dramatically reducing the rate of vertical transmission. In Chapter 4, Rita Fahrner of San Francisco General Hospital assesses the risk of occupational HIV infection to health care workers and the efficacy of antiretroviral prophylaxis for workers who experience high-risk exposure to HIV-infected blood. Bruce Walker from Harvard draws an optimistic picture in Chapter 5 of the potential for preserving HIV-specific immunity when antiretroviral therapy is initiated early in the course of acute HIV infection. He also discusses the potential for restoring or enhancing HIV-specific immunity, a prospect that could ultimately reduce the need for antiretroviral drug treatment. Judith Aberg of Washington University in St. Louis explains in Chapter 6 the effect that new potent antiretroviral drug regimens have had in North America and Europe on reconstituting immunity against AIDS-associated opportunistic infections.

The next two chapters (7 and 8) deal specifically with the newly emerging antiretroviral regimens for treating HIV infection: strategies for extending long-term efficacy after initial virologic failure (Mary Albrecht from Harvard), and complex drug interactions that occur when these agents are combined with each other and with other drugs (Bradley Kosel and Francesca Aweeka from UCSF). In Chapter 9, Michael Lederman and Hernan Valdez from Case Western Reserve University in Cleveland explain the current state of knowledge regarding cytokine and other immune-based therapies for HIV disease. Finally, in Chapter 10, Bruce Polsky from St. Lukes–Roosevelt Hospital in New York and Arthur Kim and Raymond Chung from Harvard provide an exploration of the problem of hepatitis B and C coinfection with HIV. Globally prevalent chronic hepatitis infections may ultimately be more fatal than HIV for coinfected patients.

Our heartfelt thanks and acknowledgments are extended to the authors of the *2000/2001 Review*. These overworked investigators used a considerable part of what little leisure time they had remaining for families, friends, and sleep to make their personal contributions to this volume. We are confident that their efforts will improve the care of patients with HIV disease, and we salute their unstinting commitment to the ongoing scientific and medical challenges of HIV disease.

Mark A. Jacobson
Paul A. Volberding

Contents

Contributors

Judith A. Aberg, M.D. Director of HIV Services, AIDS Clinical Trials Unit, Washington University School of Medicine, St. Louis, Missouri

Mary A. Albrecht, M.D. Assistant Professor of Medicine, Harvard Medical School, and Division of Infectious Diseases, Beth Israel Deaconess Medical Center, Boston, Massachusetts

Francesca Aweeka, Pharm.D. Associate Clinical Professor of Pharmacy, Department of Clinical Pharmacy, San Francisco General Hospital, University of California, San Francisco, San Francisco, California

Aurelio Cafaro, M.D. Senior Investigator, Laboratory of Virology, Istituto Superiore di Sanità, Rome, Italy

David D. Celentano, Sc.D., M.H.S. Professor, Department of Epidemiology, Johns Hopkins University School of Public Health, Baltimore, Maryland

Raymond T. Chung, M.D. Assistant Professor of Medicine and Medical Director, Liver Transplant Program, GI Unit, Massachusetts General Hospital and Harvard Medical School, Boston, Massachusetts

Thomas J. Coates, Ph.D.   Professor of Medicine and Epidemiology, Department of Medicine, and Director, University of California, San Francisco, AIDS Research Institute, San Francisco, California

Anke A. Ehrhardt, Ph.D.   Professor of Medical Psychology and Director, Psychiatry and HIV Center for Clinical and Behavioral Studies, New York State Psychiatric Institute and Columbia University, New York, New York

Barbara Ensoli, M.D., Ph.D.   Chief, Retrovirus Division, Laboratory of Virology, Istituto Superiore di Sanità, Rome, Italy

Rita Fahrner, R.N., M.S., N.P.   Clinical Nurse Specialist, San Francisco General Hospital Occupational Health Service, and Assistant Clinical Professor, Department of Physiological Nursing, University of California, San Francisco, San Francisco, California

Lisa M. Frenkel, M.D.   Associate Professor, Departments of Pediatrics and Laboratory Medicine, University of Washington and Children's Hospital and Regional Medical Center, Seattle, Washington

Arthur Y. Kim, M.D.   Fellow in Infectious Diseases, Massachusetts General Hospital and Harvard Medical School, Boston, Massachusetts

Bradley W. Kosel, Pharm.D.   Clinical Pharmacology Research Fellow, Drug Research Unit, San Francisco General Hospital, and Department of Clinical Pharmacology, University of California, San Francisco, San Francisco, California

Michael M. Lederman, M.D.   Professor, Division of Infectious Diseases, Department of Medicine, Case Western Reserve University and University Hospitals of Cleveland, Cleveland, Ohio

Ann J. Melvin, M.D.   Assistant Professor, Division of Pediatric Infectious Diseases, Department of Pediatrics, University of Washington and Children's Hospital and Regional Medical Center, Seattle, Washington

Bruce Polsky, M.D.   Chief, Division of Infectious Diseases, Department of Medicine, St. Luke's-Roosevelt Hospital Center, New York, New York

Hernan Valdez, M.D. Assistant Professor, Division of Infectious Diseases, Department of Medicine, Case Western Reserve University and University Hospitals of Cleveland, Cleveland, Ohio

Bruce D. Walker, M.D. Professor of Medicine, Harvard Medical School; Director, Partners AIDS Research Center, Massachusetts General Hospital; and Brigham and Women's Hospital, Boston, Massachusetts

AIDS
CLINICAL REVIEW
2000/2001

1

Human Immunodeficiency Virus Prevention: Applying the Lessons Learned

Thomas J. Coates
University of California, San Francisco, AIDS Research Institute, San Francisco, California

Anke A. Ehrhardt
New York State Psychiatric Institute and Columbia University, New York, New York

David D. Celentano
Johns Hopkins University School of Public Health, Baltimore, Maryland

1

Because most new human immunodeficiency virus (HIV) infections world-wide result from unprotected sexual intercourse with an HIV-infected person, the continued development, evaluation, and implementation of innovative behavioral strategies to reduce sexual transmission of HIV remains a high priority. An extensive body of research has produced information on effective interventions to change behavior that puts individuals at risk for HIV infection (1–3). Moreover, several studies now demonstrate the efficacy of 'social and behavioral approaches in reducing new HIV and other sexually transmitted infections (4–7). The development and choice of a particular type of behavioral intervention depends on many factors (8). The goal may be primary (prevention of infection in uninfected individuals) or secondary (prevention of secondary sequelae of HIV infection or prevention of transmission from an infected to an uninfected person). The objective of the intervention may vary from increasing knowledge, to changing attitudes, to modifying risk behaviors, to health outcomes. A variety of models has been used to frame behavioral interventions (8). These models share their focus on the variables that are central to predict and understand a particular behavior of an individual. Alternative models are community-level structural models and social

expectation models focusing to a greater extent on environmental variables
(9). Behavior change is also influenced by age, gender, and a developmental
perspective (10). These theoretical models should not be seen as competitive with each other. Their usefulness depends on the purpose of the specific
intervention.

I. INTERVENTION STRATEGIES: LEVELS OF INTERVENTION

Six levels of causation and change combine biomedical, behavioral, and
social interventions for HIV prevention: individual, dyadic/familial, institu-
tional/community, policy/legal, superstructural, and medical/technological. A
variety of hypothesized mechanisms of action (Table 1) and potential change
strategies (Table 2) is possible (11).

A. Individual and Small-Group Counseling Interventions

Recent reviews have summarized the behavioral effects of a variety of interventions among diverse populations to decrease sexual transmission of HIV

Table 1   Levels of Causation and Change Determinants of HIV Transmission

Level definition examples

Individual
  How environment is experienced and acted upon by individuals; individual
    biological states, knowledge, risk perception, self-efficacy, levels of
    intoxication, biological determinants of sexual behavior, etc.
Dyadic/familial
  How couples interact and negotiate sexual and needle-sharing behavior; how
    families communicate regarding sexual behavior; implicit and explicit "rules"
    governing power and sexual relations
Institutional/community
  Social norms, resources, and opportunities, disease prevalence, access to
    condoms, needles, health care behavior, and norms of peers
Policy/legal
  Laws and policies, paraphernalia laws, discriminatory practices, inheritance laws,
    laws and policies regarding confidentiality
Superstructural
  Social and economic structures; widely held and pervasive societal customs and
    attitudes; social and economic restraints on women

Table 2 Levels of Causation and Change Mechanisms with
Intervention Examples

Level change mechanism examples

Individual
   Educational, motivational appeals, skills building, counseling, individual or small
      group strategies, drug and alcohol treatment
Dyadic/familial
   Skills building, couples counseling with or without testing, family skills training
Institutional/Community
   Community organization and mobilization, condom marketing and distribution,
      syringe distribution, access to care, peer outreach, syringe exchange, drug and
      alcohol treatment on demand
Policy/Legal
   Legislation and policy reform, legislating syringe exchange and
      antidiscrimination, anonymous testing, movements and laws
Superstructural
   Social movements, revolution antipoverty programs

including women; gay and bisexual men (including young gay men); college
students; adolescents in school-based and non-school-based settings; men and
women in sexually transmitted disease (STD) clinics, family planning clinics,
and prison settings; and injection drug users (11–14).

Four studies in particular have demonstrated that individual or small-group
counseling, sometimes combined with STD or HIV testing and diagnosis,
can reduce risk for HIV or STD transmission. Several randomized controlled
trials have been completed that demonstrate the effectiveness of social and
behavioral interventions for reducing risk behavior and STD incidence. Three
of these investigations were conducted in the U.S. (Project RESPECT, the
National Institute of Mental Health (NIMH) Multisite HIV Prevention Trial,
and the Texas Trial), whereas three others were conducted in international
settings (the Voluntary Counseling and Testing Efficacy Study, the Thai Army
trial, and the Zimbabwe Factory Workers Study).

1. Project RESPECT

Project RESPECT (5) was a longitudinal study of HIV testing and counseling methods among 5758 HIV-uninfected heterosexual STD clinic patients.
The study involved three face-to-face interventions: two brief informational
educational messages, HIV prevention counseling with two client-centered

sessions, and enhanced counseling with four sessions. The results showed that those in the two counseling arms were significantly more likely than those in the education-only arm to use condoms 100% of the time at 3-month follow-up and were 20% less likely to have an incident STD at 6-month follow-up. At 12-month follow-up, counseling participants continued to demonstrate reduced risk for acquiring new STDs.

2. The NIMH Multisite HIV Prevention Trial

The NIMH Multisite HIV Prevention Trial (6) intervention was conducted in a small-group multiple-session ($n = 7$) modality; its focus was on building skills and changing individual behavior. This controlled trial randomized 1679 heterosexual largely low-income African-American and Hispanic STD clinic patients in same-sex groups of 5 to 15 persons over the course of a year and compared self-reported risk behavior and incident STD infections with a control group of 1855 individuals who received a 1-hour acquired immunodeficiency syndrome (AIDS) education session. This intervention trial conducted in 37 clinics in seven cities showed a significant decrease in self-reported unprotected sexual behavior and a significant increase in reported condom use in the intervention group compared with the control group at 3-, 6-, and 12-month follow-up clinic visits. In addition, the men in the intervention condition were half as likely as the men in the control group to have been diagnosed with gonorrhea during the follow-up period. No significant difference in STD infection occurred among women.

3. The Texas Trial

University of Texas Health Science Center researchers conducted a behavioral intervention program among 424 Mexican-American and 193 African-American women to determine the effect of the intervention on rates of chlamydia and gonorrhea among the participants (7). The women were assigned to either an intervention or a control group, with the intervention group receiving three small-group sessions of 3 to 4 hours designed to aid the women in determining personal susceptibility, induce behavioral change, and develop the needed skills to enact the behavioral change. Both groups received sexually transmitted disease counseling and screening. Women in the intervention group had lower infection rates at 6-month and 12-month follow-up.

4. The Voluntary Counseling and Testing Efficacy Study

The VCT (15) was a study conducted in Kenya, Tanzania, and Trinidad in which individual participants were randomly assigned to receive either client-centered HIV voluntary counseling and testing (VCT) or basic health information (HI, a culturally appropriate video on HIV). A total of 3120 individuals (1534 males and 1586 females) were recruited with an overall retention rate of 82%. Approximately 30% of males and 24% of females reported unprotected intercourse with nonprimary partners at baseline. Follow-ups at 6 and 12 months after baseline showed the percentage of individuals reporting unprotected intercourse with nonprimary partners declined significantly more for those receiving VCT than those receiving HI (males, 39% reduction in VCT vs. 13% reduction in HI; females, 43% reduction in VCT vs. 25% reduction in HI). Among those assigned to VCT at baseline, persons who were diagnosed as HIV infected were more likely to change their sexual behavior than persons diagnosed as HIV uninfected. Self-reports of behavior were positively correlated with STD incidence. Furthermore, a 40% reduction in new STDs from baseline to first follow-up occurred among men but not among women. Among both men and women, a strong relationship existed between self-reported unprotected sexual intercourse and 6 month STD incidence, both among primary partners and among casual partners.

B. Couples Interventions

Specific interventions have taken advantage of relationship dynamics in preexisting dyads or small groups. In Rwanda, women received educational information and were tested for HIV infection; the male partners of 26% of these women also received the education and testing with their female partners. At 2-year follow-up, women whose male partners had received the intervention were 50% less likely to become infected with HIV than women whose partners had not received the intervention. HIV-infected women whose partners participated were 50% less likely to contract gonorrhea during the 2-year follow-up than infected women whose partners did not participate (16). Such results suggest that the efficacy of this intervention was strengthened by engaging both partners in the intervention as a couple rather than relying on individual women to enact risk-altering behavior.

A more recent randomized controlled study of voluntary HIV counseling and testing of 429 HIV discordant heterosexual married couples in Tanzania, Kenya, and Trinidad found that sexual risk was reduced at 6-month follow-up within couples but not with extramarital partners (15). This suggests that risk was reduced within the couple that was the focus of the intervention. Moreover, at 6-month follow-up, the percentage of those reporting unprotected intercourse with their spouse was greatly reduced for HIV discordant couples (from baseline of 100% to 45% at 6 months for those with an HIV-infected man; 79% to 50% for those with an HIV-infected woman) and concordant infected couples (75% to 38%).

C.   Institutional-Level Interventions

Institutional-level interventions that locate problem behavior at an organizational level assume that individuals' behavior is influenced by organizations that they are affected by or to which they belong. Examples of organizations where HIV preventive interventions might occur include schools, bathhouses or sex clubs, churches, injection drug user shooting galleries, workplaces, and correctional facilities. Possible interventions directed at prisons include condom distribution, methadone treatment availability, needle exchange, bleach distribution, education, compulsory testing, and segregation of HIV-infected prisoners (18–20).

1.   The Thai Army Project

During 1991–1993, HIV prevalence in northern Thai military conscripts was 11–13% and HIV incidence was 2.4% per year. A matched community design evaluated a behavioral intervention that sought to reduce HIV risk among men inducted into the Thai army (20). Military units were assigned to one of three groups matched on military mission at five military reservations: 450 conscripts were in the intervention group, 681 were in adjacent military units at the same base (diffusion group) who did not receive the intensive intervention, and 414 were in isolated control units. The preventive intervention was based on theories of social influence and participation, addressing sexual aspects of conscripts' lives. Utilizing the army's formal command structure and friendship groups, the intervention focused on increasing condom use, reducing alcohol consumption and brothel patronage, and improving sexual negotiation and condom-use skills. Over the 18 months of follow-up, nine HIV infections were documented in the combined control and diffusion conditions (no significant difference, $p = 0.90$) and two were identified in the intervention group ($p = 0.358$). Incident STDs were significantly less frequent among men assigned to the intervention than the controls (relative risk, 0.15; 95% confidence interval, 0.04–0.55), after adjusting for baseline risk factors. Intensive interventions in highly structured developing-country institutions can be successful in reducing risk in settings confronting rapidly expanding heterosexual HIV epidemics. This intervention has been adopted by and sustained in the army for all Thai conscripts.

2.   The Zimbabwe Factory Project

A workplace peer education program was evaluated for its efficacy in preventing HIV incidence in 40 factories in Harare, Zimbabwe. Workplaces were randomized to HIV counseling and testing alone (control) or HIV counseling and testing plus peer education (intervention). Peer educators distributed condoms and provided HIV/STD prevention messages to their coworkers. Cohorts of workers at each factory were followed up to 3 years to measure factory-specific HIV incidence. Overall, 94 HIV seroconversions were observed over 3831 person-years (py) of observation; the incidence among intervention factories (1.9 per 100 py) was lower than in control factories (2.8 per 100 py), approaching statistical significance ($p = 0.09$). When pooled, the HIV incidence was 34% lower in intervention than control factories ($p = 0.04$). A tendency existed for HIV incidence to be inversely correlated with factory-specific level of peer education activity ($p = 0.08$). These data suggest that workplace HIV interventions, including peer education, can be successful in preventing HIV infection (D. Katzenstein, personal communication, 1999).

3. School-Based Interventions

School-based interventions have been tested extensively, especially in the developed countries. Approximately 50 published studies have used experimental or quasi-experimental designs to examine the behavioral impact of curriculum-based school and community-education programs designed specifically to reduce sexual risk-taking behavior among young adults. For statistical reasons, most of these studies measured the impact on behaviors that are logically related to HIV and STD rates: age of initiation of intercourse, frequency of sexual activity, number of sexual partners, and condom use (21, 22).

4. Abstinence-Only Programs

Abstinence-only programs focus on the importance of abstinence from sexual intercourse, typically abstinence until marriage. Either these programs do not discuss contraception or they briefly discuss contraceptive failure to provide complete protection against pregnancy and STDs. Typically, these programs are implemented in middle school or the first years of high school. Despite these common qualities, abstinence-only programs are quite heterogeneous, varying in terms of their values (postponing sex vs. abstinence until marriage), their length (five sessions vs. 2 years), and the number and type of components (instruction vs. other kinds of youth activities). Five published studies (22–26) have measured the impact of abstinence programs on the initiation of sex. None found both a consistent and significant impact on delaying the onset of intercourse, and at least one study provided strong evidence that the program did not delay the onset of intercourse. This last study evaluated a program entitled "Postponing Sexual Involvement," a five-session curriculum implemented among thousands of middle school youth in California. Despite a rigorous evaluation design and large sample sizes, the curriculum did not affect the initiation of intercourse, the frequency of sex, the number of sexual partners, use of condoms, or use of other forms of contraception. Similarly, the other five studies also failed to find a significant impact on behavior. However, all had important methodological limitations that could have obscured program impact. Thus, given the heterogeneity of abstinence-only programs and the limitations of existing studies, it is not currently known whether abstinence-only programs delay the onset of intercourse.

5. Sexuality and HIV Education Programs

These programs differ from the abstinence programs in that they discuss both condoms and other methods of contraception as methods of providing protection against STDs or pregnancy. This group includes a wide variety of programs, ranging from sex or AIDS-education programs taught on high school or university campuses to programs taught in homeless shelters and detention centers. They reflect the considerable creativity and differing perspectives of these agencies. The studies of these programs strongly support the conclusion that sexuality and HIV education curricula do not increase sexual intercourse, either by hastening the onset of intercourse, increasing the frequency of intercourse, or increasing the number of sexual partners. Of the 16 evaluations of middle school, high school, or community sexuality or HIV-education programs that measured the impact of the programs on the initiation of intercourse, none found that their respective programs significantly hastened the onset of intercourse (27–34). Similarly, none of the 11 studies that examined the impact of programs on the frequency of intercourse found a significant increase, and none of the seven studies that examined impact on number of sexual partners found a significant increase.Thus, these data clearly demonstrate that sex and HIV education programs do not significantly increase sexual activity as some people have feared. Furthermore, studies indicate that some sexuality or HIV/AIDS-education programs reduced sexual risk-taking behavior, either by delaying the onset of intercourse, reducing the frequency of intercourse, or reducing the number of sexual partners.

At least seven sexuality or HIV-education programs have particularly strong evidence indicating positive change in behavior. They include "Be a Responsible Teen," which delayed the onset of intercourse, reduced the frequency of intercourse and the number of sexual partners, and increased use of condoms (35); "Be Proud, Be Responsible," which reduced the number of sexual partners, the frequency of sex, and the frequency of sex without condoms (30); "Focus on Kids," which increased condom use (36); "Get Real about AIDS," which reduced the number of sexual partners and increased condom use (37); "Reducing the Risk," which delayed the onset of intercourse (33); and

"Safer Choices," which increased condom use and decreased the frequency of unprotected sex schoolwide (38, 39). In addition to these six curricula for teenagers, evaluations of two college HIV-prevention programs have provided credible evidence that they reduced unprotected sex by increasing condom use (39, 40), and an evaluation of a community program for young African-American women provided evidence that it increased condom use.

D. Community-Level Interventions

The premise of interventions that focus on the community level is that social norms in communities affect individuals' behavior. Preventive interventions that promote community change often use a variety of modalities to address community-level influences on risk behavior. The major advantage of these interventions is that they have the potential to reach a large number of individuals, particularly those who are likely to be influenced by their communities. In addition, such interventions may have a lasting impact on community norms, thus providing environmental support for risk reduction for individuals who may benefit most from contextual reinforcement.

In a community-based study that focused on young gay men, an HIV-prevention program used a multiple-baseline design (41). The peer-led intervention consisted of community outreach, small groups, community organizing, and a publicity campaign and was successful in reducing the amount of unprotected anal intercourse with both primary and nonprimary sexual partners. The results of the study showed a decrease in prevalence of reported unprotected anal intercourse from 41% at baseline to 30% after the intervention, including a decrease from 20.2% to 11.1% with nonprimary sexual partners. In contrast, a comparison community that was randomized not to receive the intervention demonstrated no such change. This intervention relied heavily on empowerment theory and involved young gay men in important decision making and program implementation throughout the intervention process.

Other community-level interventions have been based on the theory of Diffusion of Innovations (42, 43). Compared with gay and bisexual men who engage in risky behavior, those who engage in less-risky sexual behavior are more likely to perceive social and peer norms that condemn risky behavior (44–47). The preventive intervention is delivered through an organizational-level modality and involves recruiting popular opinion leaders from gay bars and training them in how to communicate safer sex messages to their gay peers. These opinion leaders then visibly encourage and reinforce safer sex behavior in the bars. After excluding transients and men in exclusive relationships, substantial decreases in reported HIV sexual risk behavior and increases in reported condom use in men occurred in the intervention cities 1 year after the interventions, and no such changes occurred in men in the control cities.

Media campaigns to promote condom usage have also been successful at the community level. Although media efforts often ultimately define problems at an individual level (e.g., an HIV-prevention campaign stating "Get high, get stupid, get AIDS"), the actual presence of certain media efforts in and of themselves can represent changes in community norms. In particular, in communities where condom use is not a prominent topic, mass media social marketing can intervene to promote and normalize their use. In Zaire, for example, condom sales increased from less than 1 million per year in 1987 to over 18 million in 1991 after widespread social marketing of condoms. In Switzerland, the national government implemented a nationwide HIV-prevention campaign in 1987 that included the promotion of condoms. A primary goal of the intervention was to change community norms concerning condom use to encourage their use outside of stable monogamous relationships. Telephone surveys of random samples of the general Swiss population before and after the intervention indicated that condom use with nonprimary partners has increased steadily in all age groups but that the number of reported sex partners has not (48).

E. Policy/Legal-Level Interventions

The primary concept behind interventions at the societal/cultural level is that social structures shape individuals' access to resources that enable or impede behavior change. HIV risk behavior at this level is therefore viewed as a product of societal and cultural forces that influence individuals' lives. Policy changes or large-scale sociocultural changes are most often the modality by which these influences are targeted for intervention. A major policy change occurred when the United States blood supply began to be screened for HIV in March 1985. Before that time, many individuals (particularly hemophiliacs) were infected with HIV because of the presence of HIV in the blood supply; currently, however, only 1 in 450,000 to 660,000 donations per year are infectious for HIV but are not detected by currently available screening tests (49).

In Thailand, the government enacted a policy of mandatory condom use in brothels in 1990 (The 100% Condom Program), representing a major cultural change in that country. The policy was implemented through a partnership between brothel owners, police, and public health clinics. The brothel owners ensured that customers used condoms, the police threatened brothel closure if the policy was not followed, and the clinics tracked STD infections in sex workers as an indicator of policy adherence. The results of this policy change indicate that consistent condom use increased to over 90% among sex workers, whereas STDs declined by more than 75% (54). The effect of this policy change was also evaluated by studying five cohorts of young men conscripted into the military in Thailand. This study showed that the prevalence of HIV infection was about 11% before the policy change was enacted but fell to 6.7% afterward. The study further indicated that the men's reported use of condoms during their most recent sexual contacts with sex workers increased from 61% before the policy change to 92% afterward and that the prevalence of men with a history of STD decreased from 42% to 15.2% (50–52).

II. WHERE ARE THE NEEDS?

A.   Men Who Have Sex with Men (MSM)

New infections among MSM, especially MSM of color, remain the majority of new HIV infections in the United States. Although in the United States many studies have shown efficacy of reducing sexual risk behavior among MSM, no clinical trial that directly links behavioral indicators with HIV incidence has been conducted. Within the new HIV Prevention Trials Network, Project EXPLORE is a phase II-B study of 4350 MSM recruited and randomized to two conditions in seven HIVNET MSM sites. The intervention consists of 10 counseling sessions over a 3-month period followed by at least quarterly maintenance sessions over 3 years; the control condition is standard semiannual risk-reduction counseling as implemented in the HIV Vaccine Trials Network (HIVNET) Vaccine Preparedness Study (VPS). The intervention targets condom use and breakage, alcohol and drug use, and changes in specific sexual practices. All men will be followed for 3 years with the primary outcome of behavior change and HIV incidence.

B.   Inner-City Women at High Risk for HIV Infection

The HIVNET VPS sites have documented a high HIV incidence (1.5%) among enrolled women. Within the current HIVNET structure, preparatory work for a planned randomized controlled trial of a behavioral intervention for inner-city women has been ongoing. Such a trial would be based on a body of knowledge on how to best affect risk for HIV infection among women within the context of their relationships with high-risk men. The critical aspects of such a trial will include gender specificity of the curriculum, women's sexual risk behavior within their relationships context with men, and sexual risk in combination with substance use. Such a trial will include women's methods of protection (e.g., the female condom, microbicides). Trial outcomes will include biological markers in addition to reported behavior change, such as STDs and HIV incidence.

C. Young Women in Their Teens

Adolescent and young women, both in the United States and worldwide, are a high priority for HIV-prevention research. In adolescence, behavioral and biomedical factors act synergistically to dramatically increase the risk of sexually transmitted infections and their complications among sexually active individuals (10, 53). Behaviorally, young women are at high risk because of their inexperience and lack of access to barriers for sexual intercourse. In addition, many young women tend to have male partners who are several years older and thus at increased risk for being HIV infected. Such physiological vulnerability and emotional immaturity necessitate development of effective prevention programs that lead to delay of sexual intercourse, early and consistent use of barrier methods if intercourse is initiated, and health care behaviors that foster early detection of disease.

Prevention studies with young women and their male partners are needed domestically and internationally. Based on the evidence of family planning studies around the world and HIV-prevention successes in the United States and elsewhere, such studies with adolescents need to be comprehensive and multidisciplinary, that is, they need to include developmentally appropriate sexual behavioral approaches, educational and vocational efforts, and health care delivery. The potential payoff is high, because this is a critical time in the life cycle to make lasting behavioral effects, to effect economic independence, and to prevent infection with grave consequences for recurrence, infertility, and potentially a deadly disease.

D. Populations Whose Risk Behaviors Are Influenced by Alcohol

Substantial data exist to demonstrate the association between alcohol and/or nonintravenous substance use and HIV infection in the industrialized world and the developing world. Data from several studies in Africa suggest that alcohol use is an important risk factor for both high-risk sex and HIV infection itself. Unfortunately, no research in the developing world has attempted to intervene in alcohol-using social settings to reduce incident HIV infections. By studying how HIV infection and alcohol use are intertwined among heterosexuals in the developing world, important insights into how to disrupt the alcohol and high-risk sex association will be developed and proven by empirical tests. This research will have substantial value to help prevent the growing heterosexual epidemic in developing countries, as well as in the United States.

E. HIV-Infected Persons

Despite strong support for the efficacy of VCT interventions, the fact remains that a considerable proportion of people do not alter risk behavior after HIV-1 diagnosis. In the United States and other Western societies, many people who are diagnosed with HIV-1 reduce risk of exposure to others after HIV testing and counseling (54). Even so, 40% of heterosexuals (55–56) and 50% of gay and bisexual men (63, 64) engage in unprotected sexual practices that confer risk of transmission after HIV-1 diagnosis. Many of these contacts occur with partners whose serostatus is negative or unknown. One explanation for these findings is that patterns of sexual behavior conferring risk for HIV-1 infection are highly reinforcing, strongly motivated, and enduring (57–62).

Continued sexual risk behavior in the face of HIV-1 infection has been well documented in developing African countries as well. As many as 43% of serodiscordant Rwandan couples continue to practice unprotected intercourse 2 years after HIV-1 diagnosis. Similarly, despite demonstrating behavior change after an intensive VCT with monthly booster sessions, Kamenga et al. (63) found that up to 38% of serodiscordant Zairian couples reported unprotected sexual intercourse at follow-up. In both cases, relapse to unprotected sex was highest among discordant couples in which males were the infected partner.

The Voluntary Counseling and Testing Efficacy Study (15) used univariate and multivariate analyses to identify demographic, cognitive, health, and relationship variables associated with continued sexual risk behavior among HIV-1-infected individuals. We found that women were more likely to continue unprotected vaginal intercourse with primary partners if they were married, involved in newer relationships, had more economic resources, perceived greater difficulty in negotiating condom use, and reported more relationship conflict. Men who were married, involved in newer relationships, reported fewer HIV-associated symptoms, consumed alcohol before sex, and had less concern about being HIV-1 infected were more likely to continue unprotected intercourse after diagnosis (64).

Obviously, this is an area of great concern, because no infections can occur without sexual or parenteral encounters with an HIV-infected person. Understanding better the dynamics of unsafe encounters in both the developed and developing worlds and developing interventions to address these dynamics are essential research imperatives.

III. WHAT CAN WE RECOMMEND NOW?

Expert panels and plentiful data support the potential of a variety of strategies for preventing the transmission of HIV-1. The U.S. Presidential Administration's fiscal year 2001 budget is requesting increases in funds for HIV prevention and care in the developing world of a magnitude not realized to date in the epidemic. Others (e.g., Senator Barbara Boxer from California) have proposed increases of $2 billion for the prevention of HIV disease worldwide, with half of it going to sub-Saharan Africa. Some despair, and indicate that we should wait for the vaccine and do what we can in the meantime. But the data suggest otherwise. The data point clearly to the kinds of programs that, if implemented with sufficient intensity and continuity, could break the epidemic in the developed and developing worlds.

We know what does not work: one-time education programs, abstinence-only programs, programs of testing without counseling, and programs without sufficient comprehensiveness to make a difference.

Targeted education aimed at a particular at-risk community is one critical key to inducing people to engage in preventive practices. In San Francisco, for example, information about HIV transmission and safer sex was made available at centers of gay society and in the media.

Counseling with or without testing for HIV or STDs is another strategy proven to be effective in reducing risk behaviors among both infected and uninfected individuals. *Programs in institutions such as the military, workplaces, and prisons* can be quite effective in mobilizing large populations to HIV risk reduction.

School sex education has been shown to promote safer sex and even to decrease sexual activity among young people. *Peer influence and communitiy mobilization* are excellent complements to more general education of an at-risk group. *Advertising and marketing* can also change a community norm, making condoms more acceptable to a population that may previously have avoided using them.

Easing access to condoms is another way to increase their use—both by giving them away and by making them less embarrassing to buy. A study in Washington, DC found that one third of stores still kept condoms behind the counter, forcing a prospective purchaser to request the product. Further lessening the likelihood of condoms eventually being used was resistance or condemnation encountered by adolescent girls 40% of the time when trying to buy condoms. At a drug-abuse treatment center, condoms were almost five times as likely to be taken from private restrooms as from a public waiting area. Clearly, the perception of privacy encourages the acquisition of condoms.

IV. CONCLUSION

The difficulty with HIV prevention in the world is not lack of know-how but rather lack of resolve to provide the resources necessary to get the job done and lack of political conviction to implement the strategies known to be effective. These two elements need as much work as new scientific discoveries.

REFERENCES

1. Coates TJ, Faigle M, Koijane J, Stall RD. Does HIV prevention work for men who have sex with men? Washington, DC: Office of Technology Assessment Report, U.S. Congress, 1995.

2. Interventions to Prevent HIV Risk Behaviors. NIH Consensus Development Conference. Bethesda, MD: NIH, 1997.

3. Fiscal Year 1999 National Institutes of Health Plan for HIV-Related Research. Bethesda, MD: NIH Office of AIDS Research, 1998.

4. Ehrhardt AA, Fishbein M, Washington E, Smith W, Holmes KK. The NIAID Study Group on Integrated Behavioral Research for Prevention and Control of Sexually Transmitted Diseases. Part II. Issues in designing behavioral interventions. Sex Transm Dis 1990;17:204–207.

5. Kamb M, Fishbein M, Douglas J, Rhodes F, Rogers V, Bolan G, Zenilman J, Hoxworth T, Malotte CK, Iatesta M, Kent C, Lentz A, Graziano S, Byers RH, Peterman TA. Efficacy of risk-reduction counseling to prevent human immunodeficiency virus and sexually transmitted diseases. JAMA 1998;280:1161–1167.

6. NIMH Multisite HIV Prevention Trial Group. A randomized clinical trial of small group counseling to reduce risk for HIV. Science 1998;280:1889–1894.

7. Shain RN, Piper J, Newton E, et al. A randomized, controlled trial of a behavioral intervention to prevent sexually transmitted disease among minority women. N Engl J Med 1999;340(2):93–100.

8. Fishbein M, Bandura A, Triandis HC, et al. Factors Influencing Behavior and Behavior Change: Final Report. Theorists' Workshop. Rockville, MD: NIMH, 1992.

9. Hornick R. Alternative models of behavior change. In: Wasserheit JN, Aral SO, Holmes KK, Hitchcock PJ, eds. Research Issues in Human Behavior and Sexually Transmitted Diseases in the AIDS Era. Washington, DC: American Society for Microbiology, 1992:201–218.

10. Ehrhardt AA, Wasserheit JN. Age, gender, and sexual risk behaviors for sexually transmitted diseases in the United States. In: Wasserheit JN, Aral SO, Holmes KK, Hitchcock PJ, eds. Research Issues in Human Behavior and Sexually Transmitted Diseases in the AIDS Era. Washington, DC: American Society for Microbiology, 1992:97–121.

11. Waldo C, Coates TJ. Multiple levels of analysis and intervention in HIV prevention science: exemplars and direction for new research. AIDS, in press.

12. Coates TJ, Collins C. HIV prevention: a 10-point program to protect the next generation against HIV disease. Sci Am 1998;279:76–77.

13. Coates TJ, Chesney M, Folkman S, Hulley SB, Haynes-Sanstead K, Lurie P, Marin BV, Roos L, Bunnett V, Du Wors R. Designing behavioural and social science to impact practice and policy in HIV prevention and care. Int J STD AIDS 1996;7(suppl 2):2–12.

14. Coates TJ, Bayer R, Gutzwiller F, Des Jarlais D, Kippax S, Schechter M, van den Hoek JAR. HIV prevention in developed countries. Lancet 1996;348:1143–1148.

15. Voluntary HIV-1 Counseling and Testing Efficacy Study Group. HIV-1 risk reduction among individuals and couples receiving HIV-1 voluntary counseling and testing in three developing countries: the Voluntary HIV-1 Counseling and Testing Efficacy Study. Lancet, in press.

16. Allen S, Serufilira A, Bogaerts J, et al. Confidential HIV testing and condom promotion in Africa. Impact on HIV and gonorrhea rates. JAMA 1992;268:3338–3343.

17. Des Jarlais DC, Perlis T, Friedman SR, Deren S, Chapman T, Sotheran JL, Tortu S, Beardsley M, Paone D, Torian LV, Beatrice ST, DeBernardo E, Monterroso E, Marmor M. Declining seroprevalence in a very large HIV epidemic: injecting drug users in New York City, 1991 to 1996. Am J Public Health 1998;88(12):1801–1806.

18. Dolan K, Wodak A, Penny R. AIDS behind bars: preventing HIV spread among incarcerated drug injectors [editorial]. AIDS 1995;9:825–832.

19. Nelles J, Harding T. Preventing HIV transmission in prison: a tale of medical disobedience and Swiss pragmatism. Lancet 1995;346:1507–1508.

20. Celentano D, Bond K, Lyles C, Eiumtrakul S, Gio V, Beyrer C, Chaingmai C, Nelson K, Khamboonruang C, Vaddhanaphuti C. Prevention Intervention to

Reduce Sexually Transmitted Infections; A Field Trial in the Royal Thai Army. Arch Intern Med Feb. 28, 2000; 160:536–540.

21. Youth and HIV/AIDS: an American agenda. Washington DC: Office of National AIDS Policy, 1996.

22. Kirby D. Evaluation of Education Now and Babies Later (ENABL): Final Report. Berkeley, CA: Family Welfare Research Group, School of Social Welfare, University of California at Berkeley; Scotts Valley, Calif. : Research Dept., ETR Associates; 1995.

23. Christopher FS, Roosa MW. An evaluation of an adolescent pregnancy prevention program: is "just say no" enough? Family Relations 1990;39:68–72.

24. Jorgensen SR, Potts V, Camp B. Six-month follow-up of a pregnancy prevention program for early adolescents. Family Relations 1993;42:401–406.

25. Pierre TLS, Mark MM, Kaltreider DL, Aikin KJ. A 27-month evaluation of a sexual activity prevention program in Boys & Girls Clubs across the nation. Family Relations 1995;44:69–78.

26. Roosa MW, Christopher FS. Evaluation of an abstinence-only adolescent pregnancy prevention program: a replication. Family Relations 1990;39:363–367.

27. Eisen M, Zellman GL, McAlister AL. Evaluating the impact of a theory-based sexuality and contraceptive education program. Family Planning Perspect 1990; 22:261–271.

28. Ekstrand M, Seigel D, Nido V, et al. Peer-Led AIDS Prevention Delays Initiation of Sexual Behaviors among U.S. Junior High School Students. 11th International Conference on AIDS. Vancouver, Canada, 1996.

29. Howard M, McCabe JB. Helping teenagers postpone sexual involvement. Family Planning Perspect 1990;22:21–26.

30. Jemmott JBD, Jemmott LS, Fong GT. Reductions in HIV risk-associated sexual behaviors among black male adolescents: effects of an AIDS prevention intervention. Am J Public Health 1992;82:372–377.

31. Kipke MD, Boyer C, Hein K. An evaluation of an AIDS risk reduction education and skills training ARREST program. J Adolesc Health 1993;14:533–539.

32. Kirby D. Sexuality Education: An Evaluation of Programs and Their Effects. Santa Cruz, CA: ETR/Network Publications, 1984.

33. Kirby D, Barth RP, Leland N, Fetro JV. Reducing the risk: impact of a new curriculum on sexual risk-taking. Family Planning Perspect 1991;23:253–263.

34. Kirby D, Korpi M, Adivi C, Weissman J. An impact evaluation of project SNAPP: an AIDS and pregnancy prevention middle school program. AIDS Educ Prevent 1997;9:44–61.

35. St. Lawrence JS, Brasfield TL, Jefferson KW, Alleyne E, O'Bannon RER, Shirley A. Cognitive-behavioral intervention to reduce African American adolescents' risk for HIV infection. J Consult Clin Psychol 1995;63:221–237.

36. Stanton BF, Li X, Galbraith J, Feigelman S, Kaljee L. Sexually transmitted diseases, human immunodeficiency virus, and pregnancy prevention. Combined contraceptive practices among urban African-American early adolescents. Arch Pediatr Adolesc Med 1996;150:17–24.

37. Main DS, Iverson DC, McGloin J, et al. Preventing HIV infection among adolescents: evaluation of a school-based education program. Prevent Med 1994; 23:409–417.

38. Basen-Engquist K, Parcel GS, Harrist R, et al. The safer choices project: methodological issues in school-based health promotion intervention research. J School Health 1997;67:365–371.

39. Basen-Engquist K. Evaluation of a theory-based HIV prevention intervention for college students. AIDS Educ Prevent 1994;6:412–424.

40. Fisher JD, Fisher WA, Misovich SJ, Kimble DL, Malloy TE. Changing AIDS risk behavior: effects of an intervention emphasizing AIDS risk reduction information, motivation, and behavioral skills in a college student population. Health Psychol 1996;15:114–123.

41. Kegeles SM, Hays RB, Coates TJ. The Empowerment Project: a community-level HIV prevention intervention for young gay men. Am J Public Health 1996; 86:1129–1136.

42. Kelly JA, Murphy DA, Sikkema KJ, et al. Randomized, controlled, community-level HIV-prevention intervention for sexual-risk behavior among homosexual men in U.S. cities. Community HIV Prevention Research Collaborative. Lancet 1997;350:1500–1505.

43. Rogers EM. Diffusion of Innovations. New York: Free Press, 1983.

44. Fisher JD, Misovich SJ. Evolution of college students' AIDS-related behavioral responses, attitudes, knowledge, and fear. AIDS Educ Prevent 1990;2:322–337.

45. Joseph JG, Montgomery SB, Emmons C-A, Kessler RC, et al. Magnitude and determinants of behavioral risk reduction: longitudinal analysis of a cohort at risk for AIDS. Psychol Health 1987;1:73–95.

46. Kelly JA, St. Lawrence JS, Brasfield TL, Stevenson LY, Diaz YE, Hauth AC. AIDS risk behavior patterns among gay men in small southern cities. Am J Public Health 1990;80:416–418.

47. McCusker J, Stoddard AM, Zapka JG, Zorn M, Mayer KH. Predictors of AIDS-preventive behavior among homosexually active men: a longitudinal study. AIDS 1989;3:443–448.

48. Dubois-Arber F, Jeannin A, Konings E, Paccaud F. Increased condom use without other major changes in sexual behavior among the general population in Switzerland. Am J Public Health 1997;87:558–566.

49. CDC. U.S. Public Health Service guidelines for testing and counseling blood and plasma donors for human immunodeficiency virus type 1 antigen. MMWR Morb Mortal Wkly Rep 1996;45:1–9.

50. Hanenberg RS, Rojanapithayakorn W, Kunasol P, Sokal DC. Impact of Thailand's HIV-control programme as indicated by the decline of sexually transmitted diseases. Lancet 1994;344:243–245.

51. Rojanapithayakorn W, Hanenberg R. The 100% condom program in Thailand. AIDS 1996;10:1–7.

52. Nelson KE, Celentano DD, Eiumtrakol S, et al. Changes in sexual behavior and a decline in HIV infection among young men in Thailand. N Engl J Med 1996; 335:297–303.

53. Exner TM, Seal DW, Ehrhardt AA. A review of HIV interventions for at-risk women. AIDS Behav 1997;1:93–124.

54. Weinhardt LS, Carey MP, Johnson BT, Bickham, NL. Effects of HIV counseling and testing on sexual risk behavior: a meta-analytic review of published research, 1985–1997. Am J Public Health 1999;89:1397–1405.

55. Clark RA, Kissinger P, Bedimo AL, Dunn P, Albertin H. Determination of factors associated with condom use among women infected with human immunodeficiency virus. Int J STD AIDS 1997;8:229–233.

56. Eich-Hoechli D, Niklowitz MW, Clement U, Luethy R, Opravil M. Predictors of unprotected sexual contacts in HIV-infected persons in Switzerland. Arch Sex Behav 1998;27:77–90.

57. Marks G, Cantero PJ, Simoni JM. Is acculturation associated with sexual risk behaviours? An investigation of HIV-positive Latino men and women. AIDS Care 1998;10:283–295.

58. Skurnick JH, Abrams J, Kennedy CA, Valentine SN, Cordell JR. Maintenance of safe sex behavior by HIV-serodiscordant heterosexual couples. AIDS Educ Prevent 1998;10:493–505.

59. Lemp GF, Hirozawa AM, Givertz D, Nieri GN, Anderson L, Lindegren ML, Janssen RS, Katz M. Seroprevalence of HIV and risk behaviors among young homosexual and bisexual men: The San Francisco/Berkeley young men's survey. JAMA 1994:272:449–454.

60. Posner SF, Marks G. Prevalence of high-risk sex among HIV-positive gay and bisexual men: a longitudinal analysis. Am J Prevent Med 1996;12:472–477.

61. Ekstrand ML, Coates TJ. Maintenance of safer sexual behaviours and predictors of risky sex: the San Francisco Men's Health Study. Am J Public Health 1990; 180:973–977.

62. Kelly JA, Kalichman SC. Reinforcement value of unsafe sex as a predictor of condom use and continued HIV/AIDS risk behavior among gay and bisexual men. Health Psychol 1998;17:328–335

63. Kamenga M, Ryder R, Jingu M, Mbuyi N, Mbu L, Behets F, Brown C, Heyward WL. Evidence of marked sexual behavior change associated with low HIV-1 seroconversion in 149 married couples with discordant HIV-1 serostatus: experience at an HIV counselling center in Zaire. AIDS 1991;5:61–67.

64. Forsyth A, Coates TJ, Sangiwa MG, Balmer D, Furlonge C, Gregorich S. Predictors of risky behavior among HIV-infected persons: the Voluntary HIV-1 Counseling and Testing Efficacy Study. Health Psychol, in press.

2

Novel Strategies Toward the Development of an Effective Vaccine to Prevent Human Immunodeficiency Virus Infection or Acquired Immunodeficiency Virus

Barbara Ensoli and Aurelio Cafaro

Istituto Superiore di Sanità, Rome, Italy

The inexorable spread of the human immunodeficiency virus (HIV) pandemic and the increasing deaths caused by acquired immunodeficiency syndrome (AIDS) in developing countries underscore the urgency for an effective, safe, and inexpensive vaccine against HIV. Although many attempts have been made, a candidate vaccine of proven efficacy and safety in nonhuman primate models is not yet available. This is mostly due to HIV envelope (Env) variability and to the difficulty of eliciting high titers of long-lasting neutralizing antibodies capable of blocking entry of different virus strains. Nevertheless, new strategies have been developed and new information is now available that can lead to new concepts and open new avenues to obtain an effective vaccine against HIV infection.

I. HOW AIDS VACCINE STRATEGIES HAVE EVOLVED FROM STERILIZING IMMUNITY TO THE CONTROL OF INFECTION

Over the last 15 years, most efforts in HIV vaccine development have been based on the envelope protein (Env) of HIV that is responsible for the binding and entry of the virus, with the rationale of generating neutralizing antibodies (NA) capable of inducing sterilizing immunity and protection. However, results from studies in nonhuman primate models have been largely disappointing because of the inability of such vaccines to elicit NA at titers necessary to block infection with homologous viruses or to elicit NA against viruses isolated from infected individuals (primary isolates). The reasons are several (Table 1) but are mostly related to the Env variability (1), which hampers recognition by NA that are generally directed against conformational epitopes (reviewed in Reference 2).

Moreover, partly due to the heavy glycosylation of the key envelope protein (gp120), neutralizing Env epitopes are poorly exposed even on the oligomeric form of the viral envelope (a recombinant form, conformationally indistinguishable from the spikes present on native virions). In fact, even in the course of the natural infection, titers of NA are relatively low, indicating that the relevant epitopes are poorly exposed or weakly immunogenic. However, a sterilizing immunity is conceptually possible. In this respect, experiments of passive immunization in nonhuman primates have demonstrated that NA generated during natural infection are protective (when transferred in a naive animal); however, this occurs only at very high antibody titers (3) that are approximately 1000-fold higher than those present in sera from most HIV-1-infected humans or simian/human immunodeficiency virus (SHIV)-infected monkeys (4–6). In addition, these antibodies are poorly cross-reactive (7) and therefore effective only against infection with homologous virus.

Sterilizing immunity has been obtained upon passive immunization of adult and newborn macaques with a mixture of three human monoclonal antibodies (MAb) directed against neutralizing epitopes of Env. These animals were challenged intravenously (adults) or orally (newborns) with a homologous SHIV (SHIV-*vpu*+) encoding the *env* gene of HIV-IIIB (8). Of note, the synergy among the MAbs allowed neutralization at antibody con-

Table 1 Problems in the Development of an Effective HIV Vaccine

Poor understanding of the correlates and mechanisms of protection
   against HIV
Extreme virus sequence variability due to mutations and recombinations
Rapid and persistent virus replication
Latent infection
Persistent immunity appears to require persistent antigen expression
Live attenuated viral vaccines may revert to a pathogenic form

centrations significantly lower than those needed with each MAb alone (9). The importance of infusing a mixture of antibodies also comes from another study in which protection against a mucosal challenge with the pathogenic SHIV89.6PD was greater in the group that received 3 different antibody preparations (4 out of 5 monkeys) than in the group treated with 2 (2/5) or 1 (2/4) (10). Moreover, the passively immunized monkeys that were not protected experienced a milder infection and did not develop the severe loss of CD4 cells observed in the control animals, indicating a partial containment of the infection. Notably, the level of protection was higher than that obtained after intravenous challenge (11), suggesting that antibodies are more effective when a physical barrier (i.e., the vaginal mucosa) separates the virus from target cells. Exactly where and how these antibodies neutralize the virus is presently unknown (12). Thus, sterilizing immunity is achievable, even against mucosal challenge and in the absence of antiviral secretory IgA. Nevertheless, the identification of broadly represented neutralizing epitopes and/or the induction of high titers, long-lasting NA are still major obstacles to the development of an effective sterilizing vaccine based on Env (13).

Hope comes from a new approach (14) utilizing a modified (fusion-competent) version of the native Env that, at least in mice, has induced broadly cross-reactive NA, suggesting that sterilizing immunity could be achieved with novel Env-based vaccine strategies.

The most compelling evidence that it is possible to generate a protective immune response against different HIV strains comes from studies in nonhuman primates vaccinated with live attenuated SIV and protected from heterologous challenges with highly pathogenic strains (15–18). However, ethical concerns and the appearance of revertant pathogenic viruses in vaccinees (19–21) presently hamper their use in humans (Table 1). Nevertheless, this approach provides a model to study the correlates and mechanisms of protection and supports the concept for strategies in which the gene for one or more viral antigens is expressed in the host. These include naked DNA or live vectors expressing Env alone or associated with other viral genes.

Examples of some of these strategies include modified vaccinia virus Ankara (MVA), canarypox, fowlpox, adenoviruses, and alphaviruses that are being investigated with different modalities of immunization (i.e., combined prime-boost regimens) in nonhuman primate models with SIV or SHIV (reviewed in Reference 22). These approaches have a variety of advantages, including better delivery and potency of immunization. For example, most of these vectors, as well as naked DNA, contain unmethylated CpG sequences that can also boost the innate immunity favoring a Th1-type of specific immune response and CD8-mediated antiviral activity (CAF), including beta chemokines production. This type of response appears to contribute in protection both after vaccination or during natural infection (23, 24). Moreover, live vectors can be utilized to induce a mucosal immunization, a strategy particularly important to blocking virus transmission.

Results from these approaches have provided key information for vaccine development. Although in most cases no sterilizing immunity was obtained with homologous or heterologous virus challenge, lower plasma viremia levels were observed after high-dose virus challenge. Thus, the control of infection can be achieved in the absence of NA. In most cases, protection correlated with a Th-1 type of immune response, including cytotoxic T lymphocytes (CTLs), whose relevance for protection has progressively increased as opposed to NA (25–27). Thus, new promising strategies have been formulated based on the construction of a single "minigene" encoding multiple viral major histocompatibility complex (MHC) class I restricted epitopes capable of inducing CTLs (termed polyepitope or polytope CTL) (28).

Because sterilizing immunity against different virus strains has not yet been achieved with Env-based vaccines, secondary endpoints in HIV vaccine development are acquiring more importance and have led to the concept that control of viral infection and blocking disease onset may be a more achievable goal of AIDS vaccine strategies.

In this respect, recent approaches aimed at eliciting immunity against the HIV regulatory gene products Tat, Rev, and Nef have provided exciting results. In particular, Tat (29, 30) or Tat and Rev (31) vaccination appear capable of controlling primary infection with highly pathogenic viruses, providing the first evidence of cross-protection in nonhuman primates. Similarly, immunization of macaques with a recombinant vaccinia expressing SIV-Nef generated enough cytolytic (CTLs) and monolytic (CAF) antiviral activities to control subsequent infection with a homologous strain (32). Vaccination with Tat, Rev, and Nef has also been investigated in mice (33) and in HIV-1 infected humans (34), providing evidence of safety, immunogenicity of both protein and DNA vaccination.

Such strategies target regulatory proteins that are the first to be expressed after infection and are essential for viral replication, infectivity, and pathogenesis. In particular, because of its release upon infection and its extracellular functions (35–38), Tat may represent an optimal candidate for such a strategy. Tat and Rev also have the major advantage of being highly conserved throughout viral clades (1). In addition, these strategies can be used for both preventive and therapeutic vaccination.

Another concept involves natural immunity boosted by the sole vector. This appears to contribute to protection achieved with different vaccine strategies (live attenuated, fowlpox, DNA, Tat protein; see below). Of note, the same type of immunity and antiviral activity is induced by alloimmunization (reviewed in Reference 39) that although nonvirus-specific, can strongly oppose HIV, resulting in lower susceptibility of the host to infection (40) or in a better control once the infection is established. Thus, although further studies are needed, it appears that boosting of natural immunity represents an additional and valuable tool for fighting HIV that must be explored in a greater detail.

Although many vaccine strategies are under study, this review focuses only on some of these most recent approaches.

II. LIVE ATTENUATED VACCINES: CONCEPTS TO LEARN

The best protective results against both homologous and heterologus virus challenge have been obtained in macaques with a live attenuated SIV that has the *nef* gene deleted. In these animals, persistent infection is established, but the virus replicates poorly, does not cause disease (15), and confers protection against challenge with pathogenic SIV or SHIV (16, 17, 41–43). Despite the attenuation, increased by additional deletions in *vpr* and in the negative regulatory elements, these viruses still cause disease in newborn macaques upon mucosal exposure (20) or intravenous challenge and, more importantly, in some of the vaccinated adult macaques (44, 45). In the latter, progression to disease is delayed, stressing the tight relationship between replication rate and pathogenicity. On the other hand, poorly replicating viruses such as some SHIV appear to be inefficient in conferring protection. This suggests that the replication rate affects pathogenicity but also the development of a protective immune response (46–48).

Therefore, more attenuated viruses are being generated with the rationale of determining the minimal requirements to confer protection. Of note, the progression to disease observed in a few of the vaccinated animals underscores the importance of host factors in pathogenesis and the key effect of infectious virus threshold required for progression to diseases in different individuals. However, the possibility that the virus may revert to a more pathogenic geno/phenotype is among the major concerns that prevent the use of live attenuated vaccines in humans.

Nevertheless, this approach in the animal model may help identify mechanisms by which superinfection with pathogenic strains is blocked, a very valuable aim given the poor understanding of protective immunity against HIV. In particular, experiments of passive transfer of serum from macaques vaccinated with an attenuated SIV and protected from superinfection by the wild-type viral strain does not confer protection to naive animals, ruling out a role for antibodies (49). On the other hand, neither partial depletion of CD8+ cells nor a more profound depletion of most T cells abrogate protection from superinfection (50). Thus, mechanisms other than antibodies or CD8+ CTLs are responsible for protection. The potency of such mechanim(s) in the protected animals is underscored by the lack of reactivation, upon stimulation with a recall antigen, of either the attenuated strain used for vaccination or the pathogenic strain used for challenge (51). A growing body of evidence indicates that natural immunity may be key to protection possibly through the induction of CAF, beta chemokines, and interleukin-16 secretion by $\alpha\beta$CD8+ T cells and $\gamma\delta$T cells (52–56).

III. NOVEL STRATEGIES

A. Fusion-Competent Env-Based Vaccine

The possible solution to the problems related to Env variability and induction of sterilizing immunity comes from a recent major breakthrough in the HIV research that further demonstrates the importance of basic science for vaccine development.

The definition of the crystal structure of the HIV-1 envelope has revealed new functional aspects concerning its binding to CD4 and the conformational changes it undergoes to engage the CCR5 and CXCR4 coreceptors and to subsequentely fuse to the cell membrane. It is during these transient conformational changes that new cryptic epitopes are exposed. Thus, it is conceivable that the recombinant gp160 or gp120 oligomers utilized so far for immunization, although identical to the native envelope spikes, may not expose these functional epitopes and therefore will not elicit antibodies against them.

From these considerations stemmed a completely new approach to generate broadly cross-reactive NA. LaCasse et al. (14) showed that formalin fixation of COS-7 cells expressing a dual tropic molecularly cloned Env of the B clade at the time they were starting to fuse with the human U87 glioma cells (expressing both CD4 and CCR5) results in a whole cell preparation, termed fusion-competent, in which those cryptic epitopes are exposed. Indeed, in a mouse model (transgenic for human CD4 and CCR5 to avoid the generation of an immune response against these molecules), vaccination with this fusion-competent immunogen induced antibodies that were strongly neutralizing and broadly cross-reactive, indicating that critical, and presently unknown, neutralizing epitopes are exposed only upon the transient conformational changes necessary for fusion to occur. Moreover, the capability of these antibodies to neutralize strains from several clades indicates that they recognize highly conserved epitopes, likely because of their functional role in the fusion event. Thus, these data formally prove that it is possible, at least in the mouse model, to induce antibodies that are strongly neutralizing in vitro. Of course, confirmation of these results in more suitable preclinical models such as nonhuman primates and in vivo evidence of protection are needed before considering any potential clinical application.

B. Vaccines Based on Naked DNA and Live Vectors Expressing Env Alone or Associated with Other Viral Genes (MVA, Canarypox, Fowlpox, Adenovirus, Alphaviruses)

Vectors that express viral genes may represent an alternative to live attenuated virus vaccines. In fact, expression of viral genes in the host mimics the infection with attenuated strains without their risk and should elicit a comparable immune response and efficacy. There are additional advantages of the DNA-based approaches, such as the ease of preparation, the reproducibility, the stability at room temperature, the possibility of mucosal immunization, the low cost, and the fewer inoculations needed, features that are extremely appealing when thinking of large-scale vaccination, particularly in developing countries. Moreover, it is possible to insert genes coding for molecules, such as cytokines or chemokines, in the vector which could help the immune system to mount a specific response against the nominal antigen. In addition, naked DNA and most vectors contain unmethylated CpG sequences that are commonly present in prokaryotic but not eukaryotic DNA and elicit strong natural immunity. This in turn promotes the adaptive immune response, particularly of the Th-1 type. In fact, another substantial advantage of the DNA-based approaches relies on their capability to elicit strong MHC class I restricted CTL responses, a feature almost exclusively limited to vaccines in which de novo synthesis of the immunogen occurs. This is very relevant for vaccine development because an increasing body of evidence indicates an important protective role for CTLs both after vaccination and in the course of natural infection (reviewed in Reference 57). In addition, recombinant vectors often provide priming, so that subsequent boosts with a subunit protein results in a humoral immune response of higher titer and longer duration. Moreover, the vector itself, due to its own tropism, can deliver immunogen to cells or tissues of interest. Several live viral and bacterial vectors are being used in recent protocols. Examples of strategies with MVA, canarypox, fowlpox, adenovirus, and alphaviruses are reported below.

1. Vaccinia

Vaccinia and related avipox viruses such as canarypox have been widely used for HIV vaccines. MVA has the advantage of having been safely tested in over 120,000 humans (58), allowing insertion of several genes and eliciting an immune response similar to that observed during the natural infection with the pathogen. Preexisting immunity to vaccinia because of smallpox vaccination is an issue, and boosting such a reactivity may hamper the repeated use of the vector because of immediate clearance (59–61). There are also some concerns about the potential pathogenicity of such a vector in immunocompromised hosts.

A large study conducted within a European Collaborative vaccine program with nonhuman primates has shown that intramuscular immunization of macaques with recombinant MVA vectors expressing Env and other SIV proteins (Gag/Pol, Tat, Rev, and Nef) does not confer protection upon intravenous challenge with 50 MID_{50} of the homologous pathogenic virus SIVmac251, although in some cases a reduction in viral load and a less pronounced CD4+ T-cell decline indicated a beneficial effect of the vaccination (62). These data are consistent with results from previous works (63, 64). Protection has been reported with the MVA vector alone (23), likely due to the boost of innate immunity with antiviral activity. Thus, it is conceivable that even in vaccinia-naive animals, priming with MVA may result in a strong response against the vector but not against HIV/SIV gene products. Thus, if the dominant immunogenicity of the MVA vector is confirmed, then its use for boosting rather than priming should be recommended. In fact, the strong immune response against vaccinia might be beneficial and boost antigen-specific response. Studies in monkeys are under way to address this issue, but results in the mouse model already indicate better MHC class I restricted peptide-specific T-cell induction when the animals are primed with DNA and boosted with MVA (65).

The MVA vector is also suitable for mucosal immunization, as indicated by studies in BALB/c mice immunized intrarectally with recombinant vaccinia expressing HIV gp160 (66). The immunized animals developed specific serum antibody and strong HIV-specific CTL responses. Of note, mucosal immunization generated a systemic response, overcoming the block represented by the preexisting systemic immunity to vaccinia. In addition, boosting with the same vector and by the same route was effective. The similarity of vaccinia immunity between mouse and humans suggests that a similar response should occur in humans.

2. Canarypox

Canarypox is a harmless avipox (referred to as ALVAC) used to express HIV antigens. ALVAC has already been used for several human vaccines, such as measles (virus hemagglutinin and fusion proteins), rabies virus (glycoprotein) and, more recently, to deliver the HIV-1 envelope glycoprotein (67). Like MVA, ALVAC can accomodate large amounts of foreign DNA in its genome, infect mammalian cells, and it is stable at room temperature. In contrast to MVA, ALVAC is host range restricted and does not produce infectious progeny virus in mammalian cells (67), an important safety factor especially for therapeutic vaccination in immunocompromised hosts. However, this very same feature may be responsible for the apparent lesser immunogenicity of ALVAC as compared with MVA (68). Of note, an ALVAC–Env-based vaccine is the only one currently tested in phase III trials in a canarypox/protein prime/boost regimen (reviewed in Reference 69). Although this regimen has been proved to elicit a good cellular and humoral response in humans (68, 70), its protective efficacy against infection with viruses from different clades is still an open question, hopefully to be answered by the ongoing trials.

3. Fowlpox

An attenuated fowlpox virus has been widely used in poultry to protect from infection with the wild-type pathogenic virus and recently used as a vector in vaccine studies (67). Although a recombinant fowlpox virus is 100 times less efficient than canarypox in generating protective immunity (71), recent results in macaques suggest that the use of a fowlpox vector in a prime/boost regimen may provide better immunization and protection than other approaches (72). In this study, eight different immunization protocols were compared for their ability to protect against pathogenic SHIV89.6P in rhesus macaques. The animals were primed either by intradermal injections or by gene gun delivery with DNA coding for the HIV-*env* and the SIV-*nef*, -*gag*, and -*pol* genes. Boosters were either identical to the primings or consisted in either purified Env protein or recombinant fowlpox viruses carrying HIV-*env* and SIV-*nef*, -*gag*, and -*pol* genes. The combination of intradermal DNA priming followed by recombinant pox virus boosting gave the best protection against the heterologous intravenous challenge with the SHIV89.6P. However, this challenge had been preceded by two homologous challenges with nonpathogenic SHIV-IIIB, whose impact on the subsequent heterologous challenge is yet undetermined. Of note, protection against the first of the two homologous challenges was observed also in the control group that had been primed with the empty plasmid vector and boosted with the recombinant Env protein. These animals developed the highest anti-IIIB-Env antibody titers and neutralizing activity, suggesting that antibodies were probably sufficient to protect from the first homologous challenge but not from the second one, performed 43 weeks later, when the antibody titers had declined. It is therefore conceivable that priming with the plasmid vector might have boosted the innate immunity and enhanced the response to the Env protein. It is also possible that stimulation of native immunity might have generated a first line of antiviral defense through the induction of CAF and chemokines responsible for the protection. As mentioned, however, protection against identical challenge was not observed 43 weeks later, suggesting that regardless of the mechanism, long-lasting effective immunity even against a homologous challenge is still a major problem. It will be of interest in future protocols to address the impact of the natural immunity on protection per se or on the development of an adaptive protective response after immunization.

4. Adenovirus

Adenovirus (Ad) vectors are highly promising HIV vaccine vehicles not only because they elicit good cell-mediated immunity and prime high-titered humoral immune responses, but also because the vector replicates in the epithelium of the upper respiratory tract and gut, resulting in induction of mucosal immune responses. Wild-type Ad4 and Ad7 vaccines have been used for over 25 years in the military and have proven safe and effective at preventing acute respiratory disease in recruits (73). These vaccines are easy to administer as enteric-coated capsules and are inexpensive and stable. Although preexisting immunity or induction of immunity to the vector after immunization is a concern, Ad4 and Ad7 vectors are reasonable choices for future development of HIV recombinants. Although prevalence in humans of Ad5 is significant, a recent report indicated that after cessation of the Ad4 and Ad7 military vaccine program in 1996, 66% and 73% of new military recruits lacked protective antibodies against Ad4 and Ad7, respectively. In addition, vectors of other serotypes could be developed from the 49 Ad serotypes currently identified (74).

Recent studies have demonstrated the ability of Ad4-, Ad5-, and Ad7-expressing-HIV gp160 (after boosting with the Env protein) to elicit humoral immunity and prime high titered neutralizing antibody responses in a dog model (75). Further studies indicated that a prime boost approach could elicit humoral, cellular, and mucosal Env-specific immune responses in chimpanzees (76, 77) and long-lasting immunity and protective efficacy against both homologous (78, 79) and, to a lesser extent, a high-dose heterologous (minimally passaged) nonsyncytium-inducing HIV primary isolate (80).

Priming with Ad5 host range mutant SIV*env* recombinant, followed by boosting with native SIV Env in rhesus macaques, induced viral-specific humoral, cellular, and mucosal immune responses (81) but not sterilizing immunity with a highly pathogenic SIV vaginal challenge. However, a reduced viral load was observed during the acute infection in immunized macaques (82). Notably, reduced viral burdens and slow progressor status resulted from a vaccine based only on Env. The use of multicomponent Ad recombinants should elicit even better protective efficacy, and construction of these is in the progress (83).

5. Alphaviruses

Alphaviruses are RNA viruses recently used to deliver heterologous genes for vaccine and gene therapy applications. The advantages of such vectors are their high levels of replication and gene expression, their ability to infect a variety of cell types, and the ability to manipulate cDNA clones from which infectious viral RNA can be transcribed (for review, see References 84–86). The general strategy for construction of alphavirus-based expression vectors is to substitute the genes encoding the structural proteins with a heterologous gene(s), maintaining the transcriptional control via the highly active subgenomic RNA promoter (84, 85, 87). Vector replicon RNA can be transcribed in vitro and used directly. Alternatively, the replicon RNA can be packaged into infectious vector particles by cotransfection of cultured cells with a complementing defective helper RNA, which provides the virion structural proteins in *trans*. After infection of the host, large quantities of the protein(s) are made, yet the alphavirus itself cannot replicate because it no longer contains the sequences for the structural proteins (85, 88). Sindbis virus, Venezuelan equine encephalitis virus (VEE), and Semliki Forest virus (SFV) are among the alphaviruses being exploited by using such approaches (87, 89–91).

VEE is an alphavirus of particular interest because of its tropism for the follicular dendritic cells in the lymph node, cells that are key for long-term antigen sequestration and presentation to B cells (92, 93). In addition, VEE replicon particles (91, 94) can express high levels of both glycosylated and nonglycosylated proteins. Protein expression is centered in the lymph node of the vaccinated animal, where dendritic cells are targeted for single-cycle infection either by the parental envelope proteins or by mutant envelope proteins at higher vaccine doses (95). This strategy may be important for inducing a strong immune response to HIV proteins with low intrinsic immunogenicity. In addition, mice immunized parenterally with VEE replicons are protected against influenza mucosal challenge, a feature highly desirable in sexually transmitted infections such as HIV. Immunogenicity studies in nonhuman primates showed that vaccination (six inoculations: two subcutaneous, two intravenous, two subcutaneous) with VEE replicons expressing the Gag and Env of a molecular clone (termed SIVsm H-4i) of the highly pathogenic SIVsm E660 swarm (96) induced humoral and cellular (CTL) response in three and two of the four vaccinated animals, respectively (97). When challenged intravenously with 50 MID_{50} of the pathogenic SIVsm E660, all animals became infected. However, the acute phase of infection was milder than that observed in the control animals as indicated by lower viral loads and delayed disease progression. Of note, the containment of infection correlated with the presence of both antibody titers and CTLs. These, however, were detected only in two of the four vaccinated animals, indicating that further studies are needed to optimize the immunogenicity. Not surprisingly, sterilizing immunity was not achieved despite immunization with Env, additional evidence of the poor cross-reactivity. In fact, the monkeys had been immunized with Env from a molecular clone and challenged with the virus swarm, a situation close to an heterologous challenge.

SFV represents another delivery system that allows efficient expression with only one round of infection. This approach is also suitable for mucosal immunization (98, 99). Experiments in the mouse model indicate that immunization with SFV replicons induces both a humoral and cellular immune response of the Th-1 type (99). Immunization of mice with vectors encoding influenza antigen is protective against challenge with influenza virus (99). SFV vectors expressing HIV-1 Env have been utilized for vaccination in macaques (100, 101). Although both humoral and cellular immunity were induced, sterilizing immunity upon challenge with low or highly pathogenic SHIVs was not achieved (100, 101). However, compared with nonimmunized animals, the infection was milder, as indicated by lower plasma viremia (101) and by the survival of the vaccinated animals to a lethal challenge with SHIV-PBj14 (100). For reasons already discussed, it is conceivable that immunization with HIV-1 antigens other than Env, such as the regulatory (and early) genes *tat* and *rev*, may improve the effectiveness of this approach. Indeed, priming of macaques with SFV vector expressing the SIV Tat and Rev followed by boosting with the same antigens expressed by an MVA vector resulted in an efficient control of pathogenic SIV upon intravenous challenge (31) (see following).

C. Polyepitope Vaccines

The appreciation of the importance of CD8+ CTL response in protection against HIV or SIV infection has provided the rationale for a vaccine approach based on a synthetic gene coding for partially overlapping CTL epitopes (or polyepitope) of one or more viral proteins (102–104). Among the advantages of this approach are the possibility to lower the amount of the protein to administer and to drive the immune response against the most relevant epitopes. Moreover, the inclusion of several epitopes restricted by different MHC alleles allows the elicitation of an effective CTL response in most people. In fact, eight to nine selected MHC class I-restricted epitopes would ensure the immunization of the general population if one epitope is sufficient to confer protection in each individual (105, 106).

An HIV polyepitope, termed H, that included 20 human epitopes restricted by 12 different human leukocyte antigen (HLA) alleles, 3 macaque epitopes, and 1 murine epitope to permit testing for immunogenicity in all these recipients (65) has been shown to be immunogenic in mice (107), with the best CTL induction obtained by priming with naked DNA constructs followed by MVA boosting (65). Vaccination of mice with a construct coding for both HIV and malaria epitopes, and including two mouse epitopes with distinct MHC restriction, generated CTL against both the pathogens. This demonstrates the feasibility of contemporarily generating an immune response against two unrelated pathogens and to two murine epitopes with a different MHC class I restriction (108). The immunogenicity of the polyepitope H has been further confirmed in the macaque model with a DNA prime MVA boost vaccination regimen (108). However, no protection was observed upon mucosal challenge, indicating that the selected Gag epitopes were not protective. Thus, epitope(s) selection appears to be the most critical issue for this very promising vaccine approach. Of note, the polyepitope immunogen does not elicit an antibody response. It would be of relevance to evaluate the immunogenicity and efficacy of vaccines that also elicit specific antibodies, because epitope interference or beneficial synergy between the cellular and humoral responses may both occur (109–114).

D. Vaccine Based on Regulatory Genes: *Tat, Rev, Nef*

The results from Env-based vaccine strategies have suggested that blocking virus replication and disease onset in the lack of a sterilizing immunity may represent at present a more attainable goal of AIDS vaccine development. The control of virus replication may modify the virus–host interaction favoring the host immune response providing protection and may be used for both preventive and therapeutic vaccine strategies.

Such a strategy should therefore use viral products that exert key functions in the early virus life-cycle, infectivity or pathogenicity, that are capable of inducing a broad immunity and that are conserved among the HIV clades. These includes the regulatory genes *tat*, *rev*, and *nef*.

1. Tat

The Tat protein of HIV possesses all the characteristics mentioned above and is the most studied system both in pathogenesis and vaccine development. Tat is produced early after HIV infection and is essential for virus replication and infectivity (115–117). Moreover, the Tat protein is released in the extra-cellular milieu and is taken up by the neighbor cells where it *trans*-activates virus gene expression and replication (35, 36, 38, 118, 119). Extracellular Tat also induces the expression of the chemokines receptors CCR5 and CXCR4, thus favoring the transmission of both macrophage-tropic and T lymphocyte-tropic HIV-1 strains to uninfected cells (120, 121). Tat is also involved in AIDS pathogenesis and in AIDS-associated malignancies, such as the Ka-posi's sarcoma (34, 37, 119, 122–131).

In in vivo infection, the presence of a humoral immune response against Tat correlates with the control of disease progression (129, 132–134) by the inhibition of the uptake and therefore of the effect of extracellular Tat on both HIV replication (36, 134) and T-cell immunosuppression (129). Similarly, the presence of an early anti-Tat CTL response inversely correlates with the progression to the symptomatic stage of the infection (135–137). Further, soluble Tat can induce CD8+ T-cell-mediated CTL responses by entering the MHC class I pathway (138) due to its capability of being taken up by cells (36, 38, 118) and very efficiently by antigen presenting cells (APC) through integrin receptors, which also direct cell migration to Tat (123, 130, 131; B. Ensoli, unpublished data, 1999).

Finally, Tat has well-conserved immunogenic epitopes among the different HIV-1 clades, with the exception of the O subtype (1; S. Buttò, unpublished data). Thus, although it cannot block virus entry, a Tat-based vaccine may control virus replication.

This hypothesis has been confirmed by recent studies in cynomolgus mon-keys vaccinated with a biologically active HIV-1 Tat protein (29). Six mon-keys were immunized subcutaneously with 10 μg of Tat in RIBI (three mon-keys) or alum (three monkeys) and one animal with Tat (6 μg), intradermally (ID), in the absence of adjuvants. During the following 36 weeks the ani-mals received seven to eight boosts. No toxicity (acute or chronic; local or systemic) was ever detected in the vaccinated animals throughout the immunization period. The six monkeys inoculated with Tat and RIBI or alum developed very high titers anti-Tat antibodies capable of neutralizing Tat activity and blocking virus replication *in vitro*. In contrast, the animal given Tat ID developed low and transient anti-Tat antibody titers. The anti-Tat vaccine also elicited cellular immune responses, including DTH and T-helper proliferative response to Tat and anti-Tat CD8+ T CTL secreting tumor necrosis factor alpha (TNF-α) upon antigen-specific stimulation.

At week 50 after immunization (14–18 weeks after the last boost), all animals were challenged with the SHIV89.6P, a chimeric virus that contains the *tat* gene of HIV-1 and is highly pathogenic in macaques (139). The virus stock used for the challenge was derived from a cynomolgus macaque inoculated with the original SHIV89.6P from rhesus monkeys, obtained from Dr. N. Letvin. To determine virus pathogenicity in cynomolgus and the monkey infectious doses (MID_{50}), the original virus stock obtained from the rhesus and the virus stock obtained from the cynomolgus macaques were inoculated into six and eight monkeys, respectively. High levels of viral replication, including p27 antigenemia, plasma viremia, proviral DNA, anti-SIV antibody titers, and a profound and persistent decrease in CD4 T-cell counts, were observed in all monkeys independent of the virus stock utilized, and no differences were found when the data obtained were compared with those already published by Dr. Letvin's lab, including the rate of animal death (29, 139, 140; 140a). Therefore, all vaccinated and control macaques were challenged intravenously with 10 MID_{50} of SHIV89.6P. At this time a naive control monkey was included in the protocol and inoculated with a dose threefold lower (2.8 MID_{50}) as an additional control of the virus inoculum.

After challenge, all the controls but only two of the seven Tat protein-vaccinated monkeys (one given Tat and RIBI and one Tat and alum) were infected, as indicated by the presence of high levels of p27 antigen (detected by ELISA) and viral RNA (detected by branched-DNA and quantitative-competitive RNA-polymerase chain reaction) in plasma, proviral DNA copies, cytoviremia, or positive virus isolation. In contrast, all these parameters were always negative for all the other five vaccinees up to 68 weeks postchallenge, with the exception of SIV proviral DNA, which was only sporadically and barely detected (<10 copies/μg of DNA) in a few animals. This and the presence of low and transient anti-SIV (or anti-HIV Env) antibody titers in these protected animals indicated that infection occurred but was blocked by the immune response induced by the vaccination.

Of note, anti-SIV or anti-HIV Env antibodies correlated with the level of infection. They were very high in all the control monkeys, followed by the two infected and vaccinated animals that had at least 2 logs lower titers and a delayed increase as compared with the control macaques, whereas they were very low and transient in the five protected monkeys. Consistent with the data from the virological assays, the number of CD4+ T cells remained in the normal range after the viral challenge and during all the follow-up period in the five protected monkeys, whereas it decreased considerably in all the controls and in the two vaccinated and infected macaques (29). Notably, protection correlated (100%) with the presence, before challenge, of anti-Tat-specific CTLs and with TNF-α production by CD8$^+$ T cells upon Tat stimulation but not with the presence of anti-Tat antibodies. Nevertheless, the two infected and vaccinated monkeys (that had high anti-Tat antibody titers but not CTLs) developed lower (1 log) and delayed anti-SIV antibody titers as compared with the controls, suggesting that they were exposed to a lower antigen load. Of interest, a potent and stable CAF activity was detected early after challenge in all the vaccinated and protected monkeys but not in the infected animals, including the two vaccinated macaques (D. Goletti, unpublished data, 1999). In contrast, no correlation of protection was observed with the production of beta-chemokines at postchallenge time (RANTES, MIP1α, MIP1β) (D. Goletti, unpublished data, 1999).

Thus, immunization with a biologically active Tat was safe and induced a broad immune response capable of blocking virus replication to undetectable levels, preventing the CD4 T-cell decline and disease onset. Protection correlated (100%) with a CD8-T-cell-mediated activity that includes both antigen specific CTLs and a Th-1 type cytokine production and nonantigen-specific immune responses such as CAF, suggesting that Tat vaccine can also potentiate innate immunity. The same protection data and correlates of protection have been recently obtained by a different protocol utilizing Tat DNA (B. Ensoli, unpublished data, 1999). Thus, although the Tat strategy does not block virus entry, it can efficiently control virus replication and render the natural infection "abortive." This is likely to occur against different virus strains as suggested by studies in HIV-infected Ugandan patients that although infected by different virus strains, have antibodies recognizing Tat from the clade B used in the vaccination studies (S. Buttò, unpublished data, 1999).

Although Tat protein or DNA inoculation was safe both in naive (29; B. Ensoli, unpublished data, 1999) and SHIV-infected monkeys (B. Ensoli, unpublished data, 1999), the possibility to use transdominant negative mutants of HIV-1 Tat lacking the transactivating activity but preserving the immunogenicity of the wild-type Tat was also investigated (141). Intramuscular immunization of mice with plasmids encoding two transdominant negative mutants (Tat22 and Tat22/37) (142) elicited an immune response to wild-type

Tat protein that was comparable with that induced by inoculation of wild-type Tat DNA. In particular, the humoral response was comparable to wild-type Tat protein in terms of IgG subclasses, antibody titers, epitope specificity and neutralization of the biological activities of Tat, and by the proliferation of splenocytes from the immunized mice in response (141). These mutants are currently being investigated in monkey trials.

A modified Tat, inactivated by carboxymethylation, has also been recently utilized as a vaccine. Studies in mice, rabbits, monkeys, and seronegative and seropositive humans indicated that the inactivated Tat, termed Tat toxoid, is safe and immunogenic, as assessed by measurements of antibody titers and proliferative responses (143, 144). To evaluate its efficacy, initial experiments have been performed in rhesus macaques that were vaccinated with 20–100 μg of the Tat toxoid and then challenged intrarectally with 2500 50% tissue culture infectious dose (TCID$_{50}$) of the pathogenic SHIV 89.6PD (30). In comparison with control animals, an attenuated infection was observed in vaccinated monkeys, as indicated by the reduction of p27 antigenemia and plasma viremia. In addition, the monkeys that controlled the infection (plasma viremia < 2500 copies/mL) exhibited both humoral and proliferative responses to Tat at prechallenge, suggesting that both arms of the immunity contributed to controlling disease. No information is presently available on other aspects of the cellular immune response (such as CTLs and CD8-mediated antiviral activity) to more precisely compare the Tat toxoid approach with the native Tat protein vaccine that, utilizing a biologically active Tat protein, also exploits the unique capability of Tat to be taken up by APC, to enter the MHC class I pathway of presentation, and to generate CD8+ CTLs (138). This is of importance because CTLs, but not anti-Tat antibodies, correlated with protection after vaccination with a biologically active Tat or Tat DNA in monkey trials (29; B. Ensoli, unpublished data, 1999). Nevertheless, it appears that systemic vaccination with the Tat toxoid attenuates disease upon mucosal challenge, in the apparent absence of mucosal immunity.

2. Tat and Rev

Rev is another regulatory gene expressed early after infection and essential to virus replication. As for Tat, an early immune response to Rev has been shown to correlate with long-term nonprogressor status (137). The efficacy of immunization against both *tat* and *rev* regulatory genes has been demonstrated in macaques vaccinated twice with SFV and twice with the recombinant MVA, both expressing the SIVmac32H Rev and Tat, and challenged intravenously with 50 MID$_{50}$ of SIVmac 32H (pJ5). As expected from this nonsterilizing approach, infection occurred as indicated by plasma viremia. However, plasma viremia was transient and significantly lower than in the controls, and no cell-associated viremia could be detected in the vaccinated macaques, whereas productively infected cells were easily detected in the control animals (31). However, no information is available from these initial experiments on the type of immune response elicited or on the correlates of protection. Further studies are ongoing to clarify these issues and the impact of immunization with Rev in this vaccine strategy.

3. Tat, Rev, Nef

Vaccination against all the three HIV regulatory genes *tat*, *rev*, and *nef*, has also been investigated in mice and humans. Hinkula et al. (33) were the first to demonstrate that both humoral and cellular immune responses are induced in mice (four different strains) upon immunization with cDNA plasmids encoding these HIV-1 regulatory genes with no interference being detected among these plasmids, even when plasmids encoding for the structural proteins Env and Gag were associated in the vaccination protocol. The epitope specificities of the humoral response was comparable with that obtained by vaccinating with the corresponding protein. In addition, epitope-specific T-cell responses and a Th-1 pattern of cytokine secretion were detected. The efficacy of a vaccine based on all the three regulatory gene products together and in the absence of other viral genes (i.e., *env*, *gag*) has not yet been tested in nonhuman primates. Studies in HIV-infected patients have confirmed that DNA vaccination with either *tat*, *rev*, or *nef* is safe (no evidence of increased viral load) and induces B- and T-cell responses (including CD8+ CTLs) that were absent or low before immunization (34), demonstrating the feasibility of genetic immunization to induce new immune responses in HIV-infected patients. A more recent study (145) in which the same immunization approach was combined with highly active antiretroviral treatment (HAART) confirmed the safety and immunogenicity of the vaccine, whereas the reduction of the viral load was dependent on HAART, indicating that this combination may improve the capacity of the immune system to deal with the HIV infection.

E. Alloimmunization for Anti-HIV Vaccine

A substantial body of evidence (reviewed in Reference 39) suggests that alloimmunization generates an immune response with antiviral activity that may strongly suppress HIV replication, resulting in lower susceptibility of the host to infection (40) or in better control once the infection is established. A recent study in which women were alloimmunized with their partners' mononuclear leukocytes to prevent spontaneous recurrent abortions showed a strong and long-lasting CD8-T-cell activation, with increased production of beta chemokines and soluble antiviral suppressor factors and decreased expression of the CCR5 coreceptors in both activated lymphocytes and monocytes, the major targets of HIV-1 infection (146). In vitro experiments demonstrated that all these factors contributed to the decreased susceptibility to HIV infection with both lab-adapted and primary strains. Alloimmune recognition belongs to the natural immunity (147) and has been invoked as one of the factors responsible for reduced risk of HIV vertical transmission due to increased class I disparity (148). This immune response is directed against the human HLA antigens that are exposed on the viral membrane and not against the virus, circumventing the problem of the virus variability.

A further advantage is the large number of alloreactive T cells that would respond, a proportion comprised between 1 and 10% of all T lymphocytes. Although naturally present, this alloimmunity can, in fact, be further potentiated by immunization with HLA-mismatched leukocytes (146, 149). Finally, alloimmunization is safe (150, 151). Although no evidence of in vivo protection is yet available, protection was achieved in macaques when the challenge virus was grown on xenogeneic human cells (152–156), suggesting that this may also apply to the allogeneic model in humans. The very same monkeys were not protected when rechallenged with SIV grown on allogeneic macaque cells (155, 156). However, these monkeys had not been alloimmunized. Thus, the unprimed natural alloreactivity is not sufficient per se to confer protection, as also indicated by the relative ease with which both HIV and SIV are transmitted in human and nonhuman primates, respectively. Further studies are needed to develop a protective vaccine based on the alloimmunization. However, the lessons learned with this strategy may be key to understanding the role of innate immunity in eliciting a protective response from different vaccination strategies.

IV. CONCLUSIONS AND PERSPECTIVES

A considerable amount of data have been generated in the past 15 years clarifying several aspects of HIV pathogenesis, shedding light on the inefficacy of most past vaccine approaches, and promoting the development of novel immunization strategies (Table 1). Past experience has definitively proved that regardless of the approach, HIV vaccination is safe, with the only exclusion being live attenuated viruses. Paradoxically, this is an important exclusion because attenuated viruses have been shown to provide the best protection, indicating that achievement and maintainance of effective immunity may require prolonged presentation to the immune system of multiple, native, viral antigens. Several new approaches have been generated based on this assumption, in particular those utilizing naked DNA or live viral or bacterial vectors. Antigens other than Env have been added to the list of candidate vaccines, including other structural and regulatory HIV-1 proteins. The promising results obtained in nonhuman primates with single regulatory gene vaccination (i.e., Tat) underscore the importance of targeting vital early gene products. In fact, the induction of an anti-Tat immune response has major consequences on the virus life cycle, with severe impairment of virus replication of most HIV strains that leads to a sort of "abortive" infection. It is conceivable, however, that residual minimal virus replication may still occur and may provide enough antigens to boost the anti-Tat immunity and to generate a primary immune response against all the other viral proteins, as indicated by preliminary data from Tat-vaccinated and protected monkeys (B. Ensoli, unpublished data, 1999).

All these recent approaches imply that nonsterilizing immunity would be beneficial and that cell-mediated rather than humoral immunity is protective (Table 2). Indeed, evidence in humans from the course of natural infection (157) and HAART treatment (158, 159) indicates that a low viral load correlates with maintainance of immune function and slow disease progression. Moreover, despite the present lack of clear understanding of the correlates of protection, the major protective role of cell-mediated immunity has been progressively appreciated, with a special emphasis on CD8+ CTLs (reviewed in References 57 and 160), although an important role for CD4 helper function has also been proposed (161).

Last but not the least, natural immunity appears important both for protection and for potentiating the development of adaptive immunity (39, 52–55,

Table 2 Role of Nonadaptive (Natural) and Adaptive (Antigen-Specific) Immune Responses Against HIV/SIV

	Infection		
Response	Prevention	Control	Clearance
Nonadaptive[a]	−	+(+)	−
Adaptive			
Antibody	+ + +	+ +	+/−
CD4+ T-helper cells	−	+ +	+ +
CD8+ CTLs	−	+ + (+)	+ + +

[a]Including CAF, beta chemokines, and antiviral activities mediated by natural killer T cells.

162) (Table 2). Thus, cellular immune responses, either nonadaptive or adaptive, are crucial to control and possibly to clear the viral infection. Accordingly, most strategies reported here are aimed at arming one or more of the cellular components of our defense system, the only main exception being the fusion-competent Env-based approach that might induce sterilizing immunity. In this regard, we propose that in the other Env-based vaccine strategies, HIV-1 Env may act as a decoy, driving the immune response against irrelevant and therefore nonneutralizing epitopes, whereas critical Env epitopes are hidden and exposed very shortly at the time of viral entry. Responses against other relevant viral components are inefficiently mounted because of the Env dominancy. In our view, it is conceivable that the inclusion of native Env oligomers in vaccine preparations may actually be detrimental, hampering the development of protective immunity against other viral components, such as early viral antigens (Tat, Rev, and Nef) that may play a key role in controlling viral infection. This is also suggested by trials in which all the HIV antigens have been used together (62, 163), and no protection was achieved with a low immune response to Tat and Rev. Finally, a dominant antibody response may also negatively affect the development of cellular immunity, due to epitope masking and interference with proper antigen processing and presentation (111–114, 164).

The relatively recently appreciated notion that HIV-1 infection is primarily a sexually transmitted disease has generated interest to develop immunization strategies aimed at conferring protection at the mucosal level (165). Studies in macaques have demonstrated induction of protective mucosal immunity with several approaches (SIV Env and p27 Gag; live attenuated SIV, nonpathogenic SHIV, HIV-2) (166–171). However, as for the systemic immunization, protection has been achieved mostly by infecting the animals with live attenuated viruses, with the significant exception of the approach of Lehner et al. (166) in which protection from intrarectal challenge was obtained by targeting regional lymph nodes. However, it appears more difficult to protect from a more common intravaginal challenge (172). These studies provide strong evidence that protective mucosal immunity can be induced, although safety concerns and feasibility are still unresolved issues (20, 166). Nevertheless, it appears that the recent advancements both in the comprehension of virus–host interplay and in vaccine development render the goal of prophylactic and therapeutic immunization closer.

Acknowledgments

We thank A. Lippa and F.M. Regini for editorial assistance.

REFERENCES

1. Human retroviruses and AIDS 1995. A compilation and analysis of nucleic acids and amino acid sequences. In: Myers G, Korber B, Hahn BH, Jeang KT, Mellors JW, McCutchan FE, Henderson LE, Pawlakis GN, eds. II-A-55, 56 Theoretical Biology and Biophysics, Los Alamos National Laboratory, Los Alamos, New Mexico, 1996.

2. Burton DR. A vaccine for HIV type 1: the antibody perspective. Proc Natl Acad Sci USA 1997;94:10018–10023.

3. Shibata R, Igarashi T, Haigwood N, Buckler-White A, Ogert R, Ross W, Willey R, Cho MW, Martin MA. Neutralizing antibody directed against the HIV-1 envelope glycoprotein can completely block HIV-1/SIV chimeric virus infections of macaque monkeys. Nat Med 1999;5:204–210.

4. Shibata R, Seimon C, Cho MW, Arthur LO, Nigida SM Jr, Matthews T, Sawyer LA, Schultz A, Murthy KK, Israel Z, Javadian A, Frost P, Kennedy RC, Lane HC, Martin MA. Resistance of previously infected chimpanzees to successive challenges with a heterologous intraclade B strain of human immunodeficiency virus type 1. J Virol 1996;70:4361–4369.

5. Montefiori DC, Pantaleo G, Fink LM, Zhou JT, Zhou JY, Bilska M, Miralles GD, Fauci AS. Neutralizing and infection-enhancing antibody responses to human immunodeficiency virus type 1 in long-term nonprogressors. J Infect Dis 1996;173:60–67.

6. Montefiori DC, Reimann KA, Wyand MS, Manson K, Lewis MG, Collman RG, Sodroski JG, Bolognesi DP, Letvin NL. Neutralizing antibodies in sera from macaques infected with chimeric simian-human immunodeficiency virus containing the envelope glycoproteins of either a laboratory-adapted variant or a primary isolate of human immunodeficiency virus type 1. J Virol 1998;72: 3427–3431.

7. Moore JP, Burton DR. HIV-1 neutralizing antibodies: how full is the bottle? Nat Med 1999;5:142–144.

8. Baba TW, Liska V, Hofmann-Lehmann R, Vlasak J, Xu W, Ayehnnie S, Cavacini LA, Posner MR, Katinger H, Stiegler G, Bernacky BJ, Rizvi TA, Schmidt R, Hill L, Keeling ME, Lu Y, Wright JE, Chou T, Ruprecht R. Human neutralizing antibodies of the IgG1 subtype protect against mucosal simian-human immunodeficiency virus infection. Nat Med 2000;6:200–206.

9. Li A, Katinger H, Posner MR, Cavacini L, Zolla-Pazner S, Gorny MK, Sodroski J, Chou TC, Baba TW, Ruprecht RM. Synergistic neutralization of simian-human immunodeficiency virus SHIV-vpu+ by triple and quadruple combinations of human monoclonal antibodies and high-titer anti-human immunodeficiency virus type 1 immunoglobulins. J Virol 1998;72:3235–3240.

10. Mascola JR, Stiegler G, VanCott TC, Katinger H, Carpenter C, Hanson CE, Beary H, Hayes D, Frankel S, Birx S, Lewis MG. Protection of macaques

against vaginal transmission of a pathogenic HIV-1/SIV chimeric virus by passive infusion of neutralizing antibodies. Nat Med 2000;6:207–210.

11. Mascola JR, Lewis MG, Stiegler G, Harris D, VanCott TC, Hayes D, Louder MK, Brown CR, Sapan CV, Frankel SS, Lu Y, Robb ML, Katinger H, Birx DI. Protection of macaques against pathogenic simian/human immunodeficiency virus 89.6PD by passive transfer of neutralizing antibodies. J Virol 1999;73:4009–4018.

12. Robert-Guroff M. IgG surfaces as an important component in mucosal protection. Nat Med 2000;6:129–130.

13. Burton DR, Parren PWHI. Vaccines and the induction of functional antibodies: time to look beyond the molecules of natural infection? Nat Med 2000;6:123–125.

14. LaCasse RA, Follis KE, Trahey M, Scarborough JD, Littman DR, Nunberg JH. Fusion-competent vaccines: broad neutralization of primary isolates of HIV. Science 1999;283:357–362.

15. Kestler HW 3d, Ringler DJ, Mori K, Panicali DL, Sehgal PK, Daniel MD, Desrosiers RC. Importance of the nef gene for maintenance of high virus loads and for development of AIDS. Cell 1991;65:651–662.

16. Daniel MD, Kirchhoff F, Czajak SC, Sehgal PK, Desrosiers RC. Protective effects of a live attenuated SIV vaccine with a deletion in the nef gene. Science 1992;258:1938–1941.

17. Titti F, Sernicola L, Geraci A, Panzini G, Di Fabio S, Belli R, Monardo F, Borsetti A, Maggiorella MT, Koanga-Mogtomo M, Corrias F, Zamarchi R, Amadori A, Chieco-Bianchi L, Verani P. Live-attenuated simian immunodeficiency virus prevents super-infection by cloned SIVmac251 in Cynomolgus monkeys. J Gen Virol 1997;78:2529–2539.

18. Almond NM, Heeney JL. AIDS vaccine development in primate models. AIDS 1998;12:133–140.

19. Whatmore AM, Cook N, Hall GA, Sharpe S, Rud EW, Cranage MP. Repair and evolution of nef in vivo modulates simian immunodeficiency virus virulence. J Virol 1995;69:5117–5123.

20. Baba TW, Jeong YS, Pennick D, Bronson R, Greene MF, Ruprecht RM. Pathogenicity of live, attenuated SIV after mucosal infection of neonatal macaques. Science 1995;267:1820–1825.

21. Ezzell C. The monkey's got AIDS: what now for live AIDS vaccine? J NIH Res 1997;9:21–22.

22. Liu MA. Vaccine developments. Nat Med 1998;4:515–519.

23. Hanke T, Samuel RV, Blanchard TJ, Neumann VC, Allen TM, Boyson JE, Sharpe SA, Cook N, Smith GL, Watkins DI, Cranage MP, McMichael AJ. Effective induction of simian immunodeficiency virus-specific cytotoxic T lym-

phocytes in macaques by using a multiepitope gene and DNA prime-modified vaccinia virus Ankara boost vaccination regimen. J Virol 1999;73:7524–7532.

24. Barker E, Mackewicz CE, Levy JA. Effects of TH1 and TH2 cytokines on CD8+ cell response against human immunodeficiency virus: implications for long-term survival. Proc Natl Acad Sci USA 1995;92:11135–11139.

25. Ogg GS, Jin X, Bonhoeffer S, Dunbar PR, Nowak MA, Monard S, Segal JP, Cao Y, Rowland-Jones SL, Cerundolo V, Hurley A, Markowitz M, Ho DD, Nixon DF, McMichael AJ. Quantitation of HIV-1-specific cytotoxic T lymphocytes and plasma load of viral RNA. Science 1998;279:2103–2106.

26. Schmitz JE, Kuroda MJ, Santra S, Sasseville VG, Simon MA, Lifton MA, Racz P, Tenner-Racz K, Dalesandro M, Scallon BJ, Ghrayeb J, Forman MA, Montefiori DC, Rieber EP, Letvin NL, Reimann KA. Control of viremia in simian immunodeficiency virus infection by CD8+ lymphocytes. Science 1999; 283:857–860.

27. Brodie SJ, Lewinshon D, Patterson BK, Jiyamapa D, Krieger J, Corey L, Greenberg PD, Riddel SR. In vivo migration and function of transferred HIV-1 specific cytotoxic T cells. Nat Med 1999;5:34–41.

28. Hanke T, McMichael A. Pre-clinical development of a multi-CTL epitope-based DNA prime MVA boost vaccine for AIDS. Immunol Lett 1999;66:177–181.

29. Cafaro A, Caputo A, Fracasso C, Maggiorella MT, Goletti D, Baroncelli S, Pace M, Sernicola L, Koanga-Mogtomo ML, Betti M, Borsetti A, Belli R, Åkerblom L, Corrias F, Buttò S, Heeney J, Verani P, Titti F, Ensoli B. Control of SHIV-89.6P infection of cynomolgus monkeys by HIV-1 Tat protein vaccine. Nat Med 1999;5:643–650.

30. Pauza CD, Trivedi P, Wallace M, Ruckwardt TJ, Le Buanec H, Lu W, Bizzini B, Burny A, Zagury D, Gallo R. Proceedings of the 12th Cent Gardes Meeting on Retroviruses of Human AIDS and Related Animal Diseases, Paris, France, October 25–27, 1999.

31. Osterhaus AD, van Baalen CA, Gruters RA, Schutten M, Siebelink CH, Hulskotte EG, Tijhaar EJ, Randall RE, van Amerongen G, Fleuchaus A, Erfle V, Sutter G. Vaccination with Rev and Tat against AIDS. Vaccine 1999;17: 2713–2714.

32. Gallimore A, Cranage M, Cook N, Almond N, Bootman J, Rud E, Silvera P, Dennis M, Corcoran T, Stott J, McMichael A, Gotch F. Early suppression of SIV replication by CD8+ Nef-specific cytotoxic T cells in vaccinated macaques. Nat Med 1995;1:1167–1173.

33. Hinkula J, Svanholm C, Schwartz S, Lundholm P, Brytting M, Engstrom G, Benthin R, Glaser H, Sutter G, Kohleisen B, Erfle V, Okuda K, Wigzell H, Wahren B. Recognition of prominent viral epitopes induced by immunization with human immunodeficiency virus type1 regulatory genes. J Virol 1997;71: 5528–5539.

34. Calarota S, Bratt G, Nordlund S, Hinkula J, Leandersson AC, Sandstrom E, Wahren B. Cellular cytotoxic response induced by DNA vaccination in HIV-1 infected patients. Lancet 1998;351:1320–1325.

35. Ensoli B, Barillari G, Salahuddin SZ, Gallo RC, Wong-Staal F. Tat protein of HIV-1 stimulates growth of AIDS-Kaposi's sarcoma-derived cells. Nature 1990;345:84–87.

36. Ensoli B, Buonaguro L, Barillari G, Fiorelli V, Gendelman R, Morgan RA, Wingfield P, Gallo RC. Release, uptake, and effects of extracellular HIV-1 Tat protein on cell growth and viral transactivation. J Virol 1993;67:277–287.

37. Ensoli B, Gendelman R, Markham P, Fiorelli V, Colombini S, Raffeld M, Cafaro A, Chang HK, Brady JN, Gallo RC. Synergy between basic fibroblast growth factor and HIV-1 Tat protein in induction of Kaposi's sarcoma development. Nature 1994;371:674–680.

38. Chang HC, Samaniego F, Nair BC, Buonaguro L, Ensoli B. HIV-1 Tat protein exits from cells via a leaderless secretory pathway and binds to extracellular matrix-associated heparan sulfate proteoglycans through its basic region. AIDS 1997;11:1421–1431.

39. Shearer GM, Pinto LA, Clerici M. Alloimmunization for immune-based therapy and vaccine design against HIV/AIDS. Immunol Today 1999;20:66–71.

40. Paxton WA, Martin SR, Tse D, O'Brien TR, Skurnick J, VanDevanter NL, Padian N, Braun JF, Kotler DP, Wolinsky SM, Koup RA. Relative resistance to HIV-1 infection of CD4 lymphocytes from persons who remain uninfected despite multiple high-risk sexual exposure. Nat Med 1996;2:412–417.

41. Almond N, Kent K, Cranage M, Rud E, Clarke B, Stott EJ. Protection by attenuated simian immunodeficiency virus in macaques against challenge with virus-infected cells. Lancet 1995;345:1342–1344.

42. Wyand MS, Manson KH, Garcia-Moll M, Montefiori D, Desrosiers RC. Vaccine protection by a triple deletion mutant of simian immunodeficiency virus. J Virol 1996;70:3724–3733.

43. Norley S, Beer B, Binninger-Schinzel D, Cosma C, Kurth R. Protection from pathogenic SIVmac challenge following short-term infection with a nef-deficient attenuated virus. Virology 1996;219:195–205.

44. Baba TW, Liska V, Khimani AH, Ray NB, Dailey PJ, Penninck D, Bronson R, Greene MF, McClure HM, Martin LN, Ruprecht RM. Live attenuated, multiply deleted simian immunodeficiency virus causes AIDS in infant and adult macaques. Nat Med 1999;5:194–203.

45. Connor RI, Montefiori DC, Binley JM, Moore JP, Bonhoeffer S, Gettie A, Fenamore EA, Sheridan KE, Ho DD, Dailey PJ, Marx PA. Temporal analyses of virus replication, immune responses, and efficacy in rhesus macaques immunized with a live, attenuated simian immunodeficiency virus vaccine. J Virol 1998;72:7501–7509.

46. Letvin NL, Li J, Halloran M, Cranage MP, Rud EW, Sodroski J. Prior infection with a nonpathogenic chimeric simian-human immunodeficiency virus does not efficiently protect macaques against challenge with simian immunodeficiency virus. J Virol 1995;69:4569–4571.

47. Ruprecht RM, Baba TW, Rasmussen R, Hu Y, Sharma PL. Murine and simian retrovirus models: the threshold hypothesis. AIDS 1996;10:33–40.

48. Johnson RP, Lifson JD, Czajak SC, Cole KS, Manson KH, Glickman R, Yang J, Montefiori DC, Montelaro R, Wyand MS, Desrosiers RC. Highly attenuated vaccine strains of simian immunodeficiency virus protect against vaginal challenge: inverse relationship of degree of protection with level of attenuation. J Virol 1999;73:4952–4961.

49. Almond N, Rose J, Sangster R, Silvera P, Stebbings R, Walker B, Stott EJ. Mechanisms of protection induced by attenuated simian immunodeficiency virus. I. Protection cannot be transferred with immune serum. J Gen Virol 1997;78:1919–1922.

50. Stebbings R, Stott J, Almond N, Hull R, Lines J, Silvera P, Sangster R, Corcoran T, Rose J, Cobbold S, Gotch F, McMichael A, Walker B. Mechanisms of protection induced by attenuated simian immunodeficiency virus. II. Lymphocyte depletion does not abrogate protection. AIDS Res Hum Retroviruses 1998;14:1187–1198.

51. Sernicola L, Corrias F, Koanga-Mogtomo ML, Baroncelli S, Di Fabio S, Maggiorella MT, Belli R, Michelini Z, Macchia I, Cesolini A, Cioe L, Verani P, Titti F. Long-lasting protection by live attenuated simian immunodeficiency virus in cynomolgus monkeys: no detection of reactivation after stimulation with a recall antigen. Virology 1999;256:291–302.

52. Baker E. Cell-derived anti-human immunodeficiency virus inhibitory factor. J Infect Dis 1999;179:485–488.

53. Poccia F, Battistini L, Cipriani B, Mancino G, Martini F, Gougeon ML, Colizzi V. Phosphoantigen-reactive Vgamma9Vdelta2 T lymphocytes suppress in vitro human immunodeficiency virus type 1 replication by cell-released antiviral factors including CC chemokines. J Infect Dis 1999;180:858–861.

54. Lee ME, Adams JW, Villinger F, Brar SS, Meadows M, Bucur SZ, Lackey DA 3rd, Brice GT, Cruikshank WW, Ansari AA, Hillyer CD. Molecular cloning and expression of rhesus macaque and sooty mangabey interleukin 16: biologic activity and effect on simian immunodeficiency virus infection and/or replication. AIDS Res Hum Retroviruses 1998;14:1323–1328.

55. Lee ME, Bucur SZ, Gillespie TW, Adams JW, Barker AT, Thomas EK, Roback JD, Hillyer CD. Recombinant human CD40 ligand inhibits simian immunodeficiency virus replication: a role for interleukin-16. J Med Primatol 1999;28:190–194.

56. Goletti D, Macchia I, Pace M, Leone P, Sernicola L, Maggiorella MT, Cafaro A, Baroncelli S, Verani P, Ensoli B, Titti F. Inhibition of SHIV replication by $CD8^+$ T lymphocytes from macaques immunized with live attenuated SIV: International Proceedings Division Fourth European Conference on Experimental AIDS Research, Tampere, Finland, June 18–21, 1999, pp. 85–89.

57. Brander C, Walker BD. T lymphocyte responses in HIV-1 infection: implications for vaccine development. Curr Opin Immunol 1999;11:451–459.

58. Mayr A, Danner K. Vaccination against pox diseases under immunosuppressive conditions. Dev Biol Stand 1978;41:225–234.

59. Rooney JF, Wohlenberg C, Cremer KJ, Moss B, Notkins AL. Immunization with a vaccinia virus recombinant expressing herpes simplex virus type 1 glycoprotein D: long-term protection and effect of revaccination. J Virol 1988;62: 1530–1534.

60. Cooney EL, Collier AC, Greenberg PD, Coombs RW, Zarling J, Arditti DE, Hoffman MC, Hu SL, Corey L. Safety of and immunological response to a recombinant vaccinia virus vaccine expressing HIV envelope glycoprotein. Lancet 1991;337:567–572.

61. Kundig TM, Kalberer CP, Hengartner H, Zinkernagel RM. Vaccination with two different vaccinia recombinant viruses: long-term inhibition of secondary vaccination. Vaccine 1993;11:1154–1158.

62. ELMAU Workshop "The Modified Vaccinia Ankara" in Vaccination and Immunotherapy, January 28–31, 1999.

63. Daniel MD, Mazzara GP, Simon MA, Sehgal PK, Kodama T, Panicali DL, Desrosiers RC. High-titer immune responses elicited by recombinant vaccinia virus priming and particle boosting are ineffective in preventing virulent SIV infection. AIDS Res Hum Retroviruses 1994;10:839–851.

64. Hirsch VM, Fuerst TR, Sutter G, Carroll MW, Yang LC, Goldstein S, Piatak M Jr, Elkins WR, Alvord WG, Montefiori DC, Moss B, Lifson JD. Patterns of viral replication correlate with outcome in simian immunodeficiency virus (SIV)-infected macaques: effect of prior immunization with a trivalent SIV vaccine in modified vaccinia virus Ankara. J Virol 1996;70:3741–3752.

65. Hanke T, Blanchard TJ, Schneider J, Hannan CM, Becker M, Gilbert SC, Hill AV, Smith GL, McMichael A. Enhancement of MHC class I-restricted peptide-specific T cell induction by a DNA prime/MVA boost vaccination regime. Vaccine 1998;16:439–445.

66. Belyakov IM, Moss B, Strober W, Berzofsky JA. Mucosal vaccination overcomes the barrier to recombinant vaccinia immunization caused by preexisting poxvirus immunity. Proc Natl Acad Sci USA 1999;96:4512–4517.

67. Paoletti E. Applications of pox virus vectors to vaccination: An update. Proc Natl Acad Sci USA 1996;93:11349–11353.

68. Clements-Mann ML, Weinhold K, Matthews TJ, Graham BS, Gorse GJ, Keefer MC, McElrath MJ, Hsieh RH, Mestecky J, Zolla-Pazner S, Mascola J, Schwartz D, Siliciano R, Corey L, Wright PF, Belshe R, Dolin R, Jackson S, Xu S, Fast P, Walker MC, Stablein D, Excler JL, Tartaglia J, Paoletti E, et al. Immune responses to human immunodeficiency virus (HIV) type 1 induced by canarypox expressing HIV-1MN gp120, HIV-1SF2 recombinant gp120, or both vaccines in seronegative adults. J Infect Dis 1998;177:1230–1246.

69. Mulligan MJ, Weber J. Human trials of HIV vaccines. AIDS 1999;13:S105–S112.

70. Pialoux G, Excler JL, Riviere Y, Gonzalez-Canali G, Feuillie V, Coulaud P, Gluckman JC, Matthews TJ, Meignier B, Kieny MP, et al. A prime-boost approach to HIV preventive vaccine using a recombinant canarypox virus expressing glycoprotein 160 (MN) followed by a recombinant glycoprotein 160 (MN/LAI). AIDS Res Hum Retroviruses 1995;11:373–381.

71. Taylor J, Trimarchi C, Weinberg R, Languet B, Guillemin F, Desmettre P, Paoletti E. Efficacy studies on a canarypox-rabies recombinant virus. Vaccine 1991;9:190–193.

72. Robinson HL, Montefiori DC, Johnson RP, Manson KH, Kalish ML, Lifson JD, Rizvi TA, Lu S, Hu SL, Mazzara GP, Panicali DL, Herndon JG, Glickman R, Candido MA, Lydy SL, Wyand MS, McClure HM. Neutralizing antibody-independent containment of immunodeficiency virus challenges by DNA priming and recombinant pox virus booster immunizations. Nat Med 1999;5:526–534.

73. Rubin BA, Rorke LB. Adenovirus vaccines. In: Plotkin SA, Mortimer EA Jr, eds. Vaccines. Philadelphia: W.B. Saunders, 1988:492–512.

74. Shenk T. Adenoviridae: the viruses and their replication. In: Fields BN, Knipe DM, Howley PM, Chanok RM, Melnick JL, Monath TP, Roizman B, Straus SE, eds. Fields virology, 3rd ed. Vol. 2. Philadelphia: Raven, 1996:2111–2148.

75. Natuk RJ, Chanda PK, Lubeck MD, Davis AR, Wilhelm J, Hjorth R, Wade MS, Bhat BM, Mizutani S, Lee S, Eichberg J, Gallo RC, Hung PP, Robert-Guroff M. Adenovirus-human immunodeficiency virus (HIV) envelope recombinant vaccines elicit high-titered HIV-neutralizing antibodies in the dog model. Proc Natl Acad Sci USA 1992;89:7777–7781.

76. Natuk RJ, Lubeck MD, Chanda PK, Chengalvala M, Wade MS, Murthy SC, Wilhelm J, Vernon SK, Dheer SK, Mizutani S, Lee SG, Murthy KK, Eichberg JW, Davis AR, Hung PP. Immunogenicity of recombinant human adenovirus-human immunodeficiency virus vaccines in chimpanzees. AIDS Res Hum Retroviruses 1993;9:395–404.

77. Lubeck MD, Natuk RJ, Chengalvala M, Chanda PK, Murthy KK, Murthy S, Mizutani S, Lee SG, Wade MS, Bhat BM, et al. Immunogenicity of recombinant

adenovirus-human immunodeficiency virus vaccines in chimpanzees following intranasal administration. AIDS Res Hum Retroviruses 1994;10:1443–1449.

78. Lubeck MD, Natuk R, Myagkikh M, Kalyan N, Aldrich K, Sinangil F, Alipanah S, Murthy SC, Chanda PK, Nigida SM Jr, Markham PD, Zolla-Pazner S, Steimer K, Wade M, Reitz MS Jr, Arthur LO, Mizutani S, Davis A, Hung PP, Gallo RC, Eichberg J, Robert-Guroff M. Long-term protection of chimpanzees against high-dose HIV-1 challenge induced by immunization. Nat Med 1997; 3:651–658.

79. Zolla-Pazner S, Lubeck M, Xu S, Burda S, Natuk RJ, Sinangil F, Steimer K, Gallo RC, Eichberg JW, Matthews T, Robert-Guroff M. Induction of neutralizing antibodies to T-cell line-adapted and primary human immunodeficiency virus type 1 isolates with a prime-boost vaccine regimen in chimpanzees. J Virol 1998;72:1052–1059.

80. Robert-Guroff M, Kaur H, Patterson LJ, Leno M, Conley AJ, McKenna PM, Markham PD, Richardson E, Aldrich K, Arora K, Murty L, Carter L, Zolla-Pazner S, Sinangil F. Vaccine protection against a heterologous, non-syncytium-inducing, primary human immunodeficiency virus. J Virol 1998;72:10275–10280.

81. Buge SL, Richardson E, Alipanah S, Markham P, Cheng S, Kalyan N, Miller CJ, Lubeck M, Udem S, Eldridge J, Robert-Guroff M. An adenovirus-simian immunodeficiency virus env vaccine elicits humoral, cellular, and mucosal immune responses in rhesus macaques and decreases viral burden following vaginal challenge. J Virol 1997;71:8531–8541.

82. Buge SL, Murty L, Arora K, Kalyanaraman VS, Markham PD, Richardson ES, Aldrich K, Patterson LJ, Miller CJ, Cheng SM, Robert-Guroff M. Factors associated with slow disease progression in macaques immunized with an adenovirus-simian immunodeficiency virus (SIV) envelope priming-gp120 boosting regimen and challenged vaginally with SIVmac251. J Virol 1999;73: 7430–7440.

83. Hu SL, Polacino P, Stallard V, Klaniecki J, Pennathur S, Travis BM, Misher L, Kornas H, Langlois AJ, Morton WR, Benveniste RE. Recombinant subunit vaccines as an approach to study correlates of protection against primate lentivirus infection. Immunol Lett 1996;51:115–119.

84. Huang HV. Sindbis virus vectors for expression in animal cells. Curr Opin Biotechnol 1996;7:531–535.

85. Frolov I, Hoffman TA, Pragai BM, Dryga SA, Huang HV, Schlesinger S, Rice CM. Alphavirus-based expression vectors: strategies and applications. Proc Natl Acad Sci USA 1996;93:11371–11377.

86. Strauss JH, Strauss EG. The alphaviruses: gene expression, replication, and evolution. Microbiol Rev 1994;58:491–562.

87. Xiong C, Levis R, Shen P, Schlesinger S, Rice CM, Huang HV. Sindbis virus: an efficient, broad host range vector for gene expression in animal cells. Science 1989;243:1188–1191.

88. Fries LF, Tartaglia J, Taylor J, Kauffman EK, Meignier B, Paoletti E, Plotkin S. Human safety and immunogenicity of a canarypox-rabies glycoprotein recombinant vaccine: an alternative poxvirus vector system. Vaccine 1996;14: 428–434.

89. Liljestrom P, Garoff H. A new generation of animal cell expression vectors based on the Semliki Forest virus replicon. Biotechnology 1991;9:1356–1361.

90. Bredenbeeck PJ, Frolov I, Rice CM, Huang HV. Sindbis virus expression vectors: packaging of RNA replicons by using defective helper RNAs. J Virol 1993;67:6439–6446.

91. Pusko P, Parker M, Ludwig GV, Davis NL, Johnston RE, Smith JF. Replicon-helper systems from attenuated Venezuelan equine encephalitis virus: expression of heterologous genes in vitro and immunization against heterologous pathogens in vivo. Virology 1997;239:389–401.

92. Davis NL, Brown KW, Johnston RE. A viral vaccine vector that expresses foreign genes in lymph nodes and protects against mucosal challenge. J Virol 1996;70:3781–3787.

93. Caley IJ, Betts MR, Irlbeck DM, Davis NL, Swanstrom R, Frelinger JA, Johnston RE. Humoral, mucosal, and cellular immunity in response to a human immunodeficiency virus type 1 immunogen expressed by a Venezuelan equine encephalitis virus vaccine vector. J Virol 1997;71:3031–3038.

94. Hevey M, Negley D, Pushko P, Smith J, Schmaljohn A. Marburg virus vaccines based upon alphavirus replicons protect guinea pigs and nonhuman primates. Virology 1998;251:28–37.

95. MacDonald MR, Burney MW, Resnick SB, Virgin HW IV. Spliced mRNA encoding the murine cytomegalovirus chemokine homolog predicts a beta chemokine of novel structure. J Virol 1999;73:3682–3691.

96. Hirsch VM, Dapolito G, McGann C, Olmsted RA, Purcell RH, Johnson PR. Molecular cloning of SIV from sooty mangabey monkeys. J Med Primatol 1989;18:279–285.

97. Davis NL, Caley IJ, MacDonald GH, Brown KW, Betts MR, Irlbeck DM, McGrath KM, Connel MJ, Collier ML, Nielsen A, Richmond EB, Ping LH, Dryga SA, Maughan MF, Williamson C, Morris L, Karim SSA, Fiscus SA, Olmsted R, Montefiori DC, Frelinger JA, Swanstrom R, Johnson PR and Johnston RE. SIV and HIV vaccines using VEE replicon particles. Proceedings of the 12th Cent Gardes Meeting, Paris, Oct 25–27, 1999.

98. Malone JG, Bergland PJ, Liljestrom P, Rhodes GH, Malone RW. Mucosal immune responses associated with polynucleotide vaccination. Behring Inst Mitt 1997;98:63–72.

99. Berglund P, Fleeton MN, Smerdou C, Liljestrom P. Immunization with recombinant Semliki Forest virus induces protection against influenza challenge in mice. Vaccine 1999;17:497–507.

100. Mossman SP, Bex F, Berglund P, Arthos J, O'Neil SP, Riley D, Maul DH, Bruck C, Momin P, Burny A, Fultz PN, Mullins JI, Liljestrom P, Hoover EA. Protection against lethal simian immunodeficiency virus SIVsmmPBj14 disease by a recombinant Semliki Forest virus gp160 vaccine and by a gp120 subunit vaccine. J Virol 1996;70:1953–1960.

101. Berglund P, Quesada-Rolander M, Putkonen P, Biberfeld G, Thorstensson R, Liljestrom P. Outcome of immunization of cynomolgus monkeys with recombinant Semliki Forest virus encoding human immunodeficiency virus type 1 envelope protein and challenge with a high dose of SHIV-4 virus. AIDS Res Hum Retroviruses 1997;13:1487–1495.

102. Whitton JL, Sheng N, Oldstone MB, McKee TA. A "string-of-beads" vaccine, comprising linked minigenes, confers protection from lethal-dose virus challenge. J Virol 1993;67:348–352.

103. Oldstone MB, Tishon A, Eddleston M, de la Torre JC, McKee T, Whitton JL. Vaccination to prevent persistent viral infection. J Virol 1993;67:4372–4378.

104. Thomson SA, Khanna R, Gardner J, Burrows SR, Coupar B, Moss DJ, Suhrbier A. Minimal epitopes expressed in a recombinant polyepitope protein are processed and presented to CD8+ cytotoxic T cells: implications for vaccine design. Proc Natl Acad Sci USA 1995;92:5845-5849.

105. Lalvani A, Aidoo M, Allsopp CE, Plebanski M, Whittle HC, Hill AV. An HLA-based approach to the design of a CTL-inducing vaccine against *Plasmodium falciparum*. Res Immunol 1994;145:461–468.

106. Sidney J, Grey HM, Kubo RT, Sette A. Practical, biochemical and evolutionary implications of the discovery of HLA class I supermotifs. Immunol Today 1996; 17:261–266.

107. Hanke T, Blanchard TJ, Schneider J, Ogg GS, Tan R, Becker M, Gilbert SC, Hill AV, Smith GL, McMichael A. Immunogenicities of intravenous and intramuscular administrations of modified vaccinia virus Ankara-based multi-CTL epitope vaccine for human immunodeficiency virus type 1 in mice. J Gen Virol 1998;79:83–90.

108. Hanke T, Neumann VC, Blanchard TJ, Sweeney P, Hill AV, Smith GL, McMichael A. Effective induction of HIV-specific CTL by multi-epitope using gene gun in a combined vaccination regime. Vaccine 1999;17:589–596.

109. Moskophidis D, Pircher H, Chiernik I, Odermatt B, Hengartner H, Zinkernagel RM. Suppression of virus-specific antibody production by CD8+ class I-restricted antiviral cytotoxic T cells in vivo. J Virol 1992;66:3661-3668.

110. Battegay M, Moskophidis D, Waldner H, Bründler M-A, Fung-Leung W-P, Mak TW, Hengartner H, Zinkernagel RM. Impariment and delay of neutralizing

antiviral antibody responses by virus-specific cytotoxic T cells. J Immunol 1993;151:5408–5415.

111. Watts C, Lanzavecchia A. Suppressive effect of antibody on processing of T cell epitopes. J Exp Med 1993;178:1459–1463.

112. Battegay M, Kyburz D, Hengartner H, Zinkernagel RM. Enhancement of disease by neutralizing antiviral antibodies in the absence of primed antiviral cytotoxic T cells. Eur J Immunol 1993;23:3236–3241.

113. Simitsek PD, Campbell DG, Lanzavecchia A, Fairweather N, Watts C. Modulation of antigen processing by bound antibodies can boost or suppress class II major histocompatibility complex presentation of different T cell determinants. J Exp Med 1995;181:1957–1963.

114. Seiler P, Bründler M-A, Zimmermann C, Weibel D, Bruns M, Hengartner H, Zinkernagel RM. Induction of protective cytotoxic T cell responses in the presence of high titers of virus-neutralizing antibodies: implications for passive and active immunization. J Exp Med 1998;187:649–654.

115. Arya SK, Guo C, Joseph SF, Wong-Staal F. The trans-activator gene of human T lymphotropic virus type III (HTLV-III). Science 1985;229:69–73.

116. Fisher AG, Feinberg MB, Josephs SF, Harper ME, Marselle LM, Reyes G, Gonda MA, Aldovini A, Debouk C, Gallo RC, Wong-Staal F. The trans-activator gene of HTLV-III is essential for virus replication. Nature 1986;320: 367–371.

117. Chang HK, Gallo RC, Ensoli B. Regulation of cellular gene expression and function by the human immunodeficiency virus type 1 Tat protein. J Biomed Sci 1995;2:189–202.

118. Frankel AD, Pabo CO. Cellular uptake of the Tat protein from human immunodeficiency virus. Cell 1988;55:1189–1193.

119. Barillari G, Buonaguro L, Fiorelli V, Hoffman J, Michaels F, Gallo RC, Ensoli B. Effects of cytokines from activated immune cells on vascular cell growth and HIV-1 gene expression: Implications for AIDS-Kaposi's sarcoma pathogenesis. J Immunol 1992;149:3727–3734.

120. Li CJ, Ueda Y, Shi B, Borodyansky L, Huang L, Li YZ, Pardee AB. Tat protein induces self-perpetuating permissivity for productive HIV-1 infection. Proc Natl Acad Sci USA 1997;94:8116–8120.

121. Huang L, Bosh I, Hofmann W, Sodroski J, Pardee AB. Tat protein induces human immunodeficiency virus type 1 (HIV-1) coreceptors and promotes infection with both macrophage-tropic and T-lymphotropic HIV-1 strains. J Virol 1998;72:8952–8960.

122. Viscidi RP, Mayur K, Lederman HM, Frankel AD. Inhibition of antigen-induced lymphocyte proliferation by Tat protein from HIV-1. Science 1989; 246:1606–1608.

123. Barillari G, Sgadari C, Palladino C, Gendelman R, Caputo A, Bohan Morris C, Nair BC, Markham P, Stürzl M, Ensoli B. Inflammatory cytokines synergize with the HIV-1 Tat protein to promote angiogenesis and Kaposi's sarcoma via induction of bFGF and $\alpha v\beta 3$ integrin that are required for Tat activity. J Immunol 1999;163:1929–1935.

124. Subramanyam M, Gutheil WG, Bachovchin WW, Huber BT. Mechanism of HIV-1 Tat induced inhibition of antigen-specific T cell responsiveness. J Immunol 1993;150:2544–2553.

125. Li CJ, Friedman DJ, Wang C, Metelev V, Pardee AB. Induction of apoptosis in uninfected lymphocytes by HIV-1 Tat protein. Science 1995;268:429–431.

126. Westendorp MO, Frank R, Ochsenbauer C, Stricker K, Dhein J, Walczak H, Debatin KM, Krammer PH. Sensitization of T cells to CD95-mediated apoptosis by HIV-1 Tat and gp120. Nature 1995;275:497–500.

127. Zauli G, Gibellini D, Celeghini C, Mischiati C, Bassini A, La Placa M, Capitani S. Pleiotropic effects of immobilized versus soluble recombinant HIV-1 Tat protein on CD3-mediated activation, induction of apoptosis, and HIV-1 long terminal repeat transactivation in purified CD4+ T lymphocytes. J Immunol 1996;157:2216–2224.

128. Zagury JF, Chams V, Lachgar A, et al. Mode of AIDS immunopathogenesis based on the HIV-1 gp120 and Tat-induced dysregulation of uninfected immune cells. Cell Pharmacol 1996;3:123–128.

129. Zagury D, Lachgar A, Chams V, Fall LS, Bernard J, Zagury JF, Bizzini B, Gringeri A, Santagostino E, Rappaport J, Feldman M, Burny A, Gallo RC. Interferon alpha and Tat involvement in the immunosuppression of uninfected T cells and C-C chemokine decline in AIDS. Proc Natl Acad Sci USA 1998; 95:3851–3856.

130. Barillari G, Gendelman R, Gallo RC, Ensoli B. The Tat protein of human immunodeficiency virus type-1, a growth factor for AIDS Kaposi's sarcoma and cytokine-activated vascular cells, induces adhesion of the same cell types by using integrin receptors recognizing the RGD amino acid sequence. Proc Natl Acad Sci USA 1993;90:7941–7945.

131. Barillari G, Sgadari C, Fiorelli V, Samaniego F, Colombini S, Manzari V, Modesti A, Nair BC, Cafaro A, Stürzl M, Ensoli B. The Tat protein of human immunodeficiency virus type-1 promotes vascular cell growth and locomotion by engaging the $\alpha v\beta 3$ integrins by mobilizing sequestered basic fibroblast growth factor. Blood 1999;94:663–672.

132. Reiss P, Lange JM, de Ronde A, de Wolf F, Dekker J, Debouck C, Goudsmit J. Speed of progression to AIDS and degree of antibody response to accessory gene products of HIV-1. J Med Virol 1990;30:163–168.

133. Rodman TC, To SE, Hashish H, Manchester K. Epitopes for natural antibodies of human immunodeficiency virus (HIV)-negative (normal) and HIV-positive

sera are coincident with two key functional sequences of HIV Tat protein. Proc Natl Acad Sci USA 1993;90:7719–7723.

134. Re MC, Furlini G, Vignoli M, Ramazzotti E, Roderigo G, De Rosa V, Zauli G, Lolli S, Capitani S, La Placa M. Effect of antibody to HIV-1 Tat protein on viral replication in vitro and progression of HIV-1 disease in vivo. J Acquir Immune Defic Syndr Hum Retrovirol 1995;10:408–416.

135. Venet A, Bourgault I, Aubertin AM, Kieny MP, Levy JP. Cytotoxic T lymphocyte response against multiple simian immunodeficiency virus (SIV) proteins in SIV-infected macaques. J Immunol 1992;148:2899–2908.

136. Froebel KS, Aldhous MC, Mok JY, Hayley J, Arnott M, Peutherer JF. Cytotoxic T lymphocyte activity in children infected with HIV. AIDS Res Hum Retroviruses 1994;2:83–88.

137. van Baalen CA, Pontesilli O, Huisman RC, Geretti AM, Klein MR, de Wolf F, Miedema F, Gruters RA, Osterhaus AD. HIV-1 Rev and Tat specific cytotoxic T lymphocyte frequencies inversely correlate with rapid progression to AIDS. J Gen Virol 1997;78:1913–1918.

138. Kim DT, Mitchell DJ, Brockstedt DG, Fong L, Nolan GP, Fathman CG, Engleman EG, Rothbard JB. Introduction of soluble proteins into the MHC class I pathway by conjugation to an HIV tat peptide. J Immunol 1997;159:1666–1668.

139. Reimann KA, Li JT, Veazey R, Halloran M, Park IW, Karlsson GB, Sodroski J, Letvin NL. A chimeric simian/human immunodeficiency virus type 1 isolate env causes in AIDS-like disease after in vivo passage in rhesus monkeys. J Virol 1996;70:6922–6928.

140. Karlsson GB, Halloran M, Schenten D, Lee J, Racz P, Tenner-Racz K, Manola J, Gelman R, Etemad-Moghadam B, Desjardins E, Wyatt R, Gerard NP, Marcon L, Margolin D, Fanton J, Axthelm MK, Letvin NL, and Sodroski J. The envelope glycoprotein ectodomains determine the efficiency of CD4+ T lymphocyte depletion in simian-human immunodeficiency virus-infected macaques. J Exp Med 1998;188:1159–1171.

140a. Cafaro A, Caputo A, Maggiorella MT, Baroncelli S, Fracasso C, Pace M, Borsetti A, Sernicola L, Negri D, Ten Haaft P, Betti M, Michelini Z, Macchia I, Fanales-Belasio E, Belli R, Corrias F, Buttò S, Verani P, Titti F, Ensoli B. SHIV89.6P pathogenicity in cynomolgus monkeys and control of viral replication and disease onset by HIV-1 Tat vaccine. J Med Primatol, in press.

141. Caselli E, Betti M, Grossi MP, Barbanti-Brodano G, Baldoni PG, Rossi C, Boarini C, Cafaro A, Ensoli B, Caputo A. DNA immunization with HIV-1 tat mutated in the transactivation domain induces humoral and cellular immune responses against wild-type TAT. J Immunol 1999;162:5631–5638.

142. Caputo A, Grossi MP, Bozzini R, Rossi C, Betti M, Marconi PC, Barbanti-Brodano G, Balboni PG. Inhibition of HIV-1 replication and reactivation from

latency by tat transdominant negative mutants in the cysteine rich region. Gene Ther 1996;3:235–245.

143. Gringeri A, Santagostino E, Muca-Perja M, Mannucci PM, Zagury JF, Bizzini B, Lachgar A, Carcagno M, Rappaport J, Criscuolo M, Blattner W, Burny A, Gallo RC, Zagury D. Safety and immunogenicity of HIV-1 Tat toxoid in immunocompromised HIV- 1-infected patients. J Hum Virol 1998;1:293–298.

144. Gringeri A, Santagostino E, Muca-Perja M, Le Buanec H, Bizzini B, Lachgar A, Zagury JF, Rappaport J, Burny A, Gallo RC, Zagury D. Tat toxoid as a component of a preventive vaccine in seronegative subjects. J Acquir Immune Defic Syndr Hum Retrovirol 1999;20:371–375.

145. Calarota SA, Leandersson AC, Bratt G, Hinkula J, Klinman DM, Weinhold KJ, Sandstrom E, Wahren B. Immune responses in asymptomatic HIV-1-infected patients after HIV-DNA immunization followed by highly active antiretroviral treatment. J Immunol 1999;163:2330–2338.

146. Wang Y, Tao L, Mitchell E, Bravery C, Berlingieri P, Armstrong P, Vaughan R, Underwood J, Lehner T. Allo-immunization elicits CD8+ T cell-derived chemokines, HIV suppressor factors and resistance to HIV infection in women. Nat Med 1999;5:1004–1009.

147. Clerici M, DePalma L, Roilides E, Baker R, Shearer GM. Analysis of T helper and antigen-presenting cell functions in cord blood and peripheral blood leukocytes from healthy children of different ages. J Clin Invest 1993;91:2829–2836.

148. Macdonald JC, Torriani FJ, Morse LS, Karavellas MP, Reed JB, Freeman WR. Lack of reactivation of cytomegalovirus (CMV) retinitis after stopping CMV maintenance therapy in AIDS patients with sustained elevations in CD4 T cells in response to highly active antiretroviral therapy. J Infect Dis 1998;177: 1182–1187.

149. Pinto LA, Sharpe S, Cohen DI, Shearer GM. Alloantigen-stimulated anti-HIV activity. Blood 1998;92:3346–3354.

150. Kiprov DD, Sheppard HW, Hanson CV. Alloimmunization to prevent AIDS? Science 1994;263:737–738.

151. Coulam CB, Clark DA. Immunotherapy for recurrent miscarriage. Am J Reprod Immunol 1994;32:257–260.

152. Stott EJ. Anti-cell antibody in macaques. Nature 1991;186:588–596.

153. Heeney JL, van Els C, de Vries P, ten Haaft P, Otting N, Koornstra W, Boes J, Dubbes R, Niphuis H, Dings M, Cranage M, Norley S, Jonker M, Bontrop RE, Osterhaus A. Major histocompatibility complex class I-associated vaccine protection from simian immunodeficiency virus-infected peripheral blood cells. J Exp Med 1994;180:769–774.

154. Osterhaus A, de Vries P, Heeney J. AIDS vaccine developments. Nature 1992; 355:684–685.

155.   Le Grand R, Vaslin B, Vogt G, Roques P, Humbert M, Dormont D. AIDS vaccine developments. Nature 1992;355:684.

156.   Cranage MP, Ashworth LA, Greenaway PJ, Murphey-Corb M, Desrosiers RC. AIDS vaccine developments. Nature 1992;355:685–686.

157.   Mellors JW, Rinaldo CR Jr, Gupta P, White RM, Todd JA, Kingsley LA. Prognosis in HIV-1 infection predicted by the quantity of virus in plasma. Science 1996;272:1167–1170.

158.   Autran B, Carcelain G, Li TS, Blanc C, Mathez D, Tubiana R, Katlama C, Debre P, Leibowitch J. Positive effects of combined antiretroviral therapy on CD4+ T cell homeostasis and function in advanced HIV disease. Science 1997; 277:112–116.

159.   Li TS, Tubiana R, Katlama C, Calvez V, Ait Mohand H, Autran B. Long-lasting recovery in CD4 T-cell function and viral-load reduction after highly active antiretroviral therapy in advanced HIV-1 disease. Lancet 1998;351:1682–1686.

160.   Goulder P, Rowland-Jones SL, McMichael AJ, Walker BD. Anti-HIV cellular immunity: recent advances towards vaccine design. AIDS 1999;13: S211–S236.

161.   Rosenberg ES, Walker BD. HIV type 1-specific helper T cells: a critical host defense. AIDS Res Hum Retroviruses 1998;14:S143–S147.

162.   Lehner T, Wang Y, Tao L, Bergmeier LA, Mitchell E, Doyle C. CD8-suppressor factor and beta-chemokine function as a complementary mechanism to cognate immunity. Immunol Lett 1999;66:171–176.

163.   Warren JT, Levinson MA. AIDS preclinical vaccine development: biennial survey of HIV, SIV, and SHIV challenge studies in vaccinated nonhuman primates. J Med Primatol 1999;28:249–273.

164.   Manca F, Fenoglio D, Li Pira G, Kunkl A, Celada F. Effect of antigen/antibody ratio on macrophage uptake, processing, and presentation to T cells of antigen complexed with polyclonal antibodies. J Exp Med 1991;173:37–48.

165.   Lehner T, Bergmeier L, Wang Y, Tao L, Mitchell E. A rational basis for mucosal vaccination against HIV infection. Immunol Rev 1999;170:183–196.

166.   Lehner T, Wang Y, Cranage M, Bergmeier LA, Mitchell E, Tao L, Hall G, Dennis M, Cook N, Brookes R, Klavinskis L, Jones I, Doyle C, Ward R. Protective mucosal immunity elicited by targeted iliac lymph node immunization with a subunit SIV envelope and core vaccine in macaques. Nat Med 1996;2: 767–775.

167.   Cranage MP, Whatmore AM, Sharpe SA, Cook N, Polyanskaya N, Leech S, Smith JD, Rud EW, Dennis MJ, Hall GA. Macaques infected with live attenuated SIVmac are protected against superinfection via the rectal mucosa. Virology 1997;229:143–154.

168.   Quesada-Rolander M, Makitalo B, Thorstensson R, Zhang YJ, Castanos-Velez E, Biberfeld G, Putkonen P. Protection against mucosal SIVsm challenge in

macaques infected with a chimeric SIV that expresses HIV type 1 envelope. AIDS Res Hum Retroviruses 1996;12:993–999.

169. Miller CJ, McChesney MB, Lu X, Dailey PJ, Chutkowski C, Lu D, Brosio P, Roberts B, Lu Y. Rhesus macaques previously infected with simian/human immunodeficiency virus are protected from vaginal challenge with pathogenic SIVmac239. J Virol 1997;71:1911–1921.

170. Joag SV, Liu ZQ, Stephens EB, Smith MS, Kumar A, Li Z, Wang C, Sheffer D, Jia F, Foresman L, Adany I, Lifson J, McClure HM, Narayan O. Oral immunization of macaques with attenuated vaccine virus induces protection against vaginally transmitted AIDS. J Virol 1998;72:9069–9078.

171. Putkonen P, Makitalo B, Bottiger D, Biberfeld G, Thorstensson R. Protection of human immunodeficiency virus type 2-exposed seronegative macaques from mucosal simian immunodeficiency virus transmission. J Virol 1997;71:4981–4984.

172. Miller CJ, McGhee JR. Progress towards a vaccine to prevent sexual transmission of HIV. Nat Med 1996;2:751–752.

3

Pediatric Human Immunodeficiency Virus Type 1 Infection: Updates on Prevention and Management

Ann J. Melvin and Lisa M. Frenkel
University of Washington and Children's Hospital and Regional Medical Center, Seattle, Washington

I. INTRODUCTION

Infection of children with human immunodeficiency virus type 1 (HIV-1) occurs nearly exclusively from their mothers. The fetus can be infected in utero; however, transmission occurs most often during birth or breastfeeding. Without medical intervention, between 20 and 40% of infants born to HIV-1 infected women become infected. Because of the increasing prevalence of HIV-1 infection among women of childbearing age in many areas of the world, pediatric HIV-1 infection has become a major cause of infant mortality. From studies conducted during the past 15 years, maternal and obstetrical factors associated with transmission have been identified. More recently, interventions that effectively decrease the rate of transmission have been identified. The factors associated with perinatal HIV-1 transmission and interventions that can markedly reduce the rate of mother-to-infant HIV-1 transmission are summarized, as is management of the HIV-1 exposed infant, including HIV-1 diagnosis.

II. MATERNAL AND OBSTETRICAL FACTORS ASSOCIATED WITH PERINATAL HIV-1 TRANSMISSION

A number of factors have been consistently associated with perinatal HIV-1 transmission in observational studies: breastfeeding, exposure to blood during delivery, high maternal HIV-1 viral load in blood, lack of antiretroviral prophylaxis, and lack of elective cesarean section. Factors that have been inconsistently associated with transmission include chorioamnionitis, and maternal and infant antibodies that neutralize HIV-1 and maternal vitamin A levels.

A.   Breastfeeding

HIV-1 transmission by breastfeeding was first documented from nursing mothers infected with HIV-1 from postpartum transfusions (1). A study of women who seroconverted to HIV-1 while breastfeeding showed a high rate of HIV-1 transmission (2). The infants of 9 of 16 women who seroconverted during breastfeeding were infected with HIV-1, presumably via breastfeeding. The rate of transmission through breastfeeding by chronically infected women has been estimated over time (3). Among prospectively enrolled HIV-1-infected pregnant women in Malawi, the cumulative HIV-1 infection rate of breastfeeding infants through 5, 11, 17, and 23 months of age was 3.5, 7.0, 8.9, and 10.3%, respectively. The incidence per month was estimated to be 0.7% from age 1–5 months, 0.6% from age 6 through 11 months old, and 0.3% from age 12 through 17 months old. Protective factors in this study were high maternal parity (relative risk [RR], 0.23; 95% confidence interval [CI], 0.09–0.56), and older maternal age (RR, 0.44; 95% CI, 0.23–0.84).

In a randomized study of breastfeeding versus formula feeding in Nairobi, Kenya, 44% of infant infections were attributed to breastfeeding, using an intent-to-treat analysis (4). There was a 16% (95% CI, 6.5–29) difference in the rate of HIV-1 infection, with 61 of 197 breastfed and 31 of 204 formula-fed infants infected during a median follow-up of 24 months ($p = 0.03$). Infant mortality was not different between the groups, with 45 (24%) of breastfed and 39 (20%) of formula-fed infants dying. However, formula feeding may offer a better outcome as 42% of breastfed and 30% of formula-fed infants either died or were HIV-1 infected.

Observational studies of breastfeeding women in South Africa suggest that the introduction of foods in addition to breastfeeding may increase the rate of HIV-1 transmission (5). HIV-1 infection was transmitted to 18.8% (95% CI, 12.6–24.9) of 156 never breastfed 3-month-old infants compared with 21.3% (95% CI, 17.2–25.5) of the breastfed infants. However, transmission appeared higher in infants who were also given foods (24.1%; 95% CI, 19.0–

29.2) when compared with those who were exclusively breastfed (14.5%; 95% CI, 7.7–21.4; $p = 0.03$). The authors postulate that mixed feeding may change the integrity of the intestines, reducing the barrier to HIV-1 infection, and that the protective effects provided by breast milk were less in those infants given a mixture of foods. This study, however, was not randomized, and it is not clear whether the study was biased in the distribution of maternal viral loads or obstetrical risks.

Due to social pressures and economic constraints that make formula feeding impractical and the health risks of formula feeding in certain communities, safe methods for HIV-1-infected women to breastfeed are critical to the health of many infants. Pasteurization and chemical disinfection of breast milk have been considered but are generally believed to be impractical. A study of antiviral prophylaxis of infants during breastfeeding is planned and may offer an effective yet only moderately expensive strategy for HIV-1-infected women to safely breastfeed their infants.

B.   Exposure to Maternal Blood and Virus

Obstetrical factors that result in increased exposure of the infant to maternal blood and/or secretions such as prolonged rupture of membranes (6–8) and trauma to the infant (9) have been associated with an increased risk of mother-to-child transmission of HIV-1.

Many studies have demonstrated an increased risk of mother-to-child transmission in association with increased maternal viral burden as measured by quantitative peripheral blood mononuclear cell (PBMC) coculture (10, 11), quantitative DNA polymerase chain reaction (PCR) (12), and RNA PCR (13–16). The data associating maternal p24 antigenemia with transmission have been inconsistent; some but not all studies have shown an association (15, 17, 18). Although perinatal transmission clearly decreases with lower maternal plasma HIV-1 RNA levels, transmission can occur when viral replication is below the limits of detection of the assays (14). However, effective suppression of viral replication in the pregnant women along with antiretroviral prophylaxis of her infant appears extremely effective in preventing perinatal HIV-1 transmission (15, 19, 20).

Results of the AIDS Clinical Trials Group (ACTG) 076 protocol demonstrated that while the risk of transmission increased with increasing HIV-1 plasma RNA levels, mother-to-child transmission occurred across the entire range of RNA levels and that the zidovudine (ZDV) treatment effect was seen at all RNA levels (14). A statistically significant reduction of maternal plasma HIV-1 RNA levels was associated with ZDV use in the ACTG 076 study but was of a quantity generally regarded as clinically insignificant. It was estimated that only 17% of the protective effect of ZDV was due to a reduction in maternal viral load. The mechanism of protection to the infant was, by implication, prevention of HIV-1 reverse transcription.

HIV-1 transmission has occurred when maternal viral load was below the limits of detection (14, 21); thus, an absolute maternal plasma HIV RNA level below which transmission will not occur has not been established. However, evidence of protection from HIV-1 transmission when maternal plasma HIV RNA levels were below the level of detection (< 200 copies/mL plasma) due to the use of potent antiretroviral therapies has been accumulating (19, 20, 22). These therapies have included reverse transcriptase inhibitors, such as ZDV, that pass to the fetus and provide chemoprophylaxis to the infant. None of 84 women with undetectable plasma HIV-1 RNA who participated in ACTG protocol 185 transmitted HIV-1 to their infants (15). Similarly, among 89 patients from six institutions (20) and 53 women at the University of Southern California (19) treated with highly active antiretroviral therapy (HAART), none of their 116 infants > 4 months old became infected with HIV-1. These observations provide hope that suppression of viral replication in pregnant women combined with chemoprophylaxis of their infants will prevent HIV-1 transmission.

C. Antiretroviral Prophylaxis of the Infant

The large multicenter trial that investigated the safety of ZDV during pregnancy and the efficacy of ZDV in reducing mother-to-child transmission was the ACTG 076 study (23). The trial was randomized, double blind, and placebo controlled. HIV-1-infected pregnant women were give ZDV or placebo orally for a mean of 12 weeks during pregnancy, intravenously during labor, and orally to the infant for the first 6 weeks of life. Thirteen of 180 women in the ZDV group transmitted the virus to their infants (8.3%; CI, 3.9–12.8%) compared with 40 of 183 women in the placebo group (25.5%; CI, 18.4–32.5%)—a 67% decrease in the rate of mother-to-child HIV-1 transmission. A decrease in mother-to-child HIV-1 transmission associated with the use of ZDV in pregnancy has been demonstrated in multiple other smaller observational studies (9, 13, 24–27).

ACTG Protocol 185 was initiated to determine if immunoglobulin with high levels of HIV-1-specific antibodies (HIVIG) would further reduce perinatal HIV-1 transmission compared with intravenous gamma globulin (used as a placebo). The study was stopped prematurely when an interim analysis found HIV-1 transmission to 6.0% of infants in the placebo and 4.1% in the

HIVIG groups ($p = 0.36$) (28). This event rate was too low for a difference to be detectable. In this study, HIVIG or IVIG was given in addition to medications administered for the women's own infection and for chemoprophylaxis of their infants.

Which component of the ZDV regimen used in ACTG 076 (23) (maternal oral ZDV antenatally vs. intravenous ZDV in labor vs. oral ZDV to the infant) protects the fetus/infant from HIV-1 is unknown. This is particularly relevant in developing countries where the cost of the complete ACTG 076 regimen is beyond existing resources. Several studies have suggested that a substantial protective effect can be achieved with maternal antenatal use of zidovudine (9, 25, 27). In an observational study of 188 women and 190 infants retrospectively identified at five university HIV clinics (where the women but not infants were treated with ZDV), the rate of mother-to-child transmission was 12.4% (95% CI, 8.0–18.2%) (27). When 39 women with <200 CD4 cells/μL were excluded to compare with the ACTG 076 population, the mother-to-child transmission rate (8.9%; 95% CI, 4.7, 15.0) did not differ from that observed in the ACTG 076 study (8.3%).

Analysis of perinatal transmission among HIV-1-infected women in New York state suggested that postexposure ZDV chemoprophylaxis was effective (29, 30). Among 939 HIV-1-exposed infants, viral transmission was 6.1% (95% CI, 4.1–8.9%) when ZDV treatment was begun in the woman prenatally, 10.0% (95% CI, 3.3–21.8%) when begun in the woman intrapartum, 9.3% (95% CI, 4.1–17.5%) when begun in the infant within 48 hours after birth, 18.4% (95% CI, 7.7–34.3%) when begun in the infant after 48 hours of birth, and 26.6% (95% CI, 21.1–32.7%) when no ZDV was given (29). Of the 21 infants who received ZDV within 48 hours after birth, 1 of 17 (5.9%) who received it within 12 hours of birth became infected, and 4 of 12 (25%) treated between 12 and 24 hours after birth became infected (30). This and other observational studies suggest that perinatal HIV-1 transmission was most effectively prevented by the presence of reverse transcriptase inhibitors in the fetus/infant at the time of exposure but that early postexposure chemoprophylaxis had some efficacy.

The complete ACTG 076 regimen costs approximately US$800 and is too costly to be utilized for routine prevention of perinatal HIV-1 infection in many countries where the infection is prevalent. Several comparative trials utilizing modifications of the ACTG 076 ZDV treatment regimen have been completed in Africa and Thailand. In Thailand, oral ZDV treatment of pregnant women initiated at 36 weeks gestation and administered through delivery was found to reduce HIV-1 transmission by 50.1% (95% CI, 15.4–70.6%) compared with placebo in a nonbreastfeeding population (31). The pregnant women took ZDV 300 mg twice daily for a median of 25 days before labor and a median of three ZDV 300-mg capsules given every 3 hours during labor. The infants were not given ZDV. Infection status was determined for 392 infants. Nine and four tenths percent (95% CI, 5.2–13.5%) of the ZDV and 18.9% (95% CI, 3.3–21.8%) of the placebo group were HIV-1 infected ($p = 0.006$). The transmission rate in this oral ZDV group did not differ from the ACTG 076 ZDV group, and the ZDV regimen used in Thailand cost approximately one tenth (US$80) of the former.

Three separate randomized placebo-controlled trials have studied "short-course" ZDV alone or in combination with lamivudine in breastfeeding populations in Africa. In the two studies utilizing ZDV only, the pregnant women were treated with ZDV 300 mg twice daily beginning at 36–38 weeks gestation (32, 33). During labor in one study (32), the women received ZDV 300 mg every 3 hours. In the other study (33), the women initially received ZDV 600 mg and then 300 mg every 3 hours during labor, and postpartum they received 300 mg twice daily for 7 days. The rates of transmission were 15.6% at 3 months (32) and 18% at 6 months (33). The efficacy of the two ZDV regimens were similar, 37% (95% CI, 5–63%) reduction in transmission at 3 months of age (32) and 38% (95% CI, 5–60%) at 6 months of age (33). There were four separate treatment groups in the ZDV/lamivudine study (34). The HIV-1 pregnant women in group A received both drugs beginning at 36 weeks gestation through labor, and their infants received the same drugs for a week after birth. The group B women received only intrapartum drugs with their infants receiving the same drugs for a week after birth. The group C women received only intrapartum drugs, and their infants did not receive antiretrovirals, whereas group P women received only placebo for the entire study. All groups of women breastfed their infants. The rates of HIV-1 transmission in this study when the infants were 6 weeks old were 8.6%, 10.8%, 17.7%, and 17.2%, for groups A, B, C, and P, respectively. This study clearly demonstrated that intrapartum treatment only using nucleoside analogues with short serum half-lives was not effective in the prevention of perinatal HIV-1 transmission.

In a randomized trial, a short course of nevirapine demonstrated greater protection from HIV-1 infection in a breastfeeding population than a short course of ZDV (35). In this study, HIVNET 021, nevirapine 200 mg was administered to the mother once at the time of labor, and 2 mg/kg once to their infants within 72 hours of birth in one group. In the other arm, ZDV 600 mg was initiated in the pregnant women at the beginning of labor with 300 mg administered every 3 hours thereafter until delivery. Their infants were administered ZDV 4 mg/kg twice daily for 1 week. When the infants were

14–16 weeks old, 25.1% of the ZDV- and 13.1% of the nevirapine-treated infants were HIV-1 infected ($p = 0.0006$). In addition to the remarkable potency of the nevirapine regimen, its cost (approximately US$8) will allow its implementation in many countries (Figs. 1, 2).

In two observational studies, maternal HAART, discussed above, prevented perinatal HIV-1 transmission in more that 100 mother–infant pairs (19, 20). These studies, however, were not sufficiently large enough to judge the effectiveness of HAART with confidence.

An alarming report suggested that mitochondrial dysfunction occurred with sufficient severity and frequency to pose an ethical dilemma in the use of nucleoside analogues for the prevention of perinatal HIV-1 infection (36). In contrast, a review of more than 13,000 nucleoside exposed, HIV-1-uninfected children in studies within the United States did not identify children who appear to have suffered morbidity or mortality characteristic of mitochondrial dysfunction (37). Also, 234 infants exposed to ZDV a mean of 4.2 years earlier as part of ACTG 076 have had no effect on growth or cognitive development and no deaths or cancers (38). However, two children had opthamologic abnormalities and one child a subclinical cardiomyopathy of unclear etiology.

Very little data exist concerning the safety of protease inhibitors during pregnancy and to the fetus. An increased risk of preterm delivery (33%) was observed among a small population of 16 women treated with HAART containing protease inhibitors (39). In contrast, two observational studies of significantly larger populations of protease inhibitors containing HAART did not find high rates of adverse pregnancy outcomes (19, 20).

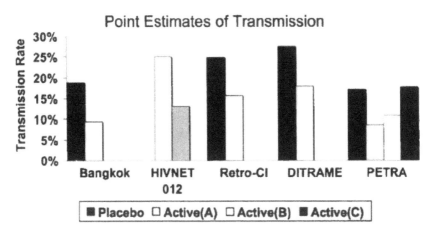

Figure 1   Overall comparison of short-course AZT AZT/3TC and NVP trial results.

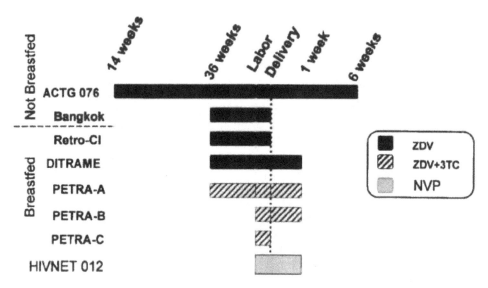

Figure 2 Comparison of timing of ACTG 076 and short-course antiretroviral regimens.

Toxicities observed in six women and their fetuses/infants participating in a phase I study of ritonavir included transient low serum glucose in the infants and a number of other temporary abnormalities that were not suspected to be due to the use of ritonavir (40). These findings emphasize the need for larger controlled studies of protease inhibitor use in pregnancy.

Although our understanding of factors related to perinatal HIV-1 transmission continues to improve, a comprehensive study of therapeutic failure has not been done. HIV-1 resistance to ZDV may diminish the protective effect of ZDV, nevirapine, and other combinations of antiretrovirals given to pregnant women for treatment and to prevent perinatal HIV-1 transmission. The development of HIV-1 resistance has been evaluated among participants in ACTG 076 and the Women and Infants Transmission Study (WITS). Virtually no resistance to ZDV was found among ACTG 076 women (41). In contrast, HIV-1 resistance to ZDV was associated with HIV-1 transmission in WITS (42), suggesting that testing maternal HIV-1 for resistance may prove useful in communities where ZDV resistance is prevalent. In two smaller studies, ZDV resistance occurred in pregnant women and was transmitted in a few cases to their infants. A study of 20 HIV-1-infected pregnant women with significant ZDV experience (mean, 52 weeks) found four women's HIV-1 had genotypic evidence of resistance to ZDV. Two of the four had high-level resistance, and one of these transmitted highly resistant virus to their infant

(43). In a separate preliminary report, genotypic resistance to ZDV occurred in 3 of 30 HIV-1-infected pregnant women (44). Two of the three women transmitted ZDV-resistant virus to their infants. An association of HIV-1 resistance with risk of transmission in women prescribed HAART has not been systematically studied. Anecdotes (45) and personal experience indicate that HIV-1 antiviral resistance, nonadherence to therapy, and a lack of prenatal care, together and alone, are all associated with risk of transmission. These factors are likely to present a challenge to obstetrical providers in the future. Fortunately, among women for whom HAART does not suppress viral replication, cesarean delivery is likely to reduce perinatal HIV-1 transmission (discussed below).

As a result of changes in the antiretroviral treatment of adults, the guidelines for antiretroviral treatment of HIV-1 infected pregnant women were modified. Previously, the regimen studied in ACTG 076 (23) was recommended. Currently, there is insufficient pharmacokinetic, safety, and efficacy data to recommend a specific regimen other than the ACTG 076 regimen. However, because lower rates of HIV-1 transmission have been associated with lower maternal viral loads and with women receiving combinations of antiretroviral agents, a discussion of current knowledge with each pregnant woman and individualization of antiretroviral regimens has been recommended (46).

D. Obstetrical Management

Until recently, the association between the mode of delivery and the risk of transmission has varied across studies. Although many studies (47, 48) reported a decreased rate of transmission after cesarean section, others did not observe this association (49). Most of these studies did not control for the duration of rupture of membranes and other factors associated with transmission of HIV-1, making comparisons between studies difficult.

A meta-analysis and a randomized trial have shown recently that HIV-1 transmission was decreased by elective cesarean section before the onset of labor. Among 8533 mother–infant pairs tracked in 15 observational studies, elective cesarean section halved the rate of perinatal transmission (adjusted odds ratio [OR], 0.43; 95% CI, 0.33–0.56) after adjustment for receipt of antiretroviral therapy, maternal stage of disease, and infant birth weight (50). Transmission was reduced by 87% with both elective cesarean section and receipt of antiretroviral therapy during the prenatal, intrapartum, and neonatal periods compared with other modes of delivery and the absence of therapy (OR, 0.13; 95% CI, 0.09–0.19). Among mother–child pairs receiving antiretroviral therapy, HIV-1 transmission occurred in 2.0% of 196 who underwent elective cesarean section and 7.3% of 1255 mothers with other modes of delivery.

A randomized comparative trial of elective cesarean section at 38 weeks gestation versus spontaneous vaginal delivery also demonstrated reduced transmission with elective cesarean section (51). In an intent-to-treat analysis, perinatal HIV-1 transmission occurred in 3 of 170 (1.8%) randomized to elective cesarean section and 21 of 200 (10.5%; $p < 0.001$) randomized to vaginal delivery. It is important to note that the women in both cohorts (50, 51) delivered for the most part before the widespread use of HAART. As was discussed above, a similar low rate of perinatal HIV-1 transmission occurs with effective antiretroviral therapy (15, 19, 20).

Morbidity associated with elective cesarean delivery has been noted to be increased among HIV-1-infected women. Morbidity in the WITS was 19% (52). In contrast, infectious morbidity in women delivering vaginally was 8% among those requiring instrumental assistance and only 4% in those with noninstrument-assisted deliveries. When multivariant analyses were applied to the data, the independent predictors of infectious complications were elective cesarean section (OR, 3; 95% CI, 1.1, 7.3), nonelective cesarean section (OR, 6; 95% CI, 3.5, 10.5), and maternal age > 30 years (OR, 1.5; 95% CI, 0.9, 2.5).

A similar degree of infectious morbidity was associated with cesarean section among women who particpated in ACTG 185 (53). Infections occurred in 26% of women who underwent an elective cesarean section (16% amnionitis/endometritis, 5% wound infections, 5% urinary tract infections) and in 40% of cesarean sections done after the onset of labor or rupture of membranes (21% amnionitis/endometritis, 8% wound infections, 11% urinary tract infections). Similar to the previous study, fewer infectious complications were also observed among women who delivered vaginally in this study. Thirteen percent of those who had a spontaneous vaginal delivery had infections (7% amnionitis/endometritis, 2% wound infections, 4% urinary tract infections) and 19% of those with assisted vaginal deliveries had infections (5% amnionitis/endometritis, 0% wound infections, 14% urinary tract infections). Interestingly, infections were not more common among those with low CD4 cells (19.5% of women with <200 CD4 and 16% of women with >200 CD4 cells). Also, in this large study, a protective effective effect of cesarean delivery was not observed, perhaps due to the low rate of transmission.

Recently, the American College of Obstetrics and Gynecology recommended that cesarean section be considered for the delivery of all infants from HIV-1-infected women. These recommendations should be communicated to and discussed with the infected pregnant women, as should the information suggesting an increased rate of complications after an operative delivery, and that suppression of viral replication in the pregnant woman appears to protect the infant from HIV-1 infection. The pregnant woman, after reviewing the current data on perinatal HIV-1 transmission with her health care providers, must decide on her antiretroviral regimen and mode of delivery.

III. ANTIRETROVIRAL THERAPY FOR HIV-1-INFECTED CHILDREN

In 1998, the Working Group on Antiretroviral Therapy and Medical Management of HIV-Infected Children published guidelines for antiretroviral treatment of HIV-infected infants and children (56) based largely on results of adult studies demonstrating virological, immunological, and clinical benefit from combination antiretroviral regimens (54) and preliminary results of Pediatric AIDS Clinical Trials Group (PACTG) protocol 338. The latter demonstrated that drug combinations including a protease inhibitor were more effective at reducing plasma HIV-1 RNA levels than a combination of two reverse transcriptase inhibitors (55). These guidelines recommend the initiation of a three-drug regimen including two reverse transcriptase inhibitors and a protease inhibitor for children with clinical and/or immunological evidence of HIV-1 disease progression and all infants less than 12 months of age (56).

Pharmacokinetic studies have suggested that children may require proportionately higher dosages of protease inhibitors to achieve comparable serum levels to adults (Table 1). Results of PACTG 377 showed the standard dosing of nelfinavir (20–30 mg/kg per dose every 8 hours) produced suboptimal serum levels in children < 25 kg (57). Improved drug levels were demonstrated with nelfinavir dosed at 55 mg/kg per dose twice daily. Similarly, pharmacokinetic analysis of ritonavir in PACTG 345 indicated that children less than 2 years of age require an increased dosage of ritonavir, 450 mg/mm^2 every 12 hours (58). Saquinavir soft-gel capsules are currently under study through PACTG 397 with a dosage of 50 mg/kg per dose every 8 hours or 50 mg/kg per dose every 12 hours when given in conjunction with nelfinavir. A dosage of 500 mg/M^2 per dose every 8 hours of indinavir capsules was suggested by Mueller et al. (59) after a dose-finding study involving 54 children. Although early studies found a high incidence of renal toxicity from indinavir use in children (60, 61), recent reports from two European centers found indinavir combinations to be well tolerated and to achieve prolonged viral suppression in children (62, 63).

Preliminary pharmacokinetic data are also available for some of the newer nucleoside and nonnucleoside reverse transcriptase inhibitors (Table 1).

Table 1 Pediatric Dosages of New Antiretroviral Agents Suggested by Recent Phase I Studies

Drug	Age	Dose
Ritonavir	≥ 1 mo to <2 yr	450 mg/M^2/dose q 12 hr
Ritonavir	≥ 2 yr	400 mg/M^2/dose q 12 hr (maximum dose of 600 mg q 12 hr)
Nelfinavir	≥ 4 mo	55 mg/kg/dose q 12 hr (maximum dose of 1500 mg q 12 hr)
Saquinavir soft-gel cap	≥ 3 yr	50 mg/kg/dose q 12 hr plus ritonavir 100 mg/M^2/dose q 12 hr (maximum dose of 1200 mg q 8 hr)
Saquinavir soft-gel cap when given with nelfinavir	≥ 3 yr	50 mg/kg/dose q 12 hr (maximum dose of 1600 mg q 12 hr)
Indinavir	≥ 3 yr	500 mg/M^2/dose q 8 hr
Efavirenz	≥ 2 yr	(wt kg/70kg)$^{0.7}$ $\times$ 600 mg q day
Abacavir	≥ 3 mo	8 mg/kg/dose q 12 hr

PACTG 382, an investigation of combination therapy including nelfinavir and efavirenz, found negligible interaction between the two agents and the dosage requirements of efavirenz capsules in children to be the same as adults. The suspension, however, was less well absorbed with drug levels being highly variable, particularly in the younger children (64, 65). A small phase I study of delavirdine found 16 mg/kg per dose given every 12 hours to older children to produce serum levels comparable with those achieved in adults (66). Abacavir, investigated through PACTG 330, dosed 8 mg/kg per dose every 12 hours produced appropriate serum levels (67). Although pharmacokinetic data for many antiretroviral agents are lacking in children < 3 months of age, several ongoing PACTG studies are performing these assays, and results should be available within the next year.

Several randomized clinical trials of combination antiretroviral therapy including protease inhibitors in children are in process, and to date the data on the use of these regimens has generally been limited to observational reports and the pharmacokinetic studies discussed above. HAART appears to be well tolerated in HIV-infected children, even in those with advanced disease (60, 68). However, although children appear to have a good immunological response to HAART, the virological response has been less encouraging with fewer than half of treated children achieving suppression of plasma HIV-1

RNA to below the level of detection in most studies (61, 69, 70). The reasons for the decreased virologic response are not entirely clear; however, difficulties with adherence (71) and failure to concurrently administer nucleoside reverse transcriptase inhibitors to which the children had not been previously exposed (61, 69, 70) may have contributed to a lack of potency. Hopefully, as new data become available on treatment of HIV-infected children with HAART, strategies will be developed to maximize the long-term efficacy of antiretroviral therapy in children.

IV. SUMMARY

A greater understanding of perinatal HIV-1 transmission has resulted in a marked decrease in the incidence of pediatric HIV-1 infection in several affluent nations. Advances in treatment have led to a decrease in HIV-1-related morbidity and mortality in some HIV-1-infected children. Studies are ongoing to determine methods to sustain the salutary effects of treatment. A goal of child advocates is to translate these advances to communities with few resources. Efforts are underway to make infant chemoprophylaxis widely available and to define strategies to reduce exposure to maternal virus. Likewise, there is the need to increase the access of children to treatment.

REFERENCES

1. Stiehm ER, Vink P. Transmission of human immunodeficiency virus infection by breast-feeding. J Pediatr 1991;118:410–412.

2. Van de Perre P, Simonon A, Msellati P, et al. Postnatal transmission of human immunodeficiency virus type 1 from mother to infant. A prospective cohort study in Kigali, Rwanda [see comments]. N Engl J Med 1991;325:593–598.

3. Miotti PG, Taha TE, Kumwenda NI, et al. HIV transmission through breastfeeding: a study in Malawi [see comments]. Jama 1999;282:744–749.

4. Nduati R. Clinical Studies of Breast Versus Formula Feeding. 2nd Conference on Global Strategies for the Prevention of HIV Transmission from Mothers to Infants. Montreal, Canada, 1999.

5. Coutsoudis A, Pillay K, Spooner E, Kuhn L, Coovadia HM. Influence of infant-feeding patterns on early mother-to-child transmission of HIV-1 in Durban, South Africa: a prospective cohort study. South African Vitamin A Study Group [see comments]. Lancet 1999;354:471–476.

6. Minkoff H, Burns DN, Landesman S, et al. The relationship of the duration of ruptured membranes to vertical transmission of human immunodeficiency virus. Am J Obstet Gynecol 1995;173:585–589.

7. Biggar RJ, Miotti PG, Taha TE, et al. Perinatal intervention trial in Africa: effect of a birth canal cleansing intervention to prevent HIV transmission. Lancet 1996; 347:1647–1650.

8. Landesman SH, Kalish LA, Burns DN, et al. Obstetrical factors and the transmission of HIV-1 from mother to child. N Engl J Med 1996;334:1617–1623.

9. Boyer PJ, Dillon M, Navaie M, et al. Factors predictive of maternal-fetal transmission of HIV-1: preliminary analysis of Zidovudine given during pregnancy and/or delivery. JAMA 1994;271:1925–1930.

10. Borkowsky W, Krasinski K, Cao Y, et al. Correlation of perinatal transmission of human immunodeficiency virus type 1 with maternal viremia and lymphocyte phenotypes. J Pediatr 1994;125:345–351.

11. Weiser B, Nachman S, Tropper P, et al. Quantitation of human immunodeficiency virus type 1 during pregnancy: relationship of viral titer to mother-to-child transmission and stability of viral load. Proc Natl Acad Sci USA 1994;91: 8037–8041.

12. Roques P, Marce D, Courpotin C, et al. Correlation between HIV provirus burden and in utero transmission. AIDS 1993;7(suppl 2):S39–S43.

13. Dickover RE, Garratty EM, Herman SA, et al. Identification of levels of maternal HIV-1 RNA associated with risk of perinatal transmission. Effect of maternal zidovudine treatment on viral load. JAMA 1996;275:599–605.

14. Sperling RS, Shapiro DE, Coombs RW, et al. Maternal viral load, zidovudine treatment and the risk of transmission of human immunodeficiendy virus type 1 from mother to infant. N Engl J Med 1996;335:1678–1681.

15. Mofenson LM, Lambert JS, Stiehm ER, et al. Risk factors for perinatal transmission of human immunodeficiency virus type 1 in women treated with zidovudine. Pediatric AIDS Clinical Trials Group Study 185 Team [see comments]. N Engl J Med 1999;341:385–393.

16. Garcia PM, Kalish LA, Pitt J, et al. Maternal levels of plasma human immunodeficiency virus type 1 RNA and the risk of perinatal transmission. Women and Infants Transmission Study Group [see comments]. N Engl J Med 1999;341: 394–402.

17. Newell ML, Dunn D, Peckham CS, Ades AE, Pardi G, Semprini AE, and the European Collaborative Study. Risk factors for mother-to-child transmission of HIV-1. Lancet 1992;339:1007–1012.

18. Scarlatti G, Lombardi V, Plebani A, et al. Polymerase chain reaction, virus isolation and antigen assay in HIV-1-antibody-positive mothers and their children. AIDS 1991;5:1173–1178.

19. Stek A, Khoury M, Kramer F, et al. Maternal and infant outcomes with highly active antiretroviral therapy during pregnancy. 6th Conference on Retroviruses and Opportunistic Infections, Chicago, IL, 1999.

20. Morris A, Zorrilla C, Vajranant M, et al. A review of protase inhibitor use on 89 pregnancies. 6th Conference on Retroviruses and Opportunistic Infections, Chicago, IL, 1999.

21. Husson RN, Lan Y, Kojima E, Venzon D, Mitsuya H, McIntosh K. Vertical transmission of human immunodeficiency virus type 1: autologous neutralizing antibody, virus load, and virus phenotype. J Pediatr 1995;126:865–871.

22. Mofenson L, Lambert J, Stiehm ER, et al. Risk factors for adverse pregnancy outcomes in HIV-infected pregnant women in PACTG 185. 6th Conference on Retroviruses and Opportunistic Infections, Chicago, IL, 1999.

23. Connor EM, Sperling RS, Gelber R, et al. Reduction of maternal-infant transmission of human immunodeficiency virus type 1 with zidovudine treatment. Pediatric AIDS Clinical Trials Group Protocol 076 Study Group [see comments]. N Engl J Med 1994;331:1173–1180.

24. Frenkel LM, Wagner LEN, Demeter LM, et al. Effects of zidovudine use during pregnancy on resistance and vertical transmission of HIV-1. Clin Infect Dis 1995;20:1321–1326.

25. Matheson PB, Abrams EJ, Thomas PA, et al. Efficacy of antenatal zidovudine in reducing perinatal transmission of human immunodeficiency virus type 1. The New York City Perinatal HIV Transmission Collaborative Study Group. J Infect Dis 1995;172:353–358.

26. Cooper ER, Nugent RP, Diaz C, et al. After AIDS clinical trial 076: the changing pattern of zidovudine use during pregnancy, and the subsequent reduction in the vertical transmission of human immunodeficiency virus in a cohort of infected women and their infants. Women and Infants Transmission Study Group. J Infect Dis 1996;174:1207–1211.

27. Frenkel L, Cowles M, Shapiro D, et al. The protective effect of zidovudine on the vertical transmission of HIV-1 appears to be primarily due to oral maternal zidovudine (ZDV) during late gestation. J Infect Dis 1996;175:971–974.

28. Stiehm ER, Lambert JS, Mofenson LM, et al. Efficacy of zidovudine and human immunodeficiency virus (HIV) hyperimmune immunoglobulin for reducing perinatal HIV transmission from HIV-infected women with advanced disease: results of Pediatric AIDS Clinical Trials Group protocol 185. J Infect Dis 1999; 179:567–575.

29. Wade NA, Birkhead GS, Warren BL, et al. Abbreviated regimens of zidovudine prophylaxis and perinatal transmission of the human immunodeficiency virus [see comments]. N Engl J Med 1998;339:1409–1414.

30. Wade N, Birkhead GS, French PT. Short course of zidovudine and perinatal transmission HIV. J Engl J Med 1999;340:1042–1043.

31. Shaffer N, Chuachoowong R, Mock PA, et al. Short-course zidovudine for perinatal HIV-1 transmission in Bangkok, Thailand: a randomised controlled trial.

Bangkok Collaborative Perinatal HIV Transmission Study Group. Lancet 1999;
353:773–780.

32. Wiktor SZ, Ekpini E, Karon JM, et al. Short-course oral zidovudine for pre-
     vention of mother-to-child transmission of HIV-1 in Abidjan, Cote d'Ivoire: a
     randomised trial. Lancet 1999;353:781–785.

33. Dabis F, Msellati P, Meda N, et al. 6-month efficacy, tolerance, and accept-
     ability of a short regimen of oral zidovudine to reduce vertical transmission of
     HIV in breastfed children in Cote d'Ivoire and Burkina Faso: a double-blind
     placebo- controlled multicentre trial. DITRAME Study Group. DIminution de
     la Transmission Mere-Enfant. Lancet 1999;353:786–792.

34. Saba J. The results of the PETRA intervention trial to prevent perinatal transmis-
     sion in Subsaharan Africa. 6th Conference on Retroviruses and Opportunistic
     Infections, Chicago, IL, 1999.

35. Guay LA, Musoke P, Fleming T, et al. Intrapartum and neonatal single-dose nevi-
     rapine compared with zidovudine for prevention of mother-to-child transmission
     of HIV-1 in Kampala, Uganda: HIVNET 012 randomised trial [In Process Ci-
     tation]. Lancet 1999;354:795–802.

36. Blanche S, Tardieu M, Rustin P, et al. Persistent mitochondrial dysfunction and
     perinatal exposure to antiretroviral nucleoside analogues [In Process Citation].
     Lancet 1999;354:1084–1089.

37. Smith ME, Group UNSRW. Ongoing nucleoside safety review of HIV exposed
     children in US studies. 2nd Conference on Global Strategies for the Prevention
     of HIV Transmission from Mothers to Infants, Montreal, CA, 1999.

38. Culnane M, Fowler M, Lee SS, et al. Lack of long-term effects of in utero
     exposure to zidovudine among uninfected children born to HIV-infected women.
     Pediatric AIDS Clinical Trials Group Protocol 219/076 Teams. JAMA 1999;281:
     151–157.

39. Lorenzi P, Masserei B, Laubereau B, et al. Safety of combined therapies in
     pregnancy. 12th World AIDS Conference, Geneva, Switzerland, 1998.

40. Scott G, Tuomala R, et al. Premature births and gestational weight in HIV-1-
     infected pregnant women. Workshop on Detection of Potential Toxicities Fol-
     lowing Perinatal Exposure to Antiretrovirals, Bethesda, MD: National Institutes
     of Health, 1999.

41. Eastman PS, Shapiro DE, Coombs RW, et al. Maternal viral genotypic zidovu-
     dine resistance and infrequent failure of zidovudine therapy to prevent perinatal
     transmission of human immunodeficiency virus type 1 in pediatric AIDS Clinical
     Trials Group Protocol 076. J Infect Dis 1998;177:557–564.

42. Colgrove RC, Pitt J, Chung PH, Welles SL, Japour AJ. Selective vertical trans-
     mission of HIV-1 antiretroviral resistance mutations. AIDS 1998;12:2281–2288.

43. Frenkel L, Manns Arcuino L, Edelstein R, et al. A study of the association of genotypic and phenotypic HIV-1 resistance to didanosine (ddI), syncytium inducing phenotype (SI), plasma RNA copy number and infectious units per million cells (IUPM) with HIV-1 disease progression in children treated with didanosine. Fifth International HIV Drug-Resistance Workshop, Whistler, B. C., 1996.

44. Weiser B, Burger H, Weislow O, Fang G, et al. AZT resistance and HIV-1 mother-to-child transmission. 3rd Conference of Retroviruses and Opportunistic Infections, Washington, DC, 1996.

45. Johnson VA, Woods C, Hamilton CD, Fiscus SA. Verticle transmission of a HIV-1 variant resistance to multiple reverse transcriptase and protease inhibitors. 6th Conference on Retroviruses and Opportunistic Infections, Chicago, IL, 1999.

46. CDC. US Public Health Service Task Force recommendations for the use of antiretroviral drugs in pregnant women infected with HIV-1 for maternal health and for reducing perinatal HIV-1 transmission in the United States. MMWR Marb Martal Wkly Rep 1998;47:1–30.

47. Kind C, Brandle B, Wyler CA, et al. Epidemiology of vertically transmitted HIV-1 infection in Switzerland: results of a nationwide prospective study. Swiss Neonatal HIV Study Group. Eur J Pediatr 1992;151:442–448.

48. Thomas PA, Weedon J, Krasinski K, et al. Maternal predictors of perinatal human immunodeficiency virus transmission. The New York City Perinatal HIV Transmission Collaborative Study Group. Pediatr Infect Dis J 1994;13:489–495.

49. Dunn DT, Newell ML, Mayaux MJ, et al. Mode of delivery and vertical transmission of HIV-1: a review of prospective studies. Perinatal AIDS Collaborative Transmission Studies. J Acquir Immune Defic Syndr 1994;7:1064–1066.

50. The International Perinatal HIV Group. The mode of delivery and the risk of vertical transmission of human immunodeficiency virus type 1—a meta-analysis of 15 prospective cohort studies [see comments]. N Engl J Med 1999;340:977–987.

51. Anonymous. Elective cesarean-section versus vaginal delivery in prevention of vertical HIV-1 transmission: a randomised clinical trial. The European Mode of Delivery Collaboration. Lancet 1999;353:1035–1039.

52. Read J, Kpamegan E, Tuomala R, et al. Mode of delivery and postpartum morbidity among HIV-infected women: The women and infants. Transmission Study (WITS). 6th Conference on Retroviruses and Opportunistic Infections, Chicago, IL, 1999.

53. Watts H, Mofenson L, Whitehouse J, et al. Complications according to mode of delivery among HIV-positive women with CD4 counts <500. 6th Conference on Retroviruses and Opportunistic Infections, Chicago, IL, 1999.

54. Hammer SM, Squires KE, Hughes MD, et al. A controlled trial of two nucleoside analogues plus indinavir in persons with human immunodeficiency virus

infection and CD4 cell counts of 200 per cubic millimeter or less. N Engl J Med 1997;337:725–733.

55. Yogev R, Stanley K, Nachman SA, et al. Virologic efficacy of ZDV + 3TC vs d4^ + ritonavir (RTV) vs. ZDV + 3TC + RTV in stable anti-retroviral experienced HIV-infected children (Pediatric ACTG Trial 338). Proceedings of the 37th Interscience Conference on Antimicrobial Agents and Chemotherapy, Toronto, Canada, 1997.

56. Working Group on Antiretroviral Therapy and Medical Management of Infants, Children and Adolescents with HIV Infection. Antiretroviral therapy and medical management of pediatric HIV infection. Pediatrics 1998;102:S1005–S1085.

57. Hayashi S, Wiznia A, Jaywardene A, et al. Nelfinavir pharmacokinetics in stable HIV positive children: the effect of weight and a comparison of BID to TID dosing. 6th Conference on Retroviruses and Opportunistic Infections, Chicago, IL, 1999.

58. Rodman J, Chadwick W, Palumbo P, Abrams E, Hsu A, Yogev R. Ritonavir (RTV) pharmacokinetics and dose requirements in HIV infected children less than two years of age. 6th Conference on Retroviruses and Opportunistic Infections, Chicago, IL, 1999.

59. Mueller BU, Sleasman J, Nelson RP Jr, et al. A phase I/II study of the protease inhibitor indinavir in children with HIV infection. Pediatrics 1998;102(1 Pt 1): 101–109.

60. Melvin AJ, Mohan KM, Manns-Arcuino LA, Edelstein RE, Frenkel LM. Clinical, virologic, and immunologic responses of children with advanced HIV-1 disease treated with protease inhibitors. Pediatr Infect Dis 1997;16:968–974.

61. Rutstein RM, Feingold A, Meislich D, Word B, Rudy B. Protease inhibitor therapy in children with perinatally acquired HIV infection. AIDS 1997;11: F107–F111.

62. Van Rossum AMC, Hartwig NG, Niesters HGM, et al. Dutch multicenter trial of HIV infected children with indinavir, zidovudine, and lamivudine: 1 year follow-up. Proceedings of the 39th Interscience Conference on Antimicrobial Agents and Chemotherapy, San Francisco, CA, 1997.

63. Vigana A, Pirollo M, Sala N, et al. Long term outcome of potent antiretroviral therapy in HIV-infected children. 6th Conference on Retroviruses and Opportunistic Infections, Chicago, IL, 1999.

64. Brundage RC, Fletcher CV, Fiske WD, et al. Pharmacokinetic of an efavirenz suspension in children. 6th Conference on Retroviruses and Opportunistic Infections, Chicago, IL, 1999.

65. Fletcher CV, Brundage RC, Fenton T, et al. Efavirenz (EFV) and nelfinavir (NFV) pharmacokinetics (PK) in HIV-infected children participating in and area under the curve (UC) controlled trial. 6th Conference on Retroviruses and Opportunistic Infections, Chicago, IL, 1999.

66. Watson D, Cox S, Carel B, Shoup R. Treatment of HIV infected children with delavirdine combined with protease inhibitors: drug levels, safety and virologic response. 6th Conference on Retroviruses and Opportunistic Infections, Chicago, IL, 1999.

67. Kline MW, Blanchard S, Fletcher CV, et al. A phase I study of abacavir (1592U89) alone and in combination with other antiretroviral agents in infants and children with human immunodeficiency virus infection. AIDS Clinical Trials Group 330 Team. Pediatrics 1999;103:e47.

68. Burchett SK, Kovacs A, Khoury M, et al. Preliminary toxicity and tolerability of 4-drug antiretroviral therapy with NRTIs, nevirapine and ritonavir in ARV-experienced children with advanced HIV disease. 6th Conference on Retroviruses and Opportunistic Infections, Chicago, IL, 1999.

69. Krogstad P, Wiznia A, Luzuriaga K, et al. Treatment of human immunodeficiency virus 1-infected infants and children with the protease inhibitor nelfinavir mesylate. Clin Infect Dis 1999;28:1109–1118.

70. Thuret I, Michel G, Chambost H, et al. Combination antiretroviral therapy including ritonavir in children infected with human immunodeficiency. AIDS 1999;13:81–87.

71. Watson DC, Farley JJ. Efficacy of and adherence to highly active antiretroviral therapy in children infected with human immunodeficiency virus type 1 [In Process Citation]. Pediatr Infect Dis J 1999;18:682–689.

4

Risk of Human Immunodeficiency Virus Infection in Health Care Workers

Rita Fahrner
San Francisco General Hospital Occupational Health Service and University of California, San Francisco, San Francisco, California

I. INTRODUCTION

Health care workers exposed to blood and other hazardous body fluids are at risk for occupational transmission of human immunodeficiency virus (HIV) with resultant infection. Since the first documented case of HIV infection after accidental needlestick exposure was reported in 1984 (1), considerable progress has been made toward developing rigorous surveillance methods and techniques that seek to explicitly define the modes of occupational HIV transmission and the degree of risk associated with discreet exposure events. Additionally, widespread efforts to improve workplace safety, educate health care workers, and reduce the risk of occupational exposure and significant advances in the science of postexposure prophylaxis for HIV exposure are ongoing.

In November 1999, the United States Department of Labor Occupational Safety and Health Administration (OSHA) issued a new OSHA instruction that updates enforcement procedures for the 1992 final rule governing occupational exposure to bloodborne pathogens (2). This bloodborne pathogen standard endeavors to eliminate or minimize occupational exposure to HIV, hepatitis B virus (HBV), and other bloodborne pathogens by encouraging the use of a combination of engineering and work practice controls, personal protective equipment, training, medical surveillance, hepatitis B vaccination, signs and labels identifying hazards, and other similar provisions. In addition, the standard mandates universal precautions for infection control and requires employers to develop a written exposure control plan and to provide postexposure evaluation and testing for all employees who have exposure incidents. The 1999 directive reflects advances in safer medical devices and knowledge about treatment, including postexposure prophylaxis for health care workers exposed to bloodborne pathogens, and stresses the importance of annual training and the use of safer devices to reduce percutaneous injuries. Currently, many states have rewritten or are in the process of rewriting their OSHA regulations to include more stringent rules mandating the use of safer medical devices, the inclusion of hepatitis C virus (HCV) as a third bloodborne pathogens for screening of both exposed health care workers and source patients, and more enhanced training of workers.

In December 1995, the results of the Centers for Disease Control and Prevention (CDC) case-control study of health care workers with percutaneous HIV exposures were published (3). This retrospective study utilizing data reported to the national surveillance systems in three countries identified four independent risk factors for transmission: deep intramuscular injections, visible blood on the needle before injury, needle used in an artery or vein, and blood from a source patient with severe acquired immunodeficiency syndrome (AIDS) (defined as death within 2 months of the exposure). A fifth factor, use of zidovudine as postexposure prophylaxis, was associated with 79% reduction in the odds of transmission. Of note, this protective benefit was comparable with that observed in a study of perinatal zidovudine prophylaxis, where treatment contributed a 67% reduction in the risk of transmission (4).

Health care workers are in fact caring for increasing numbers of HIV-infected patients as early intervention with antiretrovirals and effective chemoprophylaxis for opportunistic infections lengthen survival and thus increase the duration and number of medical interventions.

II. ANECDOTAL CASE REPORTS OF OCCUPATIONAL HIV INFECTION

As of June 1999, 55 cases of documented HIV seroconversion among health care workers have been reported to CDC and documented in their HIV/AIDS Surveillance Report (5). Documentation of seroconversion, the gold standard, occurs only when a health care worker experiences a discreet exposure to blood or another body fluid containing HIV, has negative baseline HIV markers at the time of the incident, and has sequential analysis of HIV markers demonstrating seroconversion in temporal association with the exposure. These cases furnish irrefutable evidence that occupational exposure to HIV has caused infection.

These reports also provide important knowledge about the epidemiology of occupational HIV exposure that leads to infection. Blood is unquestionably the body fluid associated with the greatest risk for occupational infection. Of the 55 cases, 50 (91%) involved blood, 3 involved concentrated virus in a laboratory setting, 1 was from visibly bloody body fluid, and 1 was from an unspecified body fluid. Twenty-five (45%) of these health care workers have developed AIDS. The absence of documented cases of HIV infection from exposure to saliva, urine, respiratory secretions, and other nonbloody body fluids is reassuring and consistent with the low titers and infrequent detection of HIV in these fluids.

Over 89% of the seroconversions (49/55) occurred as a result of needlestick or other percutaneous exposure, 2 of which had both percutaneous and mucocutaneous exposures. Mucocutaneous exposure was the route of transmission in five cases, and one had an unknown route of exposure. Because no other transmission routes have been associated with occupational infection with HIV, fears regarding the risks of inhalation of aerosolized blood or other secretions, from intact skin contact, or during close and/or sustained patient contact may begin to be alleviated. Although these modes of transmission cannot be excluded with absolute certainty, the magnitude of risk, if any, must be extremely small.

Until the CDC case-control study was reported, there had been no detailed analysis published about the aspects of specific exposures that contribute to transmission risk. The study included 31 case health care workers (reported to local, state, or national health departments) who had a documented occupational percutaneous exposure to HIV-infected blood. HIV seroconversion was temporally associated with the specific documented exposure for all, and none reported other intercurrent HIV exposure. The 679 control health care workers (derived from the CDC Needlestick Study population) had a documented occupational percutaneous exposure to HIV-infected blood but remained HIV seronegative 6 months after the exposure (3). Of the 31 case health care workers, 29 (94%) sustained hollow-bore needlesticks and 2 (7%) were injured by other sharp devices. Similarly, the control health care workers sustained 620 (91%) needlesticks (26 of these needlesticks involved solid needles) and 59 (9%) involved other sharp objects.

Documented seroconversion cases afford the greatest measure of descriptive information about occupational exposures that lead to infection but provide very little information about the true magnitude of risk. In general, health care workers as a group are not prospectively tested for HIV infection, so the true incidence of infection is not known. HIV infection is not a mandated reportable illness in most states, and it is likely that some cases have not been reported due to concerns regarding confidentiality and fears of practice restrictions. Although many AIDS experts agree that there have undoubtedly been more cases of occupational transmission in health care workers than have been reported, there is also general agreement that the magnitude of risk has not been substantially underestimated.

An additional 136 possible cases of occupational HIV transmission have been recorded since 1981 in anecdotal case reports to the CDC (5). These cases have been investigated, and no identifiable behavioral or transfusion risks have been elucidated; each health care worker reported percutaneous or mucocutaneous occupational exposures to blood or other body fluids or laboratory specimens containing HIV, but HIV seroconversion was not specifically documented as resulting from an occupational exposure. Many of these exposures occurred before serological testing was available.

Most reported occupationally acquired infections have occurred in nurses and laboratory workers: 76% in the "documented" group and 37% in the "possible" group (5). Although this phenomenon may in part reflect a bias in reporting HIV infection, nurses and laboratory workers currently may be at the highest risk for exposure because they have more direct contact with HIV-infected patients than do other categories of health care workers. As the prevalence of HIV increases in the health care environment, surgeons and other health care providers at high risk for other bloodborne infections such as HBV and HCV are likely to experience an increased incidence of exposure and subsequent infection with HIV (6). The anecdotal case reports also provide important information about the natural history of HIV disease immediately after infection. More the 50% of the infected health care workers had the onset of symptoms suggestive of acute HIV infection within several weeks of the exposure. In some cases, the development of an unexplained febrile illness prompted HIV testing and therefore detection of the infection, so it is not possible to generalize this high rate of acute symptomatology to HIV infection in general. Nevertheless, appearance of symptoms suggestive of viral illness after accidental exposure to HIV is strong evidence of infection.

Antibodies to HIV developed within 6 months in most occupationally infected health care workers. The exact time of seroconversion cannot be identified in many because testing was not performed at frequent intervals. HIV antibodies and antigen were detected as early as 3 weeks after exposure in at least one case. The available data support current recommendations for postexposure HIV testing for at least 6 months after exposure. Infection in the absence of detectable HIV antibody after 6 months is so unlikely that testing beyond this point is not recommended in most cases. The reliability of HIV antibody as an indicator of infection is supported by data from prospective studies (below) in which several hundred exposed seronegative health care workers have been followed for more than 4 years without clinical evidence of HIV infection or delayed seroconversion (7).

III. PROSPECTIVE COHORT STUDIES

The reported cases of occupational HIV infection have demonstrated the presence of risk to health care workers exposed to infected blood. However, they must not be interpreted to imply a high degree of risk. Risk assessment requires estimation of the rate of infection, that is, both the numerator (number of infected health care workers) and the denominator (number of health care workers at risk) must be prospectively measured.

The magnitude of risk from HIV exposure has been prospectively evaluated by several studies (8–10). Of the 6498 highly exposed health care workers who voluntarily enrolled in 25 prospective seroprevalence studies, 21 participants (0.32%) were established to be occupationally infected (6).

Inoculation with infected blood during accidental needlestick injury or similar injury is the only factor associated with infection in prospective study subjects to date. Risk estimates based on data from the prospective studies do not account specifically for factors that may affect the actual risk, including the amount of infected material involved, the titer of infectious virus in that material, and whether the exposed health care worker took postexposure prophylaxis. The estimated risk from mucocutaneous exposure is likely to be at least one order of magnitude lower. Although the high frequency of cutaneous contact involving intact skin precludes accurate quantitation, the risk from this type of exposure is most certainly negligible. Among dental care providers who historically have had an extremely high risk of HBV infection and who report frequent exposure to aerosolized blood and saliva and needlestick inoculations, no case of infection has been prospectively identified (11).

Other serologic markers for HIV infection have been evaluated in some of these prospective cohort studies in an attempt to further refine assessment of delayed seroconversion to HIV. Two groups analyzed data on 272 health care workers whose sera were serially tested for HIV RNA by polymerase chain reaction (PCR) (7, 12). One cohort demonstrated three positive and six indeterminate PCRs among 220 health care workers who all had negative HIV antibody results. Follow-up studies for more than 3 years failed to detect seroconversion; all were PCR negative on follow-up and none ever had p24 antigen or a positive HIV culture. In this sample, the initial PCR results likely represented false positives, a common problem with this particular laboratory test. The role of PCR in predicting seronegative latency remains unknown, but most experts agree that the test is rarely if ever indicated for exposed health care workers. Various prospective studies will continue to evaluate the usefulness of PCR and other HIV markers. At this time, HIV antibody testing remains the standard.

U.S. military seroprevalence data demonstrate that health care workers have a slightly elevated HIV antibody prevalence compared with non-health care workers but that the excess risk is accounted for by infections in never-married male medical personnel (13). However, even though over three quarters of the U.S. health care worker pool are women, there is a lower sero-prevalence in military female health care workers than males, suggesting that nonoccupational risks are likely to confound the association between health care occupation and HIV prevalence in men.

IV. PREVENTION

Primary prevention of blood or other hazardous body fluid exposure is the major focus of preventing occupational transmission of HIV and other blood-borne pathogens. The OSHA bloodborne pathogen standard has put forth a federal mandate to strongly advocate for prevention of bloodborne exposure incidents. OSHA's intent is to protect all employees at risk and authorizes coverage for any occupational bloodborne exposure (13). More than 8 million health care workers in the United States work in hospitals and other health care facilities. It is estimated that 600,000 to 800,000 percutaneous occupational exposures occur annually and that at least half of these injuries are not reported. The newly revised 1999 compliance directive of the bloodborne pathogen standard emphasizes the importance of an annual review of each employer's bloodborne pathogen exposure control plan and the use of safer medical devices to help reduce percutaneous injuries. According to OSHA, their recent focus on engineering controls is a result of massive response by health care workers and their employee organizations to OSHA's 1998 request for ideas and recommendations for reducing exposures; these front-line workers stressed their belief that many safer medical devices currently available were effective in reducing risk of occupational transmission of bloodborne pathogens but were not being provided by employers. The directive also clarifies that the standard applies to home health agencies, independent physician practices, and other noninstitutional health care facilities. It adds the most recent CDC guidelines regarding hepatitis B vaccination and postexposure treatment and follow-up for HIV and HCV exposures. It has replaced and updated appendices that now includes examples of facility committees to help with compliance, sample engineering control evaluation forms, an internet resource list, a sample exposure control plan, and appropriate CDC guidelines. The bulk of the compliance directive focuses on methods of compliance and citation guidelines.

A few states have already successfully passed bills that significantly expand the federal OSHA bloodborne pathogen standard, whereas many states have bills pending in the legislature. Other states have bills ready for study for the year 2000. These new laws seem to be focusing on better exposure surveillance through the use of sharps injury logs that document the type and brand of sharps involved and other pertinent information about each specific exposure and mandate the use of needleless systems and sharps with integral safety features.

The reality of occupational transmission of HIV among health care workers has stimulated the development of a variety of safer medical devices being promoted to decrease the risk of bloodborne exposure. Until the end of the 1980s, major concentration had been focused on developing and implementing safety guidelines that included stringent infection control precautions, safer work practices, and provisions for ongoing training to health care workers. The OSHA standard supports the concept that engineering controls, including self-sheathing needles and syringes, retractable needles, retracting intravenous stylets and needleless intravenous systems, in conjunction with safer work practices and personal protective equipment will minimize or even eliminate exposure. It has become evident that behavior change alone will not significantly decrease the rate of accidental exposure. It is difficult to demonstrate efficacy of safety devices because needlestick injuries are statistically rare events.

Most safer medical devices continue to be active rather than passive devices, and the behavior change required for proper activation of safety devices continues to be a problem. Despite a tremendous effort in educating and training health care workers about the correct use of safety devices, there continues to be poor compliance in proper activation. Unpublished data from the San Francisco General Hospital has demonstrated that less than half of safety devices discarded in sharps containers throughout the hospital have been appropriately activated; the only exception to this has been within the clinical laboratory phlebotomy service that consistently has had an activation rate of 99% (Fahrner and Gerberding, 1994–1996). One small study of sharps containers in an emergency department reported that the needle-recapping rate continues to be alarmingly frequent, occurring with 11% to 72% of the needled devices observed (14). The authors believed that this recapping rate was in fact an underestimate as they theorized that undoubtedly some of the caps fell off of the needles during handling of the containers. A multidisciplinary approach, which considers the perspectives of front-line workers, will be necessary to have a true impact on the frequency of accidental injuries.

Also, in November 1999, shortly after the dissemination of the revised OSHA 1999 bloodborne pathogen standard compliance directive, the National Institute for Occupational Safety and Health (NIOSH), a branch of the CDC, issued an alert (15). This publication was written to warn health care workers of their risk of bloodborne pathogen transmission from needlestick injuries and to request that health care workers use safety devices and safe work practices to prevent exposures. This alert includes recommendations for both employers and workers because it is clear that prevention of occupational bloodborne exposure depends on the entire health care team.

V. MANAGEMENT OF OCCUPATIONAL EXPOSURE

A specific plan for postexposure management is required by the OSHA standard and must include a procedure for immediate confidential medical evaluation and follow-up. Appropriate documentation of the route of exposure, the circumstances surrounding the exposure incident, and test results of the health care worker and the source of the exposure is necessary.

Although the pathogenesis of occupational HIV infection continues to be only partially understood, recent studies have proposed the idea of the dendritic cell as the first cell infected by an invading HIV and these cells may be important in disseminating the virus to susceptible T cells (16). Evidence has been mounting over the past few years supporting the idea that the dendritic cell is an appropriate target for postexposure treatment, and this may give one likely explanation of how postexposure prophylaxis might be effective in preventing HIV transmission.

Postexposure chemoprophylaxis was first recommended for health care workers with occupational exposure to HIV in the USPHS provisional recommendations for postexposure prophylaxis published June 1996 (17). However, at least 80% of the major U.S. medical centers had been offering zidovudine as postexposure chemoprophylaxis despite the fact that there were no efficacy data. Data from a prospective, multicenter, collaborative trial evaluating the toxicity of postexposure zidovudine demonstrated that zidovudine can be administered safely and efficiently as postexposure chemoprophylaxis for adverse exposures to HIV (11). Although no efficacy study of zidovudine was ever possible, the case-control study demonstrated an association with the use of zidovudine as postexposure prophylaxis with a decrease of 79% in the risk for HIV infection after percutaneous bloodborne exposure. This finding, the first epidemiologic evidence of real benefit to health care workers of postexposure treatment with antiretroviral medications, motivated these recommendations by the USPHS. The USPHS modified their earlier postexposure prophylaxis recommendations in May 1998 to a basic 28-day course of zidovudine and lamivudine for most HIV exposures and an expanded regimen that adds a protease inhibitor, either indinavir or nelfinavir, for higher risk exposures or when resistance to one of the recommended drugs is suspected or known (18).

Because of the increasing prevalence of zidovudine resistance among HIV-infected source patients, even in patients who have never themselves taken zidovudine, the standard of therapy has become combination therapy. Zidovudine and lamivudine appear to work synergistically and are believed to decrease the emergence of zidovudine resistance. Clinical trials of this combination in HIV-infected patients have been well tolerated, and the incidence of adverse effects has not been increased over the use of zidovudine alone. Our clinical experience has demonstrated healthy health care workers tolerate this combination therapy very well. Indinavir and nelfinavir were chosen as the best protease inhibitors to use because their potency, bioavailability, and tolerability. In our experience, health care workers have been able to continue working full-time while completing the 28-day course of postexposure prophylaxis. Health care workers who experience nausea may benefit from the use of antiemetic therapy, whereas those who have diarrhea may be helped by an antidiarrheal.

It is not known whether antiretroviral drug resistance influences risk of transmission, although there have been reported cases of drug-resistant virus being transmitted. Because many HIV-infected patients have been and are being treated with multidrug highly active antiretroviral treatment regimens and therefore are likely to have resistant virus, the issue of which drugs to choose for postexposure prophylaxis is becoming more complex. It is important to note that in perinatal transmission studies using zidovudine monotherapy, treatment was effective even though 25% to 30% of the mothers had HIV genotypes that demonstrated zidovudine resistance (16). At our institution, we have been tailoring postexposure prophylaxis to each specific exposure by noting the antiretroviral history of the source patient, the viral load data and how it relates to antiretroviral use, and genotype data when available.

Despite the most current CDC recommendations, we have been using a broader combination of drugs. We frequently use the combination of didanosine/stavudine rather than zidovudine/lamivudine with an exposure to a source patient who have been heavily treated with zidovudine/lamivudine. With exposures to patients who have been previously treated with protease inhibitors, we often use a nonnucleoside reverse transcriptase as a third drug when the exposure is particularly high risk.

There have been concerns about the use of postexposure prophylaxis during pregnancy; however, pregnancy should not prohibit the use of optimal postexposure prophylaxis (18). The decision to take postexposure prophylaxis should be made by the exposed worker after appropriate counseling regarding the risks and benefits of treatment.

Over the years, there have been well-documented cases of postexposure prophylaxis failure. Even in these times of aggressive combination postexposure prophylaxis, failures still occur. We have become more concerned with exposures to both HIV and HCV as there have been at least two cases of resultant infection with both viruses in health care workers who took combination postexposure prophylaxis. Coinfection in the source patient appears to increase risk of occupational transmission and therefore should be considered a very high-risk exposure.

Studies to assess the consequences of these new postexposure prophylaxis regimens are ongoing. The CDC maintained a postexposure prophylaxis registry for 2 years to track adverse reactions to the drug treatment. Other countries that have been active in postexposure prophylaxis, including Italy, have developed similar monitoring systems (12).

Because the process for decision making about starting postexposure prophylaxis and postexposure prophylaxis selection itself has become extremely complex, the CDC and Health Resources and Services Administration (HRSA) created the National Clinicians' Postexposure Prophylaxis Hotline (PEPline) in 1997. This free 24-hour service provides expert consultation in managing occupation exposure for clinicians across the United States and internationally. The PEPline can be reached by calling 1-888-448-4911.

VI. HIV-INFECTED HEALTH CARE WORKERS: RISKS TO PATIENTS

The 1991 Florida dental case in which five patients were documented to be HIV infected after receiving care in the same dental office brought attention to the concern regarding patient risk from HIV-infected health care providers. This has brought the issue of restricting practice of HIV-infected health care workers to public scrutiny. Experts agree that the statistical risk of transmission from infected provider to patient is extremely small—less than one in a million by most estimates. Because the risk is so remote, most medical experts also agree that the adverse effects of mandatory HIV testing of health care workers and across-the-board practice restrictions outweigh the small benefit that such policies might have. In addition to the high economic costs of counseling, testing, and replacing and retraining infected workers, such policies may in fact adversely affect access to care for HIV-infected patients.

An alternative approach is to provide the safest possible care by adhering to strict infection control guidelines and utilizing the greatest technology for preventing exposure incidents, as preventing such injuries to health care workers is the most effective way to prevent accidental exposures to patients.

VII. CONCLUSION

Health care workers continue to be at low but measurable risk for HIV infection. The degree of risk is a direct function of the prevalence of HIV in patients; the frequency of occupational exposure to blood; and the amount, duration, and route of exposure to infected blood. The magnitude of risk for infection prevails as the most significant statistic available: after accidental parenteral inoculation it is approximately 0.2% and after mucous membrane exposure or inoculation of nonintact skin it is certainly lower than the risk from needlestick exposure and too low to be detected in prospective studies of more than 6000 workers at risk for infection. No case of infection from exposure to intact skin, from aerosolization, or from exposure to nonbloody body fluids has been reported. If risk is present at all from these exposures, it is too low to be measured or quantified at the present time. The CDC case-control study has elucidated the five factors that were independently associated with risk of infection after percutaneous injury. Three of these factors (deep intramuscular injuries, visibly bloody devices, and devices used in blood vessels) are probably indicative of a higher volume of infected blood. An exposure to a terminally ill AIDS patient, defined as one who died within 2 months of the exposure, was associated with increased risk. Postexposure treatment with zidovudine was associated with a 79% decrease in the risk of HIV transmission.

It is probable that some categories of health care workers are at greater cumulative professional risk of HIV infection than others. Professionals with frequent blood exposures such as dentists, surgeons, emergency care providers, phlebotomists, nurses, and labor and delivery personnel are at highest risk for acquiring hepatitis B virus (HBV) virus infection over a lifetime of practice, particularly in areas with a high prevalence of HIV disease. Prospective studies evaluating dentists and surgeons have failed so far to demonstrate evidence of risk over relatively short follow-up intervals, but larger studies over prolonged periods of time will be necessary to adequately define the true magnitude of risk.

The absolute number of occupationally infected health care workers is likely to increase as the prevalence of HIV increases in the health care environment. Comprehensive strategies for risk reduction in health care workers must continue to include efforts to implement and enforce sensible infection control precautions and safer work practices, development and use of better safer devices and procedures, and research to evaluate the current and potential postexposure prophylactic treatments.

REFERENCES

1. Needlestick transmission of HTLV-III from a patient infected in Africa. Lancet 1984;2:1376–1377.

2. OSHA. OSHA Instruction CPL 2-2.44D: Enforcement Procedures for the Occupational Exposure to Bloodborne Pathogens. November 1999:1–68.

3. Case-control study of HIV seroconversion in health-care workers after percutaneous exposures to HIV-infected blood—France, United Kingdom, and United States, January 1988–August, 1994. MMWR Morb Mortal Wkly Rep 1995;44: 929–933.

4. Centers for Disease Control. Recommendations of the US Public Health Service task force on the use of zidovudine to reduce perinatal transmission of HIV. MMWR Morb Mortal Wkly Rep 1994;43(no RR-11):1–20.

5. Centers for Disease Control and Prevention. HIV/AIDS Surveillance Report. 1999;11:1–43.

6. Gerberding JL, Littell C, Tarkington A, et al. Risk of exposure of surgical personnel to patients' blood during surgery at San Francisco General Hospital. N Engl J Med 1990;322:1788–1793.

7. Gerberding JL, Littell C, Brown A, Ramiro N. Cumulative risk of HIV and hepatitis B (HBV) among health care workers: longterm serologic follow-up and gene amplification for latent HIV infection [abstract no. 959]. In: Programs and abstracts of the 30th Interscience Conference on Antimicrobial Agents and Chemotherapy. Atlanta, GA: American Society for Microbiology, 1990.

8. Gerberding JL. Management of occupational exposures to blood-borne viruses. N Engl J Med 1996;332:444–451.

9. Ippolito G, Puro V, De Carli G. The risk of occupational human immunodeficiency virus infection in health care workers. Italian Multicenter Study. The Italian Study Group on Occupational Risk of HIV Infection. Arch Intern Med 1993;153:1451–1458.

10. Heptonstall J, Porter K, Gill ON. Occupational HIV: Summary of Published Reports. London: Public Health Laboratory Services Communicable Disease Surveillance Centre, 1995.

11. Fahrner R, Beekmann SE, Koziol DE, Gerberding JL, Henderson DK. Safety of zidovudine (ZDV) administered as post-exposure prophylaxis to health care workers (HCW) sustaining HIV-related occupational exposures (OE) [Abstract]. In: Program and Abstracts—Interscience Conference on Antimicrobial Agents and Chemotherapy. Washington, DC, American Society for Microbiology, 1994: 133.

12. Gerberding JL. Prophylaxis for occupational exposure to HIV. Ann Intern Med 1996;125:497–501.

13. Bell DM. Human immunodeficiency virus transmission in health care settings: risk and risk reduction. Am J Med 1991;91:294S–300S.

14. Jackson MM, Mulherin S, Rickman LS. Dumpster diving in sharps disposal containers: what's really inside? Infect Control Hosp Epidemiol 1996;17:570–571.

15. National Institute for Occupational Safety and Health, CDC. NIOSH Alert: preventing needlestick injuries in health care settings. DHHS (NIOSH) Pub. No. 2000-108;1999:1–26.

16. Henderson DK. Postexposure chemoprophylaxis for occupational exposure to the human immunodeficiency virus. JAMA 1999;281:931–936.

17. Centers for Disease Control and Prevention. Update: provisional Public Health Service recommendations for chemoprophylaxis after occupational exposure to HIV. MMWR Morb Mortal Wkly Rep 1996;45:468–472.

18. Centers for Disease Control and Prevention. Public Health Service guidelines for the management of health-care worker exposures to HIV and recommendations for postexposure prophylaxis. MMWR Morb Mortal Wkly Rep 1998;47(no RR-7):1–33.

5

Can Immune Responses to Human Immunodeficiency Virus Be Preserved, Enhanced, or Restored?

Bruce D. Walker
Harvard Medical School, Massachusetts General Hospital, and Brigham and Women's Hospital, Boston, Massachusetts

I. INTRODUCTION

The past few years have seen a dramatic paradigm shift in terms of our view of viral dynamics. Whereas earlier studies had indicated that human immuno-deficiency virus (HIV) replication occurred at high levels with little influence by innate or adaptive immune responses (1–3), it is becoming increasingly clear that the viral set point is critically dependent on virus-specific immune responses that are at least partially effective in containing the virus. In fact, persons have now been identified who appear to be able to effectively contain HIV replication over 20 or more years, without the need for drug therapy and without developing HIV-related illness (4–7). Such observations suggest that effective immunity to HIV can be generated and raise the important question as to whether the immune system can be manipulated in the context of HIV infection to obtain more durable suppression of the virus. Other human virus such as Epstein-Barr virus, cytomegalovirus (CMV), and herpes simplex virus are never eradicated from the body but are held in check by effective immune responses such that they do not cause disease over the life of an immunocompetent individual. This review addresses the growing body of data indicating that HIV might also be a virus that can be contained by the immune system and addresses the possible ways in which the immune system might be preserved, enhanced, or restored to clinical benefit in this otherwise typically progressive infection.

II. COMPONENTS OF PROTECTIVE IMMUNITY IN HIV INFECTION

Early in the HIV epidemic it appeared that everyone who became infected would experience progressive and ultimately profound immune suppression and finally succumb to one or more of a variety of opportunistic infections. However, as the epidemic began to mature, cohort studies revealed a subset of infected persons who sustained normal CD4 counts and remained free of disease (4–7). Already notable, such cases entered the truly remarkable category when viral load testing became available, and it was determined that some of these individuals maintained viral loads below the limits of detection by the most sensitive assays available. Here was a group of individuals who were not only beating the odds, but they appeared to be dealing with HIV the way that many other human viruses are dealt with, namely being contained over the long term. Viral and host genetic factors that have been associated with attenuated disease progression did not appear to explain most of these cases, suggesting that it was the immune system that was actively containing the virus. It is such cases that have offered the opportunity to dissect the components of effective immunity.

There are at least three major immune responses that might be thought to contribute to immunologic control of HIV. Of these, neutralizing antibodies was one of the first to be investigated. Although published studies are somewhat contradictory (4, 8), it appeared that persons who were truly controlling HIV replication in the absence of drug therapy had weak to undetectable neutralizing antibody responses (6). Although strong reponses to virion debris could be readily demonstrated (9), the weak levels of antibodies able to neutralize primary HIV isolates suggested that it was not humoral immunity that was responsible for the containment of virus.

In addition to humoral immune responses, the adaptive immune response to viral infections typically consists of cellular immune responses as well. Notable among these are cytotoxic T lymphocytes (CTL), which kill virus infected cells (reviewed in Reference 10). When virus invades a cell, it commandeers the host cell machinery to make new virion proteins, which are then assembled into new viruses at the cell surface, bud, and go on to infect another cell and sustain the virus life cycle. At the same time these events are occurring, the infected cell is trying to signal the body's defense mechanisms that something foreign is within the cell and the cell needs to be eliminated. The specific immune recognition of infected cells is achieved by proteolytic degradation of some of the new synthesized viral proteins, which then form a complex with a developing class I molecule and are presented at the cell surface. The presence of a viral peptide, typically 8–10 amino acids in length, in the class I binding groove is a signal to the body that something foreign is in the cell, and this elicits lysis of the infected cell by CTL. This is accomplished by recognition of the viral peptide/human leukocyte antigen class I complex by the T-cell receptor on the CTL. Not only is the infected cell lysed, but the local microenvironment is bathed in soluble antiviral factors produced by the activated CTL (reviewed in Reference 11). In vitro studies show that HIV-specific CTL are extremely efficient at lysing infected cells and that this can occur before infectious virus progeny are produced (12, 13).

The role of CTL in controlling HIV replication in vivo has now been clearly demonstrated. Early studies showed the emergence of CTL responses coincident with the drop in viremia in acute HIV infection (14–16), suggesting that these cells were at least partially responsible for early containment of viremia. More recent cross-sectional studies using new flow cytometry-based assays to directly visualize and quantitate CTL responses have shown a negative association between the magnitude of CTL responses and the viral set point, again suggestive of CTL-mediated immune control (17). The most impressive data to date indicating the antiviral potency of CTL come from studies in the simian immunodeficiency virus model, in which in vivo depletion of CD8 cells leads to a dramatic increase in viremia (18, 19). Viremia subsequently declines coincident with the return of CTL, providing direct in vivo evidence of the antiviral effect of these cells. This model has also shown that immune escape from CTL may be clinically relevant (20, 21).

Given the demonstration that CTL can be extremely effective at controlling HIV replication under idealized in vitro conditions and the clear animal model evidence of an in vivo antiviral effect of these cells, a major question is why CTL ultimately fail to contain HIV in most infected persons. Animal models of chronic viral infections shed important light on this question by demonstrating that the maintenance of effective CTL responses requires the presence of virus-specific T-helper-cell responses (reviewed in Reference 22). Such cells, which recognize processed viral proteins presented in the context of a class II molecule at the cell surface, are considered to be the central orchestrator of effective antiviral immune responses. In the absence of a strong virus-specific T-helper-cell response, these animal models show that CTL activity wanes over time, and there is a lack of control of viremia in the chronic phase of infection (23–26). The most profound immunologic defect in HIV infection is the relative lack of HIV-specific T-helper cells (reviewed in Reference 22), and, as would be predicted, a loss of CTL function over time is characteristic of HIV infection (27). However, in the small subset of persons who are HIV infected and control viremia without the need for antiviral therapy, a strong T-helper-cell response has been detected (28, 29). Cross-sectional studies show a negative correlation between T-helper-cell responses and viral load, consistent with an important immunoregulatory effect of these cells (28, 29). Likewise, the relative lack of detectable numbers of these cells in infected persons with progressive infection is consistent with a lack of immune-mediated control.

III. WHY DOES THE IMMUNE SYSTEM FAIL TO CONTROL HIV?

It is likely that the lack of virus-specific T-helper cells is a central problem in generating and maintaining effective immunity in HIV infection. The lack of these cells in most infected persons might be predicted, given that HIV selectively infects activated T cells. Thus, in early HIV infection, as T-helper cells are being generated to orchestrate an effective immune response against HIV, these cells would be expected to be preferential targets for HIV. Because viral loads in primary infection are likely to be the highest of any time in the course of disease (30), the cells activated at this time would be expected to be preferentially targeted and thereby significantly decreased in number. Lack of sufficient numbers of these cells would then be expected to impair the persistence of CTL, which is what is observed in chronic HIV infection.

IV. EFFECTS OF HIGHLY ACTIVE ANTIRETROVIRAL THERAPY (HAART) ON HIV-SPECIFIC IMMUNE RESPONSES

If T-helper cells are being generated in acute infection, then treatment with potent antiviral therapy during this time might be expected to protect these cells from infection, thereby allowing for maturation of a strong T-helper-cell response. This in turn would be expected to promote maintenance of CTL function, with possible resultant control of viremia. Treatment of acute infection in fact has a dramatic effect on generation of T-helper-cell responses and provides the strongest rationale for immediate treatment of acute HIV infection (28). In our experience, all persons successfully treated in the acute stage of HIV infection have gone on to develop strong T-helper-cell responses (28, 29). These responses typically appear within 2 months of infection and persist as the virus is maintained below the limits of detection by HAART.

Anecdotal studies suggest that the immune responses induced by very early therapy may be functional and alter the progress of the infection. An example is the so-called "Berlin patient," who was treated in the early stages of acute infection (31). After an early interruption in therapy due to the development of orchitis, virus returned and therapy was reinstituted. A subsequent brief interruption in therapy was not associated with a detectable rise in viremia. He subsequently interrupted all therapy, and viremia has remained at or below the limits of detection for more that 3 years. Detailed studies of his immune function revealed the presence of strong T-helper-cell and CTL responses, as would be predicted. The course in this individual is consistent with persistent containment of viremia. One can in fact hypothesize that the early interruptions in therapy led to the boost of immunity and persistent ability to control virus. Other studies of persons who were treated early in infection and have subsequently gone on to control viremia support this hypothesis (32), which is now being tested in prospective trials. Common among these anecdotal cases is the observation of strong virus-specific immune responses, consistent with immunologic control of the virus.

V. REBUILDING THE IMMUNE SYSTEM IN CHRONIC HIV INFECTION

The existence of persons who are able to control HIV viremia in the absence of antiviral therapy indicates that the immune system can contain the virus in rare cases. The emerging immunologic data from these controllers indicates that the presence of a strong T-helper-cell response and a strong CTL response is required for this control. Emerging data in persons treated in acute infection who go on to maintain control of viremia in the absence of therapy also support a central role for CTL and T-helper cells. Immediate treatment of acute infection leads to restoration of these responses, which may be functional. Together these findings provide optimism that immune function can be augmented in the early stages of infection. The more relevant question for the huge numbers of persons who were not diagnosed and treated before seroconversion is whether functional immunity can be augmented in the chronic stage of infection.

Although firm data are lacking, there are a number of findings providing optimism for effective immune intervention even in later stage illness.

One such finding is the demonstration that persons on HAART experience progressive increases in the number of peripheral naive cells, which can potentially be educated to participate in the immune defense against pathogens (33). That truly functional immune responses can be generated in chronically infected persons is evidenced by the development of immune recovery inflammatory syndromes. These are thought to be the result of enhanced immune responses and the resultant collateral damage imposed by these that can lead to symptomatic illness. Occasionally, these inflammatory responses require that HAART is interrupted. However, with continued treatment the enhanced pathogen-specific immune function leads to clinical benefit, indicative of functionally relevant augmentation in immune function. Examples include so-called immune recovery inflammatory syndromes to CMV and tuberculosis in persons with chronic HIV infection treated with HAART. Whereas HAART has led to increased immunity against some HIV-associated pathogens, it has not led to augmentation of immunity to HIV. Immune responses to HIV have generally been observed to decrease on therapy (34, 35). This may be due to the lack of significant antigenic stimulation to prime new naive cells, thereby precluding induction of new HIV-specific immune responses.

VI. CRITICAL NEED FOR IMMUNOTHERAPY PLUS HAART IN AUGMENTING IMMUNITY TO HIV

The ability to enhance functional immunity to HIV is likely to be critically dependent on the ability to suppress HIV replication with HAART and at the same time to expose persons to HIV antigens to specifically boost virus-specific immunity. The reasons for this are twofold and include the ability of HAART to increase naive cells, and the ability to protect activated cells from becoming infected. In retrospect, these same factors reveal why immune augmentation was not successful in the pre-HAART era. On the one hand, naive cells that can be educated to recognize HIV via vaccination are expected to be a prerequisite to successful immune augmentation. HAART leads to a gradual repopulation of naive cells (33), which increase progressively over the first year or more of therapy. In the absence of HAART, these cells progressively decline. Furthermore, in the absence of HAART, activated cells that express CD4 would be expected to be preferentially infected, thus preventing meaningful repopulation with antigen-specific cells. In persons with chronic HIV infection, treatment with antiviral drug therapy might be expected to have potentially opposing effects. Although new naive cells are being generated and might be educated to become directed against HIV, the HAART-induced lack of HIV antigen leaves these cells without the required stimulus to generate HIV-specific responses. However, the prospects for therapeutic vaccination take on great potential significance in this setting, in terms of a potential means to augment effective immunity against HIV.

VII. APPROACHES TO IMMUNE ENHANCEMENT IN HIV INFECTION

The above arguments provide a strong rationale for attempts to augment immunity in infected persons and support the hypothesis that this would lead to a clinical benefit. There are a number of current approaches to augmenting immune function in HIV-infected persons. These fall in the general category of therapeutic vaccination but reflect a large number of potential approaches. These include the use of recombinant protein vaccines, recombinant live virus vector vaccines, cell-based therapies, and even judicious reexposure to one's own live virus in the way of structured treatment interruptions. Other less specific approaches, which also entail increasing virus-specific immune function, include cytokine therapies to augment the ability of cells to respond to HIV. Each of these approaches has potential benefits and risks.

Although early trials of therapeutic vaccination led to disappointing results, this entire approach has to be reexamined now that it is possible to contain viremia during the vaccination period. That the earlier studies failed to show benefit is to be expected, given the presence of infectious virus at the time that cells were being activated by vaccination. Activated CD4 cells, which based on above arguments would be key to antiviral immune control, would become preferentially infectable with HIV and thus impaired. However, in the HAART era, therapeutic vaccination is not just possible but may be a necessity. HAART will increase naive cells, but the ability of these to become educated to participate in immune control of HIV requires exposure to antigen. The antigenic threshold required to sustain cellular immune responses may be higher than the level of virus persistence in treated persons, as suggested by studies showing a decline in HIV-specific CTL responses during successful HAART treatment (34, 36).

Approaches to therapeutic immunization include presently available vaccines, some of which are already in clinical trials. Evidence that some of these vaccines may augment immunity to HIV has been presented in abstract form, providing a level of cautious optimism but by no means proving that induced responses are clinically relevant. A small trial of a whole inactivated virus vaccine resulted in the generation of significant T-helper-cell responses in recipients, even when the CD4 counts were as low as 200 (F. Valentine, personal communication, 1999). Additional trials of this vaccine, Remune, in persons treated with HAART are ongoing in the United States and Europe, and at least immunogenicity studies should be available in the next year.

The approach with whole inactivated virus vaccine may be less likely to generate CTL responses, but other approaches may. Canaypox vectors as therapeutic vaccines are already in clinical trials and are likely to be better tolerated that vaccinia virus vectors. Because these vectors produce recombinant HIV proteins intracellularly, they are likely to be processed and presented through the class I pathway, thereby leading to induction of CTL. These vectors may be less efficient at inducing T-helper-cell responses and thus combination regimens are likely to be pursued.

Cell-based therapies are another approach likely to be explored. Early trials of adoptive cell therapy have shown that CTL can home to areas of infected cells (37) but that the overall effect on viral load is marginal, perhaps because these cells do not persist well in vivo. One way in which these cells might be induced to persist for longer periods is through the coadministration of T-helper cells. Adoptive therapy studies in CMV infection have suggested that persistence of adoptively transferred cells is dependent on the presence of a critical level of T-helper-cell function (38).

It has long been known that the most potent viral vaccines are based on live replicating virus. It is this observation plus the recognition of enhanced immune responses in persons who have repeatedly interrupted antiviral therapy (31, 32) that has led to the concept of structured interruptions in therapy as a means of augmenting HIV-specific immunity. Such an approach is not without risk, both for possible acute infection syndrome and the development of antiviral drug resistance. Simultaneous interruption in all antiviral medications should lessen the development of resistance, but the washout period makes it inevitable that virus will be exposed to subtherapeutic concentrations of drug, compounded by differing half-lives of the drugs. Although this approach has generated much enthusiasm, it has yet to be shown to result in lasting immunity that is of clinical benefit.

VIII. CONCLUSIONS AND FUTURE DIRECTIONS

Emerging data provide promising preliminary answers to the questions posed in this review. Immune responses to HIV can clearly be manipulated, particularly in persons who are treated in the earliest stages of acute infection. New data indicating the central role of the immune system in determining the viral set point, and by inference in determining the long-term progression of disease, provide optimism that approaches to restore, enhance, or preserve immune function will translate into clinical benefit for infected persons. Preliminary data indeed suggest that these may be obtainable goals. The results of numerous clinical trials can be expected over the next year and hopefully will represent the next great advance in the treatment of infected persons.

REFERENCES

1. Wei X, Ghosh SK, Taylor ME, Johnson VA, Emini EA, Deutsch P, Lifson JD, Bonhoeffer S, Nowak MA, Hahn BH, Saag MS, Shaw GM. Viral dynamics in human immunodeficiency virus type 1 infection [see comments]. Nature 1995; 373:117–122.

2. Ho DD, Neumann AU, Perelson AS, Chen W, Leonard JM, Markowitz M. Rapid turnover of plasma virions and CD4 lymphocytes in HIV-1 infection [see comments]. Nature 1995;373:123–126.

3. Perelson AS, Neumann AU, Markowitz M, Leonard JM, Ho DD. HIV-1 dynamics in vivo: virion clearance rate, infected cell life-span, and viral generation time. Science 1996;271:1582–1586.

4. Cao Y, Qin L, Zhang L, Safrit J, Ho DD. Virologic and immunologic characterization of long-term survivors of human immunodeficiency virus type 1 infection [see comments]. N Engl J Med 1995;332:201–208.

5. Pantaleo G, Menzo S, Vaccarezza M, Graziosi C, Cohen OJ, Demarest JF, Montefiori D, Orenstein JM, Fox C, Schrager LK, Margolick JB, Buchbinder S, Giorgi JV, Fauci AS. Studies in subjects with long-term nonprogressive human immunodeficiency virus infection [see comments]. N Engl J Med 1995;332: 209–216.

6. Harrer T, Harrer E, Kalams SA, Elbeik T, Staprans SI, Feinberg MB, Cao Y, Ho DD, Yilma T, Caliendo AM, Johnson RP, Buchbinder SP, Walker BD. Strong cytotoxic T cell and weak neutralizing antibody responses in a subset of persons with stable nonprogressing HIV type 1 infection. AIDS Res Hum Retroviruses 1996;12:585–592.

7. Harrer T, Harrer E, Kalams SA, Barbosa P, Trocha A, Johnson RP, Elbeik T, Feinberg MB, Buchbinder SP, Walker BD. Cytotoxic T lymphocytes in asymptomatic long-term nonprogressing HIV-1 infection. Breadth and specificity of the response and relation to in vivo viral quasispecies in a person with prolonged infection and low viral load. J Immunol 1996;156:2616–2623.

8. Montefiori DC, Pantaleo G, Fink LM, Zhou JT, Zhou JY, Bilska M, Miralles GD, Fauci AS. Neutralizing and infection-enhancing antibody responses to human immunodeficiency virus type 1 in long-term nonprogressors. J Infect Dis 1996; 173:60–67.

9. Burton DR. A vaccine for HIV type 1: the antibody perspective. Proc Natl Acad Sci USA 1997;94:10018–10023.

10. Brander C, Walker BD. T lymphocyte responses in HIV-1 infection: implications for vaccine development. Curr Opin Immunol 1999;11:451–459.

11. Yang OO, Walker BD. CD8+ cells in human immunodeficiency virus type I pathogenesis: cytolytic and noncytolytic inhibition of viral replication. Adv Immunol 1997;66:273–311.

12. Yang OO, Kalams SA, Rosenzweig M, Trocha A, Jones N, Koziel M, Walker BD, Johnson RP. Efficient lysis of human immunodeficiency virus type 1-infected cells by cytotoxic T lymphocytes. J Virol 1996;70:5799–5806.

13. Yang OO, Kalams SA, Trocha A, Cao H, Luster A, Johnson RP, Walker BD. Suppression of human immunodeficiency virus type 1 replication by CD8+ cells: evidence for HLA class I-restricted triggering of cytolytic and noncytolytic mechanisms. J Virol 1997;71:3120–3128.

14. Koup RA, Safrit JT, Cao Y, Andrews CA, McLeod G, Borkowsky W, Farthing C, Ho DD. Temporal association of cellular immune responses with the initial control of viremia in primary human immunodeficiency virus type 1 syndrome. J Virol 1994;68:4650–4655.

15. Borrow P, Lewicki H, Hahn BH, Shaw GM, Oldstone MB. Virus-specific CD8+ cytotoxic T-lymphocyte activity associated with control of viremia in primary human immunodeficiency virus type 1 infection. J Virol 1994;68:6103–6110.

16. Borrow P, Lewicki H, Wei X, Horwitz MS, Peffer N, Meyers H, Nelson JA, Gairin JE, Hahn BH, Oldstone MB, Shaw GM. Antiviral pressure exerted by HIV-1-specific cytotoxic T lymphocytes (CTLs) during primary infection demonstrated by rapid selection of CTL escape virus [see comments]. Nat Med 1997; 3:205–211.

17. Ogg GS, Jin X, Bonhoeffer S, Dunbar PR, Nowak MA, Monard S, Segal JP, Cao Y, Rowland-Jones SL, Cerundolo V, Hurley A, Markowitz M, Ho DD, Nixon DF, McMichael AJ. Quantitation of HIV-1-specific cytotoxic T lymphocytes and plasma load of viral RNA. Science 1998;279:2103–2106.

18. Schmitz JE, Kuroda MJ, Santra S, Sasseville VG, Simon MA, Lifton MA, Racz P, Tenner-Racz K, Dalesandro M, Scallon BJ, Ghrayeb J, Forman MA, Montefiori DC, Rieber EP, Letvin NL, Reimann KA. Control of viremia in simian immunodeficiency virus infection by CD8+ lymphocytes. Science 1999;283: 857–860.

19. Jin X, Bauer DE, Tuttleton SE, Lewin S, Gettie A, Blanchard J, Irwin CE, Safrit JT, Mittler J, Weinberger L, Kostrikis LG, Zhang L, Perelson AS, Ho DD. Dramatic rise in plasma viremia after CD8(+) T cell depletion in simian immunodeficiency virus-infected macaques. J Exp Med 1999;189:991–998.

20. Evans DT, O'Connor DH, Jing P, Dzuris JL, Sidney J, da Silva J, Allen TM, Horton H, Venham JE, Rudersdorf RA, Vogel T, Pauza CD, Bontrop RE, DeMars R, Sette A, Hughes AL, Watkins DI. Virus-specific cytotoxic T-lymphocyte

responses select for amino-acid variation in simian immunodeficiency virus Env and Nef. Nat Med 1999;5:1270–1276.

21. Goulder PJ, Walker BD. The great escape—AIDS viruses and immune control [news]. Nat Med 1999;5:1233–1235.

22. Kalams SA, Walker BD. The critical need for CD4 help in maintaining effective cytotoxic T lymphocyte responses [comment]. J Exp Med 1998;188:2199–2204.

23. Battegay M, Moskophidis D, Rahemtulla A, Hengartner H, Mak TW, Zinkernagel RM. Enhanced establishment of a virus carrier state in adult CD4+ T-cell-deficient mice. J Virol 1994;68:4700–4704.

24. Matloubian M, Concepcion RJ, Ahmed R. CD4+ T cells are required to sustain CD8+ cytotoxic T-cell responses during chronic viral infection. J Virol 1994; 68:8056–8063.

25. von Herrath MG, Yokoyama M, Dockter J, Oldstone MB, Whitton JL. CD4-deficient mice have reduced levels of memory cytotoxic T lymphocytes after immunization and show diminished resistance to subsequent virus challenge. J Virol 1996;70:1072–1079.

26. Zajac AJ, Blattman JN, Murali-Krishna K, Sourdive DJ, Suresh M, Altman JD, Ahmed R. Viral immune evasion due to persistence of activated T cells without effector function [see comments]. J Exp Med 1998;188:2205–2213.

27. Klein MR, van Baalen CA, Holwerda AM, Kerkhof Garde SR, Bende RJ, Keet IP, Eeftinck-Schattenkerk JK, Osterhaus AD, Schuitemaker H, Miedema F. Kinetics of Gag-specific cytotoxic T lymphocyte responses during the clinical course of HIV-1 infection: a longitudinal analysis of rapid progressors and long-term asymptomatics. J Exp Med 1995;181:1365–1372.

28. Rosenberg ES, Billingsley JM, Caliendo AM, Boswell SL, Sax PE, Kalams SA, Walker BD. Vigorous HIV-1-specific CD4+ T cell responses associated with control of viremia [see comments]. Science 1997;278:1447–1450.

29. Kalams SA, Buchbinder SP, Rosenberg ES, Billingsley JM, Colbert DS, Jones NG, Shea AK, Trocha AK, Walker BD. Association between virus-specific cytotoxic T-lymphocyte and helper responses in human immunodeficiency virus type 1 infection. J Virol 1999;73:6715–6720.

30. Kahn JO, Walker BD. Acute human immunodeficiency virus type 1 infection. N Engl J Med 1998;339:33–39.

31. Lisziewicz J, Rosenberg E, Lieberman J, Jessen H, Lopalco L, Siliciano R, Walker B, Lori F. Control of HIV despite the discontinuation of antiretroviral therapy [letter]. N Engl J Med 1999;340:1683–1684.

32. Ortiz GM, Nixon DF, Trkola A, Binley J, Jin X, Bonhoeffer S, Kuebler PJ, Donahoe SM, Demoitie MA, Kakimoto WM, Ketas T, Clas B, Heymann JJ, Zhang L, Cao Y, Hurley A, Moore JP, Ho DD, Markowitz M. HIV-1-specific immune responses in subjects who temporarily contain virus replication after

discontinuation of highly active antiretroviral therapy [see comments]. J Clin Invest 1999;104:R13–R18.

33. Autran B, Carcelain G, Li TS, Blanc C, Mathez D, Tubiana R, Katlama C, Debre P, Leibowitch J. Positive effects of combined antiretroviral therapy on CD4+ T cell homeostasis and function in advanced HIV disease [see comments]. Science 1997;277:112–116.

34. Kalams SA, Goulder PJ, Shea AK, Jones NG, Trocha AK, Ogg GS, Walker BD. Levels of human immunodeficiency virus type 1-specific cytotoxic T-lymphocyte effector and memory responses decline after suppression of viremia with highly active antiretroviral therapy. J Virol 1999;73:6721–6728.

35. Ogg GS, Jin X, Bonhoeffer S, Moss P, Nowak MA, Monard S, Segal JP, Cao Y, Rowland-Jones SL, Hurley A, Markowitz M, Ho DD, McMichael AJ, Nixon DF. Decay kinetics of human immunodeficiency virus-specific effector cytotoxic T lymphocytes after combination antiretroviral therapy. J Virol 1999;73:797–800.

36. Ogg GS, Kostense S, Klein MR, Jurriaans S, Hamann D, McMichael AJ, Miedema F. Longitudinal phenotypic analysis of human immunodeficiency virus type 1-specific cytotoxic T lymphocytes: correlation with disease progression. J Virol 1999;73:9153–9160.

37. Brodie SJ, Lewinsohn DA, Patterson BK, Jiyamapa D, Krieger J, Corey L, Greenberg PD, Riddell SR. In vivo migration and function of transferred HIV-1-specific cytotoxic T cells [see comments]. Nat Med 1999;5:34–41.

38. Walter EA, Greenberg PD, Gilbert MJ, Finch RJ, Watanabe KS, Thomas ED, Riddell SR. Reconstitution of cellular immunity against cytomegalovirus in recipients of allogeneic bone marrow by transfer of T-cell clones from the donor [see comments]. N Engl J Med 1995;333:1038–1044.

6

Reconstitution of Immunity Against Opportunistic Infections in the Era of Potent Antiretroviral Therapy

Judith A. Aberg
Washington University School of Medicine, St. Louis, Missouri

I. INTRODUCTION

The availability and application of potent new antiretroviral agents to human immunodeficiency virus (HIV)-infected individuals has dramatically altered the natural history of acquired immunodeficiency virus (AIDS)-related complications. Since the introduction of potent antiretroviral therapy, the incidence of opportunistic infections (OIs) has been reported to dramatically decrease, although the incidence of OIs actually started to decline before highly active antiretroviral therapy (HAART); presumably due to earlier interventions such as prophylaxis and nucleoside therapy plus improved clinical recognition and care for OIs (1–4). Unusual manifestations of common OIs such as localized mycobacterium avium complex (MAC) lymphadenitis and cytomegalovirus (CMV) vitritis have emerged as a result of improvements in the immune function (5, 6). Paradoxical worsening of tuberculosis also has been reported to occur more frequently when HAART is initiated concomitantly with antituberculous therapy (7, 8). The outcome of some previously refractory OIs such as cryptosporidiosos, azole-resistant thrush, progressive multifocal leukoencephalopathy, wasting, and Kaposi's sarcoma has improved as a result of HAART (9). In addition, HAART has been associated with reductions in AIDS-related mortality, days of hospitalization, and the incidence of new OIs (10). What is it about HAART that has so altered this epidemic? What do we know about immune reconstitution after HAART?

Studies (11–13) suggest that the initial rise seen in the blood absolute CD4+ T-cell count after 4–6 weeks of HAART is due to expansion of the circulating lymphoid cells excluding natural killer cells. A much more gradual increase of naive T cells occurs over the next few years. Conflicting laboratory data exist as to whether restoration of immune function occurs (11, 12, 14–16). Multiple studies are currently in development and in progress to examine the function of CD4+ T cells after HAART via cytokine induction and lymphoproliferative assays using specific antigens. The Adult AIDS Clinical Trials Group (ACTG) funded by the National Institute of Allergy and Infectious Diseases has three trials in progress to examine the immunological and clinical implications of discontinuing maintenance therapy in opportunistic CMV, MAC, and histoplasmosis disease. Investigators at the University of California, San Francisco are examining the discontinuation of maintenance therapy for cryptococcal meningitis. Several studies by the ACTG and the Community Programs for Clinical Research of AIDS are currently underway evaluating the discontinuation of prophylaxis for MAC and *Pneumocystis carinii* pneumonia (PCP) in patients in whom the CD4+ T-cell count has increased above the recommended guideline for prophylaxis (i.e., CD4+ T-cell count < 50 cells/μL for MAC and <200 cells/μL for PCP; Table 1). The United States Public Health Service/Infectious Disease Society of America (USPHS/IDSA) recently released their 1999 guidelines that have been updated to consider the discontinuation of primary prophylaxis in patients who have had a sustained increase in their CD4+ T-cell count rather than the previous recommendation to maintain prophylaxis based on the nadir CD4+ T-cell count (17) (Table 2).

Despite the availability of HAART, OIs continue to occur. The intent of this chapter is to review the current guidelines for the prevention of the major OI pathogens and address whether it is safe to withdraw prophylaxis in HIV-infected patients who have achieved presumed immune reconstitution. I review several specific pathogens and discuss both the clinical and scientific evidence supporting immune reconstitution.

II. PCP

PCP continues to be a significant cause of morbidity and mortality in patients with AIDS despite the availability of effective prophylaxis and HAART. Pre-

Table 1 Clinical Trials Evaluating the Discontinuation of Prophylaxis or Maintenance Therapy

Trial sponsor	Target accrual	Schema
ACTG 360	300	Prospective observational study of development of CMV in patients who have had CD4 < 50 within past 24 mos and no history of active CMV disease
ACTG 362	636	MAC prophylaxis study: azithromycin versus placebo in patients whose CD4 counts were once <50 and are now >100 on HAART
CPCRA 048	850	Similar to ACTG 362 but also evaluating risk of bacterial pneumonia
ACTG 379	125	Discontinuation of CMV maintenance therapy in patients diagnosed with this OI
ACTG 393	50	Discontinuation of MAC maintenance therapy in patients diagnosed with this OI
ACTG 888	250	Discontinuation of primary and secondary PCP prophylaxis
ACTG 5038	50	Discontinuation of Histoplasmosis maintenance therapy
CFAR	10	Discontinuation of Cryptococcal meningitis maintenance therapy

ACTG, AIDS Clinical Trials Group (ACTG 360, 362, and 888 primary prophylaxis arm have been fully accrued and are closed to enrollment); CPCRA, Community programs for Clinical Research of AIDS; CFAR, Center for AIDS Reasearch Pilot Study at UCSF.

viously categorized as a protozoan, *P. carinii* is now categorized as a fungus. Unfortunately, *P. carinii* still cannot be cultivated in the laboratory; hence there remains significant confusion in the literature on the nomenclature that describes the forms that are visualized on stains.

P. carinii is cleared from the lung of 75% of patients within 1 year after diagnosis of PCP, suggesting that latency is unlikely and that infection arises from an exogenous source. On the other hand, there is a high seroprevalence of antipneumocystis antibodies present in young children; therefore, one cannot exclude the possibility of reactivation of latent disease (18). *P. carinii* can be isolated from the environment by means of a spore trap and identified by polymerase chain reaction (PCR). Given that *P. carinii* cannot be cultivated, it is not known if these forms identified by PCR are infectious. Molecular typing suggests that repeated episodes of PCP are most likely related to acquisition of different strains rather than reactivation. *P. carinii* is known to

Table 2 Primary Prophylaxis for Opportunistic Infections in HIV-Infected Adults

Pathogen	Indication	First choice	Alternatives
PCP	CD4+ T-cell count < 200/μL or oropharyngeal candidiasis or unexplained fever ≥ 2 wks or previous episode of PCP	TMP/SMX DS 1 tab p.o. q.d.	Dapsone 50 mg po b.i.d. or dapsone 100 mg p.o. q.d. or pentamidine aerosolized 300 mg q.m. or atovaquone 1500 mg p.o. q.d.
MAC	CD4+ T-cell count < 50/μL	Clarithromycin 500 mg p.o. b.i.d. or azithromycin 1200 mg p.o. q.w.	Rifabutin 300 mg p.o. q.d. (Must be dose-adjusted if given with HIV protease inhibitors)
CMV[a]	CD4+ T-cell count < 50/μL and positive CMV IgG antibody	Ganciclovir 1 g p.o. t.i.d. or fundoscopic monitoring	None
Toxoplasmosis gondii	CD4+ T-cell count < 100/μL and positive toxoplasma IgG antibody	TMP/SMX DS 1 tab p.o. q.d.	TMP/SMX SS 1 tab p.o. q.d. or dapsone 50 mg p.o. q.d plus pyrimethamine 50 mg p.o. q.w. plus leucovorin 25 mg p.o. q.w. or atovaquone 1500 mg p.o. q.d.
Systemic mycoses	No definitive recommendations		

[a]Not recommended for most patients; indicated for use only in unusual circumstances.

be host species specific, suggesting that human infection is unlikely to be a zoonosis. Whether *P. carinii* can be transmitted person to person is unknown; therefore, current recommendations are that hospitalized patients with PCP do not require respiratory isolation.

Although most patients who develop PCP are unaware of their HIV status at time of PCP diagnosis, approximately 15% of PCP cases occur in patients who do not fulfill the current criteria for prophylaxis. Prophylaxis for PCP should be initiated for all HIV-infected individuals with CD4+ T-cell count < 200 cells/μL, unexplained fever (>100°F or 37.7°C) for ≥2 weeks, history of oral candidiasis, or previous episode of PCP. A retrospective chart review of over 33,000 HIV-infected patients by Kaplan et al. (19) revealed that an AIDS-defining illness or non-*P. carinii* pneumonia (PCP) constituted independent risk factors for PCP in addition to those noted by the USPHS/IDSA.

Trimethoprim-sulfamethoxazole (TMP/SMX) is the preferred prophylactic agent at a dose of one double-strength (DS) tablet daily. In addition to its proven efficacy and low cost, TMP/SMX reduces the incidence of toxoplasmosis and bacterial infections (20–22). Single-strength tablets may also be effective and may be better tolerated (17). Alternative prophylaxis include TMP/SMX DS t.i.w., dapsone 50 mg p.o. b.i.d. or 100 mg p.o. daily or atovaquone 1500 mg p.o. daily or aerosolized pentamidine 300 mg monthly. Patients who are at risk for toxoplasmosis and intolerant of TMP/SMX should be offered dapsone 50 mg p.o. daily plus pyrimethamine 50 mg and leucovorin 25 mg weekly or atovaquone 1500 mg p.o. daily with or without pyrimethamine.

Patients who are intolerant of TMP/SMX should be rechallenged. Gradual initiation of TMP/SMX may improve its tolerability. In ACTG 268 (23), patients were randomized (double blind) to receive either TMP/SMX suspension (1 mL for 3 days, then 2 mL for 3 days, then 5 mL for 3 days, then 10 mL for 3 days, then 20 mL) or to initiate prophylaxis with one DS daily. Adverse reactions such as fever and/or skin rash were reported in 34% started on DS daily compared with 16% on gradual initiation. Reducing the TMP/SMX dose to single strength or three times a week may improve tolerance as well. Patients absolutely intolerant of TMP/SMX should be prophylaxed with dapsone. Patients intolerant of TMP/SMX and dapsone should be prophylaxed with aerosolized pentamidine or atovaquone. Results of ACTG 277/CPCRA034 (24) comparing atovaquone 1500 mg p.o. daily with dapsone 100 mg p.o. daily in patients intolerant of SMX/TMP revealed similar efficacy in both prevention of PCP and survival. Dapsone was associated with more hypersensitivity complaints, whereas atovaquone was associated with more gastrointestinal complaints. Although clindamycin/primaquine is an effective therapeutic alternative, this regimen has not been adequately studied for prophylaxis. Other proposed investigational prophylactic agents include azithromycin, benzimidazoles, and 8-aminoquinolones; however, given the diminished incidence of PCP and the excellent overall efficacy of currently U.S. Food and Drug Administration-approved therapies, no clinical trails evaluating these agents are in progress.

Prophylaxis failure is unusual in patients whose CD4+ T-cell count is >75 cells/μL. Most failures of prophylaxis are associated with CD4+ T-cell count < 50 cells/μL, nonadherence, and regimens other than TMP/SMX. Kazanjian et al. (25) reported that patients receiving TMP/SMX or dapsone were more likely to develop *P. carinii* dihydropteroate synthase (DHPS) gene mutations than those not receiving prophylaxis. Despite the presence of this mutation, these patients responded to therapy with TMP/SMX; hence, the role of resistance in breakthrough PCP is unknown. Helweg-Larsen et al. (26) reported DHPS gene mutations were more commonly seen in patients who developed PCP while on prophylaxis and were associated with a poorer prognosis than those patients who did not have DHPS gene mutations.

PCP prophylaxis should be offered to all pregnant women. TMP/SMX is the preferred agent of choice; however, aerosolized pentamidine may be offered during the first trimester due to theoretical concerns of teratogenicity.

Schneider et al. (27) from the Netherlands reported the successful discontinuation of PCP primary prophylaxis in 62 patients and PCP secondary prophylaxis in 16 patients whose CD4+ T-cell counts were greater than 200 cells/μL on HAART. At the time of discontinuation of PCP prophylaxis, the mean CD4+ T-cell count was 346 cells/μL and the viral load was below the limits of detection in 61 patients. None of the patients have developed PCP after 7–14 months. Two patients did restart PCP prophylaxis when their CD4+ T-cell count declined to <200 cells/μL.

In the EuroSIDA study (28), a prospective observational cohort study in 52 centers in Europe and Israel, 319 patients discontinued primary PCP prophylaxis and 59 patients discontinued secondary PCP prophylaxis after a median of 10 months on HAART. The median CD4+ T-cell counts were 274 cells/μL and 270 cells/μL, respectively. None of the patients developed PCP during 247 person-years of follow-up.

Antinori et al. (29) reported the preliminary results of an open controlled randomized trial on the discontinuation of PCP prophylaxis in patients whose CD4 counts > 200 cells/μL for at least 3 months. A total of 607 patients were prospectively followed, 300 of whom were randomized to stop PCP prophylaxis. During a median follow up of 6.7 months (range, 1–15) and a total of 340 person-years, no episodes of PCP were observed.

Lopez et al. (30) also conducted a prospective, open, controlled, randomized trial evaluating 488 patients of which 247 were randomized to stop PCP prophylaxis. There were no reported episodes of PCP after a median of 11.3-month follow-up.

In addition to the above reports, there have been multiple abstracts presented suggesting that both primary and secondary prophylaxis may be safely withdrawn in HIV-infected patients whose CD4+ T-cell counts rise above 200 cells/μL on HAART (31–33).

The USPHS 1999 draft guidelines state, "While the optimal criteria for discontinuation remain to be defined, providers may wish to discontinue prophylaxis when patients have a sustained CD4+ T-lymphocyte count > 200 cells/μl for at least 3–6 months." There are no data to guide recommendations for reinstitution of primary prophylaxis or the discontinuation of secondary prophylaxis. One should strongly consider the reinstitution of prophylaxis when a patient's CD4 count starts to decline and definitely restart if either the CD4 percent falls < 14% or CD4 count < 200 cells/μL as per the initial recommendations. It is unclear what the risk of developing PCP is when virologic failure precedes the decline in CD4 count. In patients whose CD4 nadirs were <200 cells/μL and are experiencing virologic rebound or never achieved full HIV viral load suppression with CD4 counts > 200 cells/μL, one may want to consider reinitiating or continuing prophylaxis based on the results of Center for Disease Control and Prevention's Adult and Adolescent Spectrum of Disease Project, which suggests that viral load is an independent predictor of the development of OI's (34).

III. MAC

Disseminated infection with MAC is one of the most common life-threatening opportunistic infections affecting patients with AIDS (35, 36). Approximately 40% of patients will develop MAC within 2 years of the diagnosis of AIDS if no prophylaxis is given (36–38). Disseminated MAC (dMAC) infection is a cause of serious morbidity, including intractable fever, night sweats, fatigue, diarrhea, and wasting, and retrospective studies indicate that AIDS patients with dMAC have a shorter survival than matched patients without dMAC (39–41).

Prophylaxis for MAC is recommended for all patients with CD4+ T-cell counts of less than 50 cells/μL. The selection of drug(s) for a patient should be based on efficacy, adverse events, cost, resistance, and drug interactions. Clarithromycin, azithromycin, and rifabutin have each been shown to reduce the risk of the development of dMAC (38, 42–44). Based on reviews of the trials available at the time of publication of the USPHS/IDSA guidelines, clarithromycin 500 mg p.o. b.i.d. or azithromycin 1200 mg p.o. every week were chosen as the preferred agents as being more effective than rifabutin 300 mg p.o. every day for the prevention of MAC. Subsequently, a French study (45) reported a similar breakthrough rate of MAC in patients receiving rifabutin prophylaxis comparable with the macrolides. Macrolides still remain the preferred drug of choice because of the increased drug interactions associated with rifabutin. Azithromycin and rifabutin is more efficacious than either drug alone (38) but is associated with increased side effects, cost, and drug interactions.

Since antiretroviral therapy became available in clincial practice, localized lesions including endobronchial, cutaneous abscesses, osteomyelitis, and lymphadenitis have been reported (46–49). One report described an isolated cavitary pulmonary MAC without bacteremia in an HIV patient with a CD4+ T-cell count of 302 (50). The patient was treated with clarithromycin, ethambutol, and rifabutin with resolution of the chest x-ray and symptoms. Another case series documented five patients with HIV disease who developed pulmonary MAC without dissemination (51). Two patients had CD4+ T-cell counts above 220, but history of prior CD4 counts and antiretroviral therapy were not described. Patients were treated for 10 months without relapse with clarithromycin, ethambutol and/or rifabutin. In a case series by Race et al. (52), five patients were admitted with high fevers, leucocytosis, and lymph node enlargement 1–3 weeks after starting indinavir. Lymph node biopsies revealed MAC. Symptoms resolved with combination MAC treatment. Phillips et al. (5) reported similar findings in several patients who developed MAC lymphadenitis within 12 weeks of initiating HAART, which they attributed to the augmentation of the cellular immune responses to mycobacterial antigens that "unmasks" subclinical MAC infection.

Paradoxical worsening, on the other hand, occurs when pathogen-specific immunity results in a presumed inflammatory response directed at the specific antigens released. Paradoxical worsening has a long history predating AIDS and was originally reported in patients being treated for tuberculosis (53) as the development or worsening of lymphadenopathy and exacerbation of cerebral tuberculomas and adult respiratory distress syndrome. However, paradoxical worsening of tuberculosis has been reported to occur more frequently when HAART is initiated concomitantly with antituberculous therapy (7, 8). In such patients, antiretroviral therapy was started between 2 and 40 days before symptoms were manifest. Reactions included fevers, lymphadenopathy, worsening chest x-rays, and extrapulmonary lesions. These all eventually resolved with continuation of antituberculosis medications, although some patients require the use of steroids.

The preliminary results of ACTG 362 (54), a randomized placebo-controlled trial of azithromycin prophylaxis for the prevention of MAC in subjects with increases of CD4 counts > 100 cells/μL, revealed two MAC events occurred in 321 patients randomized to placebo. No MAC events occurred in the 322 patients randomized to continue prophylaxis. Although these data suggest that it is safe to withdraw MAC prophylaxis in patients who have had sustained CD4 increases > 100 cells/μL, we do need to recognize the possibility that these atypical manifestations can still occur when patients do have sustained elevations of their CD4+ T cells. The two patients with MAC events in this trial differ from those previously reported as both had been on stable HAART with a sustained increases CD4+ T-cell count and suppressed viral load for several months before development of symptoms. It is also interesting to note that both events involved localized spinal infections with MAC. There has been only one other report of a spinal infection with MAC occurring in an AIDS patient, and this patient had advanced HIV disease with concomitant lymphoma (55). In contrast, there have been multiple case reports of localized spine infections secondary to MAC in HIV-negative patients either receiving steroids or without known cause of immunosuppression (56–61).

It is hypothesized that infection with MAC starts with colonization of the gastrointestinal or respiratory tract. A localized infection occurs with intermittent MAC bacteremia, leading to seeding of other organs, particularly the reticuloendothelial system. MAC proliferates in these islands of infection until mycobacterial burden is so high as to spill over as bacteremia (37, 40, 62–64). Disk space infection usually arises from hematogenous spread either by arterial seeding or through the vertebral venous plexus (Batson's plexus). It is reasonable to assume that in these patients with a CD4 count nadir of <50, MAC may have already seeded the disk space and remained dormant for a prolonged period before reactivating, a common scenario in tuberculosis infections.

To understand these patients' clinical course in the face of a high CD4+ T-cell count, it is useful to review what is known so far about immune reconstitution after initiating HAART. As HIV advances, there is a loss of CD4+ naive cells with CD4+ memory cells (the T-cells activated by exposure to antigen in the recent past) predominating. When compared with naive T cells, memory cells are more rapidly dividing and may have more avid binding to tissues. In the case series of focal mycobacterial lymphadenitis described by Race et al. (52) when HAART was initiated, immunotyping of two patients revealed that most cells were memory CD4+ T cells (92% and 98%) despite increased CD4+ T-cell counts after HAART. Connors et al. (65) found that after initiating HAART, naive T cells increased only if they were present before initiation of therapy. These data suggest that although antiretroviral and immune based therapies can dramatically increase CD4+ T cells, the original CD4+ T-cell repertoire may only be partially restored.

With HAART, there may be a selective reconstitution of CD4+ memory T cells specific for MAC. These may be preferentially expanded with a resultant exuberant inflammatory response around the established infection site. Cytokine flow cytometry analysis of one patient's lymphocytes documented that he could produce interferon-gamma, interleukin-12, and tumor necrosis factor-alpha responses to MAC antigen (R.B. Pearce, personal communication, 1999).

Aberg et al. (66) at the University of California, San Francisco reported four patients who discontinued MAC therapy after receiving 12 months of a macrolide based antimycobacterial regimen and whose CD4 count rose above 100 cells/μL while on HAART. None of the patients had signs or symptoms of MAC, plus each had a sterile bone marrow aspirate culture and sterile peripheral blood cultures before discontinuing their antimycobacterial therapy to ensure there was no evidence of subclinical infection. None of these patients have had recurrence of MAC after 8–13 months. Since the time of this publication, none of the four patients had a recurrence of MAC after 24–29 months (J. Aberg, personal communication, 1999). ACTG 393, a study similar to the pilot described above, is ongoing. No preliminary data are available at this time.

Although the optimal criteria for discontinuation of MAC prophylaxis remain to be defined, it is reasonable to consider discontinuing prophylaxis in patients with a sustained CD4+ T-lymphocyte count > 100 cells/μL (e.g., >3–6 months and sustained suppression of HIV plasma RNA). There are no data to guide recommendations for reinstitution of primary prophylaxis or the discontinuation of secondary prophylaxis. Clarithromycin should not be used during pregnancy. Azithromycin plus ethambutal are the preferred drugs for secondary prophylaxis in pregnancy.

IV. CMV

CMV end-organ disease affected up to 40% of patients with AIDS in the pre-HAART era. In approximately 85% of cases of AIDS-related CMV disease, the retina is affected, and in less than 15% it manifests as gastrointestinal disease. Infection of the central nervous system is uncommon, although autopsy series suggest it may be underdiagnosed. CMV disease occurring at higher CD4+ T cell counts and associated with unusual presentations (submaxillary lymphadenitis, pseudotumor colitis, and pneumonitis) have been reported (67, 68). Since HAART became available, the incidence of CMV disease has dramatically declined. Jacobson et al. (69) at San Francisco General Hospital did report a slight increase in the incidence of CMV retinitis at their institution during 1998. Of more interest was the fact that 5 of 10 new cases in 1998 occurred in patients who failed to have immunological and complete virological responses despite 7–16 months on HAART. Of the 14 cases diagnosed in 1997–1998, retinitis healed in those patients receiving anti-CMV therapy who had good immunological and virological responses to HAART, whereas patients who did not have good immunological/virological responses on HAART developed early reactivation and progression of their CMV retinitis.

HIV-infected individuals with CD4+ T-cell counts < 50 cells/μL and CMV seropositivity are known to be at risk of developing CMV disease. Currently, the only approved therapy for prophylaxis is oral ganciclovir 1 g p.o. t.i.d. In the first prospective randomized study (70) comparing oral ganciclovir to placebo, the frequency of CMV disease was reduced by 49% and the rate of positive culture was reduced from 55% in the placebo arm to <20% in the ganciclovir arm. In addition, less zone 1 disease (within 1500 μm of optic nerve head or 3000 μm of the fovea) and a trend for improved survival was noted among ganciclovir recipients. Unfortunately, oral ganciclovir has poor bioavailability, is problematic for patients in terms of the number of pills to be taken daily, has risk of significant adverse reactions including neutropenia, and is very costly. It has not been shown that oral ganciclovir prophylaxis results in improved survival or visual preservation compared with frequent clinical monitoring and early diagnosis/treatment. There has been much interest in delineating which patients would benefit the most from prophylaxis. Many investigators (71–75) have presented data suggesting detection or quantitation of CMV blood viral load (either PCR amplified CMV DNA or CMV antigen detected in peripheral leukocytes) might have clinical utility in predicting the risk of CMV disease and monitoring response to therapy. If reliable, such markers could be used to target those patients most likely to develop disease and spare others the cost and toxicities of anti-CMV intervention. In these individuals with detectable CMV DNA in the plasma, therapy would be preemptive rather than prophylactic. Several potent oral anti-CMV agents are currently in phase I/II trials. Until such prophylactic strategies prove to be efficacious, the USPHS/IDSA has recommended that oral ganciclovir may be considered in patients with CD4+ T-cell counts < 50 cells/μL and who are CMV seropositive; however, ganciclovir-induced neutropenia, anemia, conflicting reports of efficacy, lack of proven survival benefit, risk of developing ganciclovir-resistant CMV, and cost are among the issues that should be considered in decisions about whether to institute prophylaxis in individual patients.

At the Interscience Conference on Antimicrobial Agents and Chemotherapy in September 1997, Torriani et al. (76) at the University of California, San Diego reported eight patients that discontinued CMV maintenance therapy for CMV retinitis (CMVR) after long periods of nonprogression. The median CD4+ T-cell count at time of CMVR was 39 cells/μL and median days on HAART was 398. At the time of discontinuation of CMV maintenance therapy, the median CD4+ T-cell count was 172 cells/μL (range, 63–404) and the mean plasma viremia was 68,000 (range, <200–508,000). No individuals progressed after a mean follow-up of 146 days (range, 72–205). CD4+ T-cell counts remained elevated (mean, 198 cells/μL) despite six of eight patients having detectable viral load (mean, 40,000; range, 409–423,000). Follow-up data on these eight patients presented at the 5th Conference on Retroviruses and Opportunistic Infections in February 1998 (77, 78) revealed that none of the eight patients showed any recurrence of disease (median, 300 days). This suggests that HAART might restore CMV-specific immunity even in patients without complete suppression of plasma viremia.

Subsequently, the San Diego investigators (79) reported the lack of reactivation of CMVR in 11 patients who had discontinued CMV therapy and had sustained elevations in CD4+ T-cell counts; however, three patients did experience relapse when their CD4+ T-cell counts dropped below 50 cells/μL (F. Torriani, personal communication, 1999).

Tural et al. (80) from Spain reported long-lasting remission (9–12 months) of CMVR in seven patients who had discontinued CMV maintenance therapy after 3 months of a protease inhibitor-containing antiretroviral regimen resulting in CD4+ T-cell counts greater than 150 cells/μL and an HIV viral load < 200 copies/mL.

Preliminary evidence by Komanduri et al. (16) suggest that CMV antigen-specific CD4+ lymphocytes responses measured by flow cytometry may correlate with clinical outcome. They noted that patients who were HIV-positive and had quiescent CMV retinal disease on HAART had similar responses to patients who were HIV positive and CMV IgG antibody positive. The presence of active CMVR correlated with the loss of CMV-specific CD4+ responses. Similarly, Torriani et al. (77) reported a clinical correlation between in vitro lymphoproliferative responses to CMV antigen in AIDS patients with quiescent CMV disease on HAART as described above.

Li et al. (81) reported a patient with CMV viremia and lacking CMV-specific CD4+ responses who became aviremic with restoration of CMV-specific CD4+ responses after 3 months of HAART. This reactivity against CMV antigen persisted along with CMV-negative blood cultures for a period of 18 months post-HAART at time of publication. This 3-month delay in the development of CMV-specific CD4+ responses may account for the atypical manifestations previously reported when patients develop CMV disease within the first weeks of starting HAART (6, 82).

Per the 1999 USPHS draft guidelines, discontinuation of CMV maintenance therapy may be considered in patients with a sustained (e.g., >3–6 month) increase in CD4 count to >100–150 cells/μL on HAART. Such decisions should be made in consultation with an ophthalmologist and should take into account such factors as the magnitude and duration of CD4+ T-lymphocyte increase, magnitude and duration of viral load suppression, anatomic location of the retinal lesion, vision in the contralateral eye, and feasibility of regular ophthalmic monitoring. Maintenance therapy should not be discontinued in patients with extraocular CMV disease. There are insufficient data to guide recommendations for reinstitution of anti-CMV treatment, although it may be reasonable to restart therapy when the CD4 count has decreased to <50–100 cells/μL.

V. TOXOPLASMOSIS

Toxoplasmic encephalitis (TE) is the most common cause of focal brain disease in patients with AIDS. The incidence of TE is dependent on the prevalence of *Toxoplasma gondii* in the general population in a geographic region. Approximately 5–10% of AIDS patients in the United States who are seropositive for *T. gondii* will develop TE (83). Given the risk of reinfection with a different strain, seropositive and seronegative patients should be advised of preventive measures to avoid infection with *T. gondii*. These measures include eating only well-cooked red meats, changing a cat's litter box daily so oocysts are discarded before maturation, and proper hand washing after contact with soil that may have been contaminated with cat feces.

Chemoprophylaxis should be initiated if a patient has a CD4+ T-cell count < 100 cells/μL and is seropositive for IgG antibody to *T. gondii* and is not already receiving a regimen for PCP prophylaxis that is also effective for toxoplasmosis. Current recommended prophylaxis is either TMP/SMX DS one tablet daily or dapsone 50 mg daily/pyrimethamine 50 mg weekly/leucovorin 25 mg weekly or atovaquone 1500 mg daily. Efficacy of clindamycin/pyrimethamine or macrolides for prophylaxis is unknown.

It is unlikely that a large clinical trial to withdraw chronic suppressive therapy will be conducted due to the low overall incidence; however, it is expected that we will be able to infer the relative safety of withdrawing primary prophylaxis for toxoplasmosis by meta-analysis of all the primary prophylaxis withdrawal trials for PCP. Until such time, the USPHS guidelines recommends that there are insufficient data to warrant discontinuation of primary or secondary toxoplasmosis prophylaxis.

VI. SYSTEMIC MYCOSES

The efficiency of utilizing azoles as primary prophylaxis for systemic mycoses is unclear. Specific questions remain unanswered. At what dose or what duration is protection optimal? Are there certain patient characteristics that would support the use of primary prophylaxis in certain subgroups? The overall incidence of serious fungal infections is low and careful monitoring may be more cost effective. Further studies are needed to determine if certain risk factors or predictive factors exist to support the use of an azole as primary prophylaxis. There is concern that prolonged usage of an azole may result in acquired resistance to that azole. In addition, drug-related adverse reactions and drug–drug interactions need to be considered. Until further studies are performed, the clinical utility of fluconazole or itraconazole as primary prophylaxis for systemic mycoses is unknown. Currently, two studies are ongoing evaluating the safety of withdrawing chronic suppressive therapy in patients with disseminated histoplasmosis and cryptococcosis. No data are available at this time. Until such time, the USPHS guidelines recommends that there are insufficient data to warrant discontinuation of secondary prophylaxis.

VII. SUMMARY

Critical questions remain unanswered regarding the safety and efficacy of withdrawing primary and secondary prophylaxis in the context of HAART-associated immune reconstitution. What are the mediators of first phase cellular increases? Will continued HIV suppression result in continued immune restoration? And what are the immunological consequences of viral rebound despite HAART in patients whose CD4 counts remain elevated? Can immunity, once lost, be restored by reintroduction of antigens such as by tetanus or pneumococcal vaccination? Can immunoassays predict who will relapse or reactivate an OI? Is it possible to eradicate infections such as MAC, cryptococcosis, and histoplasmosis? Certainly, one can never eradicate CMV infection but can immunoassays predict who will have disease reactivate?

Unfortunately, various studies have reported contradicting results regarding the immunological response in vitro to specific antigens. Until these immunoassays become standardized and validated, it is unclear if immunoassays will be predictive of who would be at risk of development of disease or relapse. Therefore, until such time, clinicians may want to initiate and maintain primary prophylaxis in HIV-infected individuals as recommended by the USPHS/IDSA guidelines based on the nadir CD4+ T-cell count at least until studies have clearly demonstrated whether the increased CD4+ T-cell response attributed to HAART does in fact confer protection against these pathogens. Although for some OIs it does appear safe to withdraw primary prophylaxis and probably secondary prophylaxis, the decision to stop prophylaxis or maintenance therapy should be a joint decision by the patient and clinician based on the risks and benefits of stopping the therapy and the availability of close clinical monitoring for evidence of disease.

REFERENCES

1. CAESAR Committee. Randomised trial of addition of lamivudine or lamivudine plus loviride to zidovudine-containing regimens for patients with HIV-1 infection: the CAESAR trial. Lancet 1997;349:1413–1421.

2. Moore RD, Chaisson RE. Natural history of opportunistic disease in an HIV-infected urban clinical cohort. Ann Intern Med 1996;124:633–642.

3. Hogg RS, Heath KV, Yip B, Craib KJ, O'Shaughnessy MV, Schechter MT, Montaner JS. Improved survival among HIV-infected individuals following initiation of antiretroviral therapy. JAMA 1998;279:450–454.

4. McCutchan A, Bozette S, Shapiro M, Turner B, Asch S, Gifford A, Keseey J. Lifetime prevalence of opportunistic infections in a nationally representative sample (HCSUS) of HIV-infected persons in care. Abstract 13238, 12th World AIDS Conference, Geneva, June 1998.

5. Phillips P, Kwiatkowski MB, Copland M, Craib K, Montaner J. Mycobacterial lymphadenitis associated with the initiation of combination antiretroviral therapy. J Acquir Immune Defic Syndr Hum Retrovirol 1999;20:122–128.

6. Jacobson MA, French M. Altered natural history of AIDS-related opportunistic infections in the era of potent combination antiretroviral therapy. AIDS 1998; 12(suppl A):S157–S163.

7. Narita M, Ashkin D, Hollender ES, Pitchenik AE. Paradoxical worsening of tuberculosis following antiretroviral therapy in patients with AIDS. Am J Respir Crit Care Med 1998;158:157–161.

8. Chien JW, Johnson JL. Paradoxical reactions in HIV and pulmonary TB. Chest 1998:114:933–936.

9. Currier JS, Havlir DV. New Insights into HIV-Related Complications (Highlights from the 5th Conference on Retrovirus and Opportunistic Infections Feb 1998).

International AIDS Society—USA Improving the Management of HIV Disease 1998;6:14–18.

10. Palella FJ Jr, Delaney KM, Moorman AC, Loveless MO, Fuhrer J, Satten GA, Aschman DJ, Holmberg SD. Declining morbidity and mortality among patients with advanced human immunodeficiency virus infection. N Engl J Med 1998; 338:853–860.

11. Autran B, Carcelain G, Li TS, Blanc C, Mathez D, Tubiana R, Katlama C, Debre P, Leibowitch J. Positive effects of combined antiretroviral therapy on CD4+ T cell homeostasis and function in advanced HIV disease. Science 1997;277: 112–116.

12. Lederman MM, Connick E, Landay A, Kuritzkes DR, Spritzler J, St Clair M, Kotzin BL, Fox L, Chiozzi MH, Leonard JM, Rousseau F, Wade M, Roe JD, Martinez A, Kessler H. Immunologic responses associated with 12 weeks of combination antiretroviral therapy consisting of zidovudine, lamivudine, and ritonavir: results of AIDS Clinical Trials Group Protocol 315. J Infect Dis 1998; 178:70–91.

13. Pakker NG, Notermans DW, de Boer RJ, Roos MT, de Wolf F, Hill A, Leonard JM, Danner SA, Miedema F, Schellekens PT. Biphasic kinetics of peripheral blood T cells after triple combination therapy in HIV-1 infection: a composite of redistribution and proliferation. Nat Med 1998;4:208–214.

14. Angel JB, Kumar A, Parato K, Filion LG, Diaz-Mitoma F, Daftarian P, Pham B, Sun E, Leonard JM, Cameron DW. Improvement in cell-mediated immune function during potent anti-human immunodeficiency virus therapy with ritonavir plus saquinavir. J Infect Dis 1998;177:898–904.

15. Liebmann J, Huang X, Fan Z, Mellors J, Al-Shboul Q, McMahon D, Riddler S, Day R, Chen W, Bazmi A, Rinaldo C. Highly Active Antiretroviral Therapy Results in Delayed Enhancement of CD4+ T cell Reactivity to Mitogen and Recall Antigens, but not HIV-1Antigens. Abstract 169 Presented at 5th Conference on Retroviruses and Opportunistic Infections, 1998. Chicago, IL.

16. Komanduri KV, Viswanathan MN, Wieder ED, Schmidt DK, Bredt BM, Jacobson MA, McCune JM. Restoration of cytomegalovirus-specific CD4+ T-lymphocyte responses after ganciclovir and highly active antiretroviral therapy in individuals infected with HIV-1. Nat Med 1998;4:953–956.

17. 1999 USPHS/IDSA Guidelines for the Prevention of Opportunistic Infections in Persons with Human Immunodeficiency Virus. May 14, 1999, Draft 5.

18. Ng VL, Yajko DM, Hadley WK. Extrapulmonary pneumocystosis. Clin Micro Rev 1997;10:401–418.

19. Kaplan JE, Hanson D, Jones J. Risk factors for Primary PCP in HIV-Infected Adolescents and Adults in the U.S.: Should History of AIDS-Defining Illness be Included in the Criteria for PCP Prophylaxis? Abstract 691 Presented at 4th Conference on Retroviruses and Opportunistic Infections, 1997, Washington DC.

20. Carr A, Tindall B, Brew BJ, Marriott DJ, Harkness JL, Penny R, Cooper DA. Low-dose trimethoprim-sulfamethoxazole prophylaxis for toxoplasmic encephalitis in patients with AIDS. Ann Intern Med 1992;117:106–111.

21. Ioannidis JPA, Cappelleri JC, Skolnick PR, Lau J, Sacks HS. A meta-analysis of the relative efficacy and toxicity of *Pneumocystis carinii* prophylactic regimens. Arch Intern Med 1996;156:177–188.

22. Dirienzo, G, van der Horst C, Frame P, et al. Prevention of Bacterial infection in AIDS: A Randomized Trial of Three Agents. Abstract 537, 35th Annual Meeting of the Infectious Disease Society of America, San Francisco, 1997.

23. Para MF, Dohn M, Frame P, Becker S, Finkelstein D, Walawander A. ACTG 268 Trial-Gradual Initiation of TMP/SMX as Primary Prophylaxis for *Pneumocystis carinii* pneumonia (PCP). Abstract 694, Presented at 4th Conference on Retroviruses and Opportunistic Infections, 1997, Washington DC.

24. El-Sadr WM, Murphy RL, Yurik TM, Luskin-Hawk R, Cheung TW, Balfour HH Jr, Erg R, Hooton TM, Kerkering TM, Schutz M, van der Horst C, Hafner R. Atovaquone compared with dapsone for the prevention of Pneumocystis carinii pneumonia in patients with HIV infection who cannot tolerate trimethoprim, sulfonamides, or both. N Engl J Med 1998;339:1889–1895.

25. Kazanjian P, Locke A, Hossler PA, Lane BR, Bartlett MS, Smith JW, Cannon M, Meshnick SR. Pneumocystis carinii mutations associated with sulfa and sulfone prophylaxis failures in AIDS patients. AIDS 1998;12:873–878.

26. Helweg-Larsen J, Benfield TL, Eugen-Olsen J, Lundgren JD, Lundgren B. Mutations in the *Pneumocystis carinii* Dihydropteroate Synthase Gene as Virulence Factor in AIDS-Associated PCP. Abstract 49 at the 39th Interscience Conference on Antimicrobial Agents and Chemotherapy. San Francisco 1999.

27. Schneider MME, Borleffs JCC, Stolk RP, Jaspers CA, Hoepelman AI. Discontinuation of prophylaxis for *Pneumocystis carinii* pneumonia in HIV-1 infected patients treated with highly active antiretroviral therapy. Lancet 1999;353:201–203.

28. Weverling GJ, Mocroft A, Ledergerber B, Kirk O, Gonzales-Lahoz J, d'Arminio Monforte A, Proenca R, Phillips AN, Lundgren JD, Reiss P. Discontinuation of *Pneumocystis carinii* pneumonia prophylaxis after start of highly active antiretroviral therapy in HIV-1 infection. Lancet 1999;353:1293–1298.

29. Antinori A, Borghi V, Concia E, DeRienzo B, Govoni A, Mongiardo N, Mussini C, Pezzitti P, Bonazzi L, Cerri M, Chido F, d'Arminio Monforte A, De Luca A. An Open Controlled Randomized Trial on the Discontinuation of Primary PCP Prophylaxis among HIV-infected Individuals Whose CD4 Count Returned to a level Greater than 200 Cells/mm^3 after HAART:CIOP Study. Abstract 1165 at the 39th Interscience Conference on Antimicrobial Agents and Chemotherapy. San Francisco 1999.

30. Lopez JC, Miro JM, Pena JM, Podzamczer D. Discontinuation of PCP Prophylaxis is Safe in HIV-Infected Patients After Immunological Recovery with HAART. Results of the Gesida 04/98 Study. Abstract LB-24 at the 39th Interscience Conference on Antimicrobial Agents and Chemotherapy. San Francisco 1999.

31. Ravaux I, Quinson AM, Chadapaud S, Gallais H. Discontinue Primary and Secondary Prophylaxis Regimens in Selected HIV-Infected Patients Treated with HAART. Abstract I-203, 38th Interscience Conference of Antimicrobial Agents and Chemotherapy, San Diego 1998.

32. Vazquez EG, DeGorgolas M, Delgado RG, Guerrero MLF. Is PCP Prophylaxis Needed in Patients on Highly Active Antiretroviral Therapy with Increasing CD4 Count? Abstract I-204, 38th Interscience Conference of Antimicrobial Agents and Chemotherapy, San Diego 1998.

33. Yangco BG, Von Bargen JC, Moorman AC. Can PCP Prophylaxis Be safely Discontinued among Clinically Improving HIV Patients? Abstract I-262, 38th Interscience Conference of Antimicrobial Agents and Chemotherapy, San Diego 1998.

34. Kaplan JE, Hanson DL, Dworkin MS, Jones JL. HIV Plasma RNA, an Independent Predictor of Opportunistic Infections in HIV-Infected Persons. Abstract 124 at the 39th Interscience Conference on Antimicrobial Agents and Chemotherapy. San Francisco 1999.

35. Horsburgh CR. *Mycobacterium avium* complex infection in the acquired immunodeficiency syndrome. N Engl J Med 1991;324:1332–1338.

36. Nightingale SD, Byrd LT, Southern PM, Jockusch JD, Cal SX, Wynne BA. Incidence of *Mycobacterium avium-intracellulare* complex bacteremia in HIV-positive patients. J Infect Dis 1992;165:1082–1085.

37. Chaisson RE, Moore RD, Richman DD, Keruly J, Creagh T, Zidovudine Epidemiology Study Group. Incidence and natural history of *Mycobacterium-avium* complex in patients with advanced human immunodeficiency virus disease treated with zidovudine. Am Rev Respir Dis 1992;146:258–259.

38. Havlir DV, Dube MP, Sattler FR, Forthal DN, Kemper CA, Dunne MW, Parenti DM, Lavelle JP, White AC, Witt MD, Bozzette SA, McCutchan JA for the California Collaborative Treatment Group. Prophylaxis against disseminated *Mycobacterium avium* complex with weekly azithromycin, daily rifabutin, or both. N Engl J Med 1996;335:392–398.

39. Horsburgh CR, Havlik JA, Ellis DA, Kennedy E, Fann SA, Dubois RE, Sumner ET. Survival of Patients with acquired immune deficiency syndrome and disseminated *Mycobacterium avium* complex infection with and without antimycobacterial chemotherapy. Am Rev Respir Dis 1991;144:557–559.

40. Jacobson MA, Hopewell, PC, Yajko DM, Hadley WK, Lazarus E, Mohanty PK, Modin GW, Feigal DW, Cusick PS, Sande MA. Natural history of Disseminated

Mycobacterium avium complex infection in AIDS. J Infect Dis 1991;164:994–998.

41. Hoover DR, Graham NMH, Bacellar H, Murphy R, Visscher B, Anderson R, McArthur J. An epidemiologic analysis of *Mycobacterium avium* complex disease in homosexual men infected with human immunodeficiency virus type 1. Clin Infect Dis 1995;20:1250–1258.

42. Pierce M, Crampton S, Henry D, Heifets L, La Marca A, Montecalvo M, Wormser GP, Jablonowski H, Jemsek J, Cynamon M, Yangco BG, Notario G, Craft JC. A randomized trial of clarithromycin as prophylaxis against disseminated *Mycobacterium avium* complex infection in patients with advanced acquired immunodeficiency syndrome. N Engl J Med 1996;335:384–391.

43. Benson CA, Cohn DL, Williams P, the ACTG 196/CPCRA 009 Study Team. A Phase III prospective, randomized, double-blind study of the safety and efficacy of clarithromycin (CLA) vs. rifabutin (RBT) vs. CLA+RBT for prevention of Mycobacterium avium complex (MAC)disease in HIV + patients with CD4 counts less than 100 cells/microliter. Abstract 205, Presented at the 3rd Conference on Retroviruses and Opportunistic Infections, 1996, Washington DC.

44. Oldfield EC 3rd, Fessel WJ, Dunne MW, Dickinson G, Wallace MR, Byrne W, Chung R, Wagner KF, Paparello SF, Craig DB, Melcher G, Zajdowicz M, Williams RF, Kelly JW, Zelasky M, Heifets LB, Berman JD. Once weekly azithromycin therapy for prevention of Mycobacterium avium complex infection in patients with AIDS: a randomized, double-blind, placebo-controlled multicenter trial. Clin Infect Dis 1998;26:611–619.

45. Maslo C, Bure-Rossier A, Girard PM, Gholizadeh Y, Lebrette MG, Rozenbaum W. Clinical and bacteriologic impact of rifabutin prophylaxis for *Mycobacterium avium* complex infection in patients with human immunodeficiency virus infection. Clin Infect Dis 1997;24:344–349.

46. Packer SJ, Cesario T, Williams JH. Mycobacterium avium complex infection presenting as endobronchial lesions in immunosuppressed patients. Ann Intern Med 1988;109:389–393.

47. Sheppard DC, Sullam PM. Primary septic arthritis and osteomyelitis due to *Mycobacterium avium* complex in a patient with AIDS. Clin Infect Dis 1997; 25:925–926.

48. Miller RS, Thomas SJ, Hospenthal DR, Oster CN. Isolated *Mycobacterium avium* complex osteomyelitis in a patient with AIDS. Abstract 574, 35th Annual meeting of the Infectious Diseases Society of America, San Francisco, September 1997.

49. Barbaro DJ, Orcutt VL, Coldiron BM. Mycobacterium avium-mycobacterium intracellulare infection limited to the skin and lymph nodes in patients with AIDS. Rev Infect Dis 1989;11:625–628.

50. Alisky JM, Schlesinger L. Isolated cavitary pulmonary mycobacterium avium complex infection in a patient with AIDS. Clin Infect Dis 1998;27:1542–1543.

51. Hocqueloux L, Lesprit P, Herrmann JL, de La Blanchardiere A, Zagdanski A, Decazes J-M, Modai J. Pulmonary mycobacterium avium complex disease without dissemination in HIV-infected patients. Chest 1998;113:542–547.

52. Race EM, Adelson-Mitty J, Kriegel G, Barlam TF, Reimann KA, Letvin NL, Japour AJ. Focal mycobacterial lymphadenitis following initiation of protease-inhibitor therapy in patients with advanced HIV-1 disease. Lancet 1998;351:252–255.

53. Chloremis CB, Padiatellis C, Zoumboulakis D, Yannakos D. Transitory exacerbation of fever and roentgenographic findings during treatment of tuberculosis in children. Am Rev Tuberc 1955;72:527–536.

54. Currier JS, Williams PL, Koletar S, Murphy RL, Cohn S, Heald A, Knirsch C, Taylor J, Coloqhoun D, Nevin T, Hafner R, McCutchan JA. A Randomized, Placebo-Controlled Trial of Azithromycin Prophylaxis for the Prevention of MAC in Subjects with Increases in CD4 Cells on Antiretroviral Therapy. Abstract LB-23 at the 39th Interscience Conference on Antimicrobial Agents and Chemotherapy. San Francisco 1999.

55. Moulignier A, Eliasewicz M, Mikol J, Polivka M, Thiebaut JB, Dupont B. Spinal cord compression due to concomitant primary lymphoma and *Mycobacterium avium-intracellulare* infection of the paravertebral muscles in an AIDS patient. Eur J Clin Microbiol Infect Dis 1996;15:891–893.

56. Sato Y, Tamura K, Seita M. Multiple osteomyelitis due to Mycobacterium avium with no pulmonary presentation in a patient of sarcoidosis. Intern Med 1992;31:489–492.

57. Weiner BK, Love TW, Fraser RD. *Mycobacterium avium intracellulare*: vertebral osteomyelitis. J Spinal Disord 1998;11:89–91.

58. Uldry PA, Bogousslavsky J, Regli F, Chave JP, Beer V. Chronic *Mycobacterium avium* complex infection of the central nervous system in a nonimmunosuppressed woman. Eur Neurol 1992:32:285–288.

59. Kawaguchi H, Torii Y, Senda Y, Totani Y, Suzuki M, Ooshika H, Wakayama H, Ito Y, Noguchi M. A case of generalized disseminated atypical mycobacteriosis caused by *M. avium* complex with a giant gravitation abscess. Kekkaku 1994:69:77–82.

60. Brodkin H. Paraspinous abscess with *Mycobacterium avium-intracellulare* in a patient without AIDS. South Med J 1991;84:1385–1386.

61. Sarria JC, Chutkan NB, Figueroa JE, Hull A. Atypical mycobacterial vertebral osteomyelitis: case report and review. Clin Infect Dis 1998;26:503–505.

62. Inderlied CB, Kemper CA, Bermudez LEM. The *Mycobacterium avium* complex. Clin Micro Rev 1993;6:266–310.

63. Kemper CA, Havlir DV, Bartok AE, Kane C, Camp B, Lane N, Deresinski SC. Transient bacteremia due to *Mycobacterium avium* complex in patients with AIDS. J Infect Dis 1994;170:488–493.

64. Hafner R, Inderlied CB, Peterson DM, Wright DJ, Standiford HC, Drusano G, Muth K. Correlation of quantitative bone marrow and blood cultures in AIDS patients with disseminated Mycobacterium avium complex infection. J Infect Dis 1999;180:438–447.

65. Connors M, Kovacs JA, Krevat S, Gea-Banacloche JC, Sneller MC, Flanigan M, Metcalf JA, Walker RE, Falloon J, Baseler M, Feuerstein I, Masur H, Lane HC. HIV infection induces changes in CD4+ T-cell phenotype and depletions within the CD4+ T-cell repertoire that are not immediately restored by antiviral or immune-based therapies. Nat Med 1997;3:533–540.

66. Aberg JA, Yajko, DM, Jacobson MA. Eradication of disseminated *Mycobacterium avium* complex (DMAC) in four patients after twelve months anti-mycobacterial therapy and response to highly active antiretroviral therapy (HAART). J Infect Dis 1998;178:1446–1449.

67. Jacobson MA, Zegans M, Pavan PR, O'Donnell JJ, Sattler F, Rao N, Owens S, Pollard R. Cytomegalovirus retinitis after initiation of highly active antiretroviral therapy. Lancet 1997;349:1443–1445.

68. Gilquin J, Piketty C, Thomas V, Gonzales-Canali G, Belec L, Kazatchkine MD. Acute cytomegalovirus infection in AIDS patients with CD4 counts above 100 x 10(6) cells/l following combination antiretroviral therapy including protease inhibitors AIDS 1997;11:1659–1660.

69. Jacobson MA, Stanley H, Holtzer C, Margolis T, Cunningham E. Natural History and Outcome of New AIDS-Related CMV Retinitis Cases Diagnosed in the Era of Highly Active Antiretroviral Therapy. Abstract 1159 at the 39th Interscience Conference on Antimicrobial Agents and Chemotherapy. San Francisco 1999.

70. Spector SA, McKinley GF, Lalezari J, Samo T, Andruczk R, Follansbee S, Sparti PD, Havlir DV, Simpson G, Buhles W, Wong R, Stempien M. Oral ganciclovir for the prevention of cytomeglovirus disease in persons with AIDS. N Engl J Med 1996;334:1491–1497.

71. Spector SA, Wong R, Hsia K, Pilcher M, Stempien MJ. Plasma cytomegalovirus (CMV) DNA load predicts CMV disease and survival in AIDS patients. J Clin Invest 1998;101:497–502.

72. Hansen KK, Ricksten A, Hofmann B, Norrild B, Olofsson S, Mathiesen L. Detection of cytomegalovirus DNA in serum correlates with clinical cytomegalovirus retinitis in AIDS. J Infect Dis 1994;170:1271–1274.

73. Spector SA, Hsia K, Crager M, Pilcher M, Cabral S, Stempien MJ. Cytomegalovirus (CMV) DNA load is an independent predictor of CMV disease and survival in advanced AIDS. J Virol 1999;73:7027–7030.

74. Rasmussen L, Morris S, Zipeto D, Fessel J, Wolitz R, Dowling A, Merigan TC. Quantitation of human cytomegalovirus DNA from peripheral blood cells of human immunodeficiency virus-infected patients could predict cytomegalovirus retinitis. J Infect Dis 1995;171:177–182.

75. Bowen EF, Sabin CA, Wilson P, Griffiths PD, Davey CC, Johnson MA, Emery VC. Cytomegalovirus (CMV) viraemia detected by polymerase chain reaction identifies a group of HIV-positive patients at high risk of CMV disease. AIDS 1997;11:889–893.

76. Torriani FJ, MacDonald JC, Karevellas M, Freeman WR. Lack of Progression after Discontinuation of Maintenance Therapy for Cytomeglovirus Retinitis in AIDS Patients Responding to Highly Active Antiretroviral Therapy. Abstract I-33 presented at the 37th Interscience Conference of Antimicrobial Agents and Chemotherapy, Ontario 1997.

77. Torriani FJ, Havlir DV, Freeman WR, Durand D, Schrier R. Proliferative responses Against CMV in AIDS Patients on HAART and with Healed CMV Retinitis Who Stopped Maintenance Therapy. Abstract 747 presented at 5th Conference on Retroviruses and Opportunistic Infections, Chicago 1998.

78. Freeman WR, MacDonald JC, Torriani FJ, Karavellas M. Opthalmologic Manifestations of Immune Recovery in AIDS Patients on HAART Therapy. Abstract 757 presented at 5th Conference on Retroviruses and Opportunistic Infections, Chicago 1998.

79. Macdonald JC, Torriani FJ, Morse LS, Karavellas MP, Reed JB, Freeman WR. Lack of reactivation of cytomegalovirus (CMV) retinitis after stopping CMV maintenance therapy in AIDS patients with sustained elevations in CD4 T cells in response to highly active antiretroviral therapy. J Infect Dis 1998;177:1182–1187.

80. Tural C, Romeu J, Sirera G, Andreu D, Conejero M, Ruiz S, Jou A, Bonjoch A, Ruiz L, Arno A, Clotet B. Long-lasting remission of cytomegalovirus retinitis without maintenance therapy in human immunodeficiency virus-infected patients. J Infect Dis 1998;177:1080–1083.

81. Li TS, Tubiani R, Fillet AM, Autran B, Katlama C. Negative result of cytomegolvirus blood culture with restoration of CD4$^+$ T-cell reactivity to cytomegalovirus after HAART in an HIV-infected patient. J Acquir Immune Def Syndr Hum Retroviral 1999;20:514–516.

82. Karavellas MP, Plummer DJ, Macdonald JC, Torriani FJ, Shufelt CL, Azen SP, Freeman WR. Incidence of immune recovery vitritis in cytomegalovirus retinitis patients following institution of successful highly active antiretroviral therapy. J Infect Dis 1999;179:697–700.

83. Luft BJ, Remington JS. Toxoplasmic encephalitis in AIDS. Clin Infect Dis 1992; 15:211–222.

7

Salvage Therapy for Patients Failing their Current Antiretroviral Regimen

Mary A. Albrecht

Harvard Medical School and Beth Israel Deaconess Medical Center, Boston, Massachusetts

I. BACKGROUND

Selected combination treatment regimens for human immunodeficiency virus (HIV) infection have rapidly evolved over the past few years in response to recent sentinel advances in the field of HIV therapeutics. Further insights into mechanisms of disease pathogenesis and viral dynamics (1–6), the expanding number of currently available U.S. Food and Drug Administration-approved agents with enhanced potency derived from distinct antiretroviral classes, and the advent of increasingly more refined viral load monitoring assays (7–12) have afforded substantial progress in the treatment of HIV infection.

The current rationale for initiation of potent antiretroviral therapy in early HIV infection has been largely based on the following characteristics of HIV replication: high viral turnover rate with up to 10 billion virions generated and cleared daily (1–3), the potential for frequent base pair substitutions occurring in the viral genome due to inherently error-prone viral RNA replication (4), and the existence of second and third phases of viral decay (13, 14) and a reservoir of resting latently HIV-infected memory CD4 lymphocytes that may serve as an ongoing source of replication-competent HIV (13).

Plasma viral load has been linked to HIV disease progression in the Multicenter AIDS Cohort Study that demonstrated the level of viremia served as the most significant predictor of death and progression to acquired immunodeficiency syndrome (AIDS) over a 10-year observation period; a threefold rise in baseline viral load conferred a 1.57 increased relative hazard of death (15).

With the widespread availability of viral load assays (limit of quantitation (LOQ) < 50 copies/mL) with lower threshold detection limits, treatment response has more recently been evaluated by viral load endpoints rather than by clinical events. These developments have essentially redefined the approach to HIV therapy with the recent use of increasingly more potent combination regimens that are initiated at earlier stages of HIV infection with the aim of achieving maximal viral suppression to below the limit of detection and conferring a durable treatment response.

The current guidelines for HIV therapy recommend dual nucleoside analogues (nucleoside reverse transcriptase inhibitors [NRTIs]) in combination with a protease inhibitor (PI) agent (16, 17) as the initial treatment regimen. In clinical trials, triple combination PI-containing regimens have resulted in sustained viral suppression (plasma HIV RNA < 500 copies/mL) in 60–90% of protease inhibitor-naive patients (18, 19). Durable suppression of viral load < 20 copies/mL through 52 weeks has also been demonstrated in treatment-naive patients who received potent triple combination therapy featuring a nonnucleoside reverse transcriptase inhibitor (NNRTI), nevirapine, plus dual nucleoside analogue therapy containing zidovudine (ZDV) and didanosine (ddI) (20). The widespread use of PI-based combination regimens has also had a favorable impact on HIV disease progression as shown by a dramatic decline in AIDS-related morbidity and mortality of up to 60–85% compared with the pre-PI era (21–24).

In the Merck 035 trial, suppression of plasma HIV RNA < 500 copies/mL in ZDV-experienced patients with CD4 counts between 50 and 400/mm^3 was achieved in >80% of patients in the triple indinavir (IDV)-containing arm (ZDV/lamivudine [3TC]/IDV) for up to 1 year (18). The synchronous use of a triple-drug PI-containing regimen has furthermore been shown to provide superior suppression of viral load compared with sequential introduction of NRTI and PI agents: 78% of patients in the simultaneous initiation of ZDV/3TC/IDV arm achieved HIV RNA < 500 copies/mL at 100 weeks compared with only 30–45% of patients in the ZDV/3TC and IDV arms (25). Although triple-based PI regimens have demonstrated impressive success in attaining durable viral load suppression in treatment-naive patients in clinical trials conducted to date, 10–20% of patients experience virologic failure with the initial PI-based regimen (26). The reasons for such treatment failure are complex. Patients with advanced HIV disease stage such as those enrolled in the AIDS Clinical Trials Group (ACTG 320) and Merck 039 trials (19, 27) with high baseline viral load and depressed CD4 counts (<50 cells/mm^3) have demonstrated typically lower response rates (45–85%) after the introduction of triple-drug PI-containing combination therapy. Impaired drug adherence (28), pharmacokinetic interactions in complex combination regimens resulting in subtherapeutic plasma drug levels (29–31), lack of potency in selected regimens due to potential drug antagonism (32), prior extensive antiretroviral treatment or a history of sequential monotherapy, and the emergence of drug resistance (33–44) have been implicated as factors contributing to treatment failure. Patients in clinical practice often demonstrate lower response rates to PI combination regimens than those observed in subjects participating in clinical trials; complex regimens with high pill burden, inconvenient and/or frequent dosing schedules, and dietary and fluid restrictions have been more difficult to adapt to a practice setting compared with an intensively monitored clinical trial, which may partially explain the higher rates of observed treatment failure.

Disturbing trends of higher rates of virologic failure approaching 35–44% have recently been reported (26, 45) in both unselected and prospective patient cohorts being treated with highly active antiretroviral therapy (HAART). The high rates of treatment failure observed in clinical trials underscore the urgent need to develop more effective salvage therapy regimens.

The nadir in plasma HIV RNA achieved after initiation of a PI-based regimen was shown by Kempf et al. (46) to be highly predictive of the durability of virologic response, whereas baseline RNA and magnitude of RNA decline from baseline were not highly associated. Suppression of plasma viral load below 50 copies/mL correlates with greater reductions in HIV RNA levels in lymphoid tissue and is associated with restricted evolution of resistance mutations in this compartment (47). The selection of the initial combination regimen in any given patient is therefore critical to ensure treatment success with the primary goal of attaining maximal and durable suppression of viral load.

Failure of initial combination therapy will adversely influence the virologic response observed with the second-line treatment regimen. Selecting compact initial combination regimens that feature potent activity, convenient dosing schedules, minimal drug interactions, and decreased potential of long-term toxicities will enhance patient adherence and minimize the potential for viral rebound and progressive acquisition of resistance mutations. The approach to alternative therapy for patients who experience viral rebound on potent combination therapy is a focus of intense investigation due to the increased rates of treatment failure being reported in extensively treated patients with fewer alternative options currently available.

II. DEFINING VIROLOGIC FAILURE

The definition of virologic failure is likely to include more stringent HIV RNA level criteria as the newer viral load assays being developed feature lower threshold cutoff values. Durability of viral suppression at 18–24 months in several pivotal trials, such as the INCAS trial (48), was shown to be significantly greater in patients who maintained HIV RNA levels below 20 copies/mL compared with patients whose plasma viral loads were in the range of 20–500 copies/mL.

In a study conducted by Natarajan et al. (49), HIV RNA was detected both in peripheral blood mononuclear cells and lymphoid tissue samples derived from individuals being treated with highly potent combination regimens (19 months duration) who maintained suppression of plasma viral load to below 50 copies/mL for at least 6 months. PI-treated patients who maintained plasma HIV RNA < 20 copies/mL for a mean of 25 months demonstrated superior suppression of HIV replication in lymphoid tissue as shown by *in situ* hybridization and cocultivation assays compared with patients with undetectable plasma viral loads treated with nucleoside analogues alone (50). Related studies (51, 52) indicate that current triple combination regimens may be only partially suppressive of HIV replication in peripheral blood mononuclear cells and in the lymphoreticular compartment. Because the primary goal of HIV treatment remains complete and durable suppression of viral load with restoration of the normal immune response, any confirmed viral rebound above the level of detection (i.e., >50 copies/mL) will be increasingly interpreted as treatment failure.

The criteria defining virologic failure featured in recent treatment guidelines submitted in the report of the NIH Panel to define principles of therapy (17) were as follows:

Less than 0.5–0.75 log reduction in plasma HIV RNA by 4–8 weeks after initiation of therapy,

Failure to achieve plasma HIV RNA levels below the limit of detection within 4–6 months after starting treatment,

Viral rebound: repeated detection of virus in plasma after having demonstrated suppression to undetectable levels, suggesting the development of resistance,

Any confirmed increase, defined as threefold or greater, in viral load from the nadir of plasma HIV RNA not attributable to intercurrent infection, vaccination, or test methodology,

Persistently declining CD4 cell counts measured on at least two separate occasions,

Clinical deterioration while on antiretroviral therapy (ART), such as the development of AIDS-related opportunistic infections or wasting, which may signal treatment failure. In patients with advanced HIV infection at the time of initiation of ART, however, selected opportunistic infections may develop despite having achieved adequate viral suppression due to the still depressed CD4 cell count. In this subset of patients, the development of opportunistic infections may not necessarily indicate virologic failure on the given ART regimen but may reflect the persistently immunosuppressed status of the patient who has not sustained a robust CD4 cell count increase.

Once virologic failure has been confirmed, it is essential to identify the factors that might be implicated in treatment failure such as impaired absorption with inadequate drug levels; unfavorable drug–drug interactions, inadequate potency of the initial regimen (i.e., dual NRTI therapy), poor drug adherence, and emergence of resistance.

Assessment of adherence has, to date, been difficult to accurately determine but remains a critical focus of further investigation in clinical trials. Serum PI trough concentrations were recently compared with self-reported adherence questionnaires in predicting virologic outcome in a prospective study that enrolled 149 patients; serum evidence of adherence was observed in 122 patients (82%), of whom 83% achieved suppression of viral load (2 $\log_{10}$ RNA decline in naive patients; 1 $\log_{10}$ RNA decline in experienced patients). Serum evidence of adherence was significantly associated with viral response ($p = 0.000005$) and with self-reported adherence ($p = 0.0005$); serum PI concentration (90% sensitivity and 43% specificity) was a better tool than the self-reported adherence (29).

III. WHEN TO SWITCH THERAPY

Once virologic failure has been confirmed, a switch to alternative therapy should be considered. Reasons for treatment failure need to be identified before any change in therapy: marginal adherence to ART, limited absorption with inadequate plasma drug concentrations, inadequate potency of the initial regimen, or development of drug resistance should be assessed. If adherence to the current regimen has been uniformly good, the timing of the switch is then contingent upon the number of readily available treatment options remaining for a given patient.

For patients who experience virologic failure with their initial combination regimen, a switch to alternative therapy should optimally be undertaken early at a lower plasma viral load to minimize the risk of acquiring additional resistance mutations. Lower HIV RNA levels at the time of the switch and the addition of new NRTIs at the time of the switch have both been predictive of a more durable response to the alternative (i.e., salvage) regimen (53, 54). In extensively treated patients, failure on a given PI-containing regimen may preclude an immediate switch due to the development of cross-resistance to other PI agents.

Patients experiencing viral rebound on their second or third PI-containing regimen may still derive clinical benefit while continuing the same therapy with preserved CD4 cell count increases persisting up to 48 weeks (53, 55). In selected patients with extensive prior ART whose clinical status remains stable and whose CD4 cell increase is sustained despite virologic failure, a more conservative approach to subsequent therapy options may be appropriate, such as continuation of the same regimen (53, 56). The decision to switch therapy needs to be individualized and must take into account the potential reasons for treatment failure, ability of the patient to remain adherent on revised therapy, tolerability of the new regimen, and the availability of treatment options that feature either new drugs and/or classes of drugs that do not exhibit cross-resistance to previously used agents on the failing regimen.

IV. DEVISING SALVAGE THERAPY

There are currently 16 agents derived from three different antiretroviral drug classes that are either approved or in expanded clinical development for treatment of HIV infection (Table 1). An expanding array of initial and salvage combination regimens are being used in standard practice or undergoing evaluation in clinical trials.

Combination drug regimens often need to be revised in patients who develop adverse toxicity, intolerance, or who exhibit poor adherence (16). In patients whose plasma HIV RNA remains suppressed on serial viral load monitoring, substitution of a single new agent in the regimen is frequently done to manage selected toxicities or to avoid unfavorable drug–drug interactions. When revising therapy in patients with documented drug failure, however, current practice guidelines recommend that at least two new drugs and, optimally, that all drugs in a failing regimen are changed (16, 17). Thus

Table 1 Antiretroviral Agents

Approved antiretroviral agents	Expanded clinical development
Nucleoside analogue reverse transcriptase inhibitors	Nucleotide analogue reverse transcriptase inhibitors
Zidovudine (ZDV)	Adefovir dipivoxil
Zalcitabine (ddC)	
Didanosine (ddI)	
Stavudine (d4T)	
Lamivudine (3TC)	
Abacavir	
Nonnucleoside reverse transcriptase inhibitors	
Delavirdine	
Nevirapine	
Efavirenz	
Protease inhibitors	Protease inhibitors
Saquinavir	ABT-378
Ritonavir	
Indinavir	
Nelfinavir	
Amprenavir	

far, most salvage therapy regimens have largely been targeted to address confirmed virologic failure in patients receiving an initial PI-containing regimen.

With the advent and increasingly widespread use of potent PI-sparing treatment strategies as the initial combination regimen in treatment-naive individuals, more diverse salvage therapy strategies that feature the optimal sequencing of different classes of agents and that exploit pharmacokinetic interactions with novel drug combinations that allow for alternative more compact regimens with once daily dosing schedules will be required. The current practice guidelines outlining initiation of antiretiroviral therapy (16, 17) in which a PI plus two NRTIs is the standard regimen in treatment-naive individuals may soon be revised based on recent results from several pivotal clinical trials featuring triple-drug PI-sparing combination therapy.

The extended follow-up from two such trials is as follows. The DMP 266-006 trial (57), an open-label study comparing the antiviral activity and tolerability of efavirenz (EFV)/ZDV/3TC versus EFV/IDV versus IDV/ZDV/3TC, featured an initial cohort of 450 HIV-infected patients (85% treatment naive) with baseline HIV RNA and CD4 counts of 4.78 $\log_{10}$ copies/mL and 341 cells/mm^3, respectively. Week 48 results were recently reported by Staszewski et al. (58). The EFV/ZDV/3TC arm ($n = 147$) demonstrated superior viral load suppression at 72 weeks compared with the IDV/ZDV/3TC ($n = 146$) arm (60% < 50 copies/mL vs. 40% < 50 copies/mL, respectively). In an extended cohort of 1266 patients randomized to these three arms, time to treatment failure (confirmed viral rebound > 400 copies/mL) was significantly longer in the EFV/ZDV/3TC arm ($p = 0.0001$) compared with the control IDV/ZDV/3TC arm.

The phase III, randomized, placebo-controlled, comparative trial (CNA 3005) evaluated the efficacy and tolerability of an abacavir (ABC)-based triple nucleoside regimen (ABC/ZDV/3TC) versus a standard triple PI/dual NRTI (IDV/ZDV/3TC) regimen in 562 treatment-naive HIV-infected patients with baseline median HIV RNA and median CD4 counts of 4.85 $\log_{10}$ and 359 cells/mm^3, respectively. Week 48 results were recently reported (58). Patients were stratified by entry viral load (HIV RNA > 10,000–100,000 vs. HIV RNA > 100,000). At week 48, both arms demonstrated equivalent viral load response: in the intent to treat (ITT) analysis, 51% patients in each arm achieved HIV RNA < 400 copies/mL. No significant differences were noted in treatment response at week 48 between the ABC and IDV arms in the stratified lower viral load group, but in the HIV RNA > 100,000 stratified group, 45% of patients in the IDV arm compared with only 31% of patients in the ABC arm achieved HIV RNA < 50 copies/mL. In time to rebound (HIV RNA > 400 copies/mL) ITT analyses, however, no significant differences were noted between treatment arms in the stratified viral load groups.

Guidelines have previously been developed for devising alternative therapy in the setting of virologic failure with a PI-containing regimen (16, 17) based in part on available clinical trial data. More general recommendations for devising salvage therapy for patients with confirmed viral rebound on a current ART regimen are outlined in Table 2. These guidelines (16, 17) emphasize that stringent adherence to several important principles will facilitate the approach to selecting effective alternative treatment in patients with suspected drug failure.

The key principles that pertain to devising salvage therapy are as follows:

Avoid adding a single drug to a failing regimen, which essentially constitutes sequential montherapy; at least two new drugs should be used, and if feasible, the entire regimen should be replaced with at least three new drugs.

In patients who have achieved partial viral suppression on their current regimen and who have limited treatment options to confer adequate potency, the continuation of the prior regimen may still provide clinical benefit and remains a reasonable approach.

Table 2 Devising Salvage Therapy

Current combination regimen	Alternative salvage regimens
2 NRTIs +	2 *new* NRTIs +
NFV[a]	IND or RTV or APV; dual PI RTV/SQV; RTV/IDV; NNRTI + *new* PI: IDV, RTV, APV
RTV[a]	NFV or APV; dual PI: APV/IDV, RTV/IDV or RTV/SQV; NNRTI + *new* PI: NFV or APV
IDV[a]	NFV or APV, dual PIs: APV/NFV, RTV/SQV/RTV/IDV; NNRTI + *new* PI: NFV or APV
SQV[a]	NFV, IDV, APV; dual PI APV/NFV, APV/IDV, RTV/IDV, RTV/SQV; NNRTI + *new* PI: NFV, APV, IDV
APV[a]	NFV, IDV, SQV; dual PI: SQV/RTV, RTV/IDV, SQV/RTV; NNRTI + *new* PI: IDV, NFV, SQV
2 NRTIs + NNRTI	2 *new* NRTIs + PI; *or* 1 *new* NRTI + dual PI
2 NRTIs	2 *new* NRTIs + PI *or* 1–2 *new* NRTIs + NNRTI + PI

[a]Protease inhibitor (PI) agents: NFV, nelfinavir; RTV, ritonavir; IDV, indinavir; SQV, saquinavir; APV, amprenavir. NRTIs, nucleoside analog reverse transcriptase inhibitors; NNRTIs, nonnucleoside reverse transcriptase inhibitors.

Source: Guidelines for the use of antiretrovirol agents in HIV-infected adults and adolescents. MMWR 1998; 47(RR5):43–82

Dual PI regimens and regimens that feature combinations of PIs with selected NNRTI agents, nevirapine or delavirdine, have thus far not been extensively evaluated; these regimens may serve as salvage therapy in patients with limited options due to drug intolerance and/or potential drug resistance.

Avoid using new drugs in the revised regimen that exhibit cross-resistance to drugs that the patient has previously been exposed to in prior regimens: avoid switching from ritonavir to indinavir or vice versa in setting of drug failure and avoid switching from nevirapine to delavirdine or vice versa because high-level cross-resistance is likely.

When devising new combination therapy, avoid resuming an agent, such as ZDV, which was featured in a prior drug regimen that ultimately failed.

Drug resistance strains can be replaced with wild-type drug-sensitive strains after stopping the given drug; upon resuming the previously used agent, however, drug resistance can rapidly reemerge upon repeat exposure. (Adapted from MMWR 1998;47:(RR-5):43–82.)

V. SALVAGE THERAPY IN PATIENTS FAILING PI-CONTAINING REGIMENS: CLINICAL TRIAL RESULTS

A. PI-Containing Salvage Regimens

1. IDV/NRTIs after Saquinavir (SQV) Failure

The *ACTG 333* study was a 24-week, open-label, randomized clinical trial (59) that evaluated viral load response after switching PI therapy in 72 patients with baseline median viral load and median CD4 count of 4.3 $\log_{10}$ copies/mL and 222 cells/mm^3 respectively, who had at least 48 weeks exposure (median duration SQV hard gel capsule [hgc] was 112 weeks) to SQV hgc in combination with other ART agents (Table 3). Patients were randomized to SQV soft gel capsule (sgc), IDV, or continuation of SQV hgc; background ART remained stable. At week 8, the SQV sgc arm and the IDV arm had sustained -0.23 $\log_{10}$ ($p = 0.016$) and -0.58 $\log_{10}$ ($p < 0.001$) declines, respectively, in HIV RNA levels, whereas the SQV hgc arm did not sustain any decrease in viral load. This study indicated that prior PI therapy with confirmed virologic failure may blunt or attenuate viral load response after switching to a second PI agent.

2. Nelfinavir (NFV)/Adefovir/EFV/ABC after IDV/NRTI Failure

The *ACTG 372b* trial (60) was factorially designed to evaluate the comparative efficacy of ABC versus approved NRTIs and of NFV vs. placebo on and background of newly administered EFV and adefovir (ADF) in NNRTI-naive patients who had confirmed virologic failure (HIV RNA $\geq$ 500 copies/mL) while receiving IDV/ZDV or d4T/3TC (Table 3). Ninety-four patients with baseline HIV RNA of 39,102 copies/mL and CD4 196 cells/mm^3 were randomized to one of four arms: ABC/EFV/ADF/NFV, ABC/EFV/ADF/NFV placebo, NRTIs/EFV/ADF/NFV, or NRTIs/EFV/ADF/NFV placebo. Arms were stratified by screening HIV RNA levels: $\leq$15,000 versus >15,000 copies/mL. The primary study endpoint was defined as HIV RNA $\geq$ 500 copies/mL at week 16. Efficacy analyses (ITT) included primary factorial comparisons of ABC versus NRTIs and of NFV versus NFV placebo. By HIV RNA stratum, 13 (43%) and 50 (81%) patients with screening HIV RNA levels of $\leq 15,000$ and $>15,000$ copies/mL, respectively, had HIV RNA > 500 copies/mL at week 16 ($p < 0.001$). By factorial comparison, at week 16, 19 (45%) and 10 (24%) patients in the NFV-containing and NFV-placebo arms, respectively, demonstrated HIV RNA < 500 copies/mL ($p = 0.046$), and 16 (37%) and 13 (32%) patients in the ABC-containing and NRTI-containing arms, respectively, had HIV RNA < 500 copies/mL ($p = 0.623$). Primary endpoint (HIV RNA ≥ 500 copies/mL) rate was significantly greater in the higher HIV RNA stratum. NFV provided superior viral suppression compared with NFV placebo, whereas abacavir was no different from other NRTIs (in combination with EFV and ADF) in this heavily NRTI-experienced patient population. NFV, in combination with EFV, ADF, and nucleoside analogues, was shown to achieve early success (43% success rate) in patients with early breakthrough on IDV.

3.   Amprenavir (APV)/ABC/EFV after PI Failure

CNA 2007 was an open-label, phase II, single-arm trial (61) evaluating combination salvage therapy with APV/ABC/EFV in 101 patients in whom virologic failure (screening HIV RNA ≥ 500 copies/mL) had developed on a stable (at least 20 weeks) PI-based regimen (Table 3). Prior NRTI (except ABC), NNRTI, and PI exposure were allowed. Of 101 patients who enrolled, 90 completed 16 weeks of study therapy. Patients were highly treatment experienced: 87% of these 90 patients had >2 years prior ART. At baseline, 71% of isolates had more than five reverse transcriptase (RT)-associated (NRTI and NNRTI) mutations. Most isolates had at least five PI-associated mutations at baseline; the most frequent mutations observed in protease gene were L63P (86%), L10/V/F/R (72%), L90M (72%), A71V/T (64%), and M46I/L (57%). Phenotypic resistance assays for nucleoside analogues at baseline showed that 19–90% of isolates were NRTI resistant. Also, 45% of isolates were APV resistant and 72–84% of isolates were resistant to SQV, IDV, NFV, and ritonavir (RTV). In regard to NNRTIs, 10 of 20 (50%) and 21 of 53 (40%) EFV- and nevirapine (NVP)-experienced patients, respectively, had reduced susceptibility to EFV and NVP.

At week 16, 34% of 65 patients achieved either a 1 $\log_{10}$ decline in plasma HIV RNA levels or HIV RNA < 400 copies/mL. The highest proportion of patients with HIV RNA < 400 copies/mL at week 16 was observed in NNRTI-naive patients whose baseline viral load was <4.6 $\log_{10}$ copies/mL. Patients with at least three ZDV-associated mutations plus M184V RT genotypic mutations had an inferior viral load response. Baseline plasma viral load ($p = 0.005$) and phenotypic resistance to EFV ($p = 0.006$) or to ABC ($p = 0.006$) were strongly predictive of virologic response. Five (56%) of 9 subjects with baseline isolates susceptible to all three drugs (ABC/EFV/APV)

Table 3 Clinical Trial Results for PI-Based Salvage Regimens

Study	Prior therapy	Regimen/ arm	No. Patients	Baseline HIV RNA (log 10 copies/mL)	Baseline CD4 (/μL)
Single PI					
ACTG 333	SQV hgc	SQVsgc+RTIs IDV+RTIs SQVhgc+RTIs	72	4.3	222
ACTG 372b	IDV+ZDV (or d4T)/3TC	EFV/ADF+: ABC ABC/NFV NRTIs/NFV NRTIs	94	4.6	196
CNA2007	PI, NNRTI experienced; ABC naive	APV/ABC/EFV	101		
Dual PI					
RTV/SQV (Tebas)	NFV+RTIs	RTV/SQV+RTIs	26	4.7	222
RTV/SQV (Zolopa)	NFV+RTIs	RTV/SQV+NRTIs and/or NNRTIs	97	4.5	259
RTV/SQV (Deeks)	IDV or RTV+RTIs	RTV/SQV+2 RTIs	18	4.4	172
NFV/SQV+EFV (Duval)	PI/RTIs	NFV/SQV/EFV+RTIs	10	5.1	122
ACTG 359	IDV+RTIs	SQVsgc/RTV or SQVsgc/NFV+: ADF DLV ADF+DLV	277	4.5	229
RTV/IDV	PI	RTV/IDV+RTIs	28	5.5	196
ABT-378					
M97-765	PI; NNRTI naive	ABT-378+NVP+ NRTIs	70	4.0	349

Table 3   (*Continued*)

Follow-Up (wk)	HIV RNA change (copies/mL)	CD4+ change	Comments
24; week 8 results	0.23 $\log_{10}$ $-0.0.58$ $\log_{10}$ No change	37 22	Long-term SQVhgc exposure attenuates response to 2nd PI
16	45% and 24% < 500 copies/mL for NFV vs. NFV placebo ($p = 0.046$); 37% and 32% < 500 copies/mL for ABC vs. RTIs ($p = 0.62$)	60 14 36 36	CNS symptoms, ≥ grade 2 proteinuria, and rash seen: 18%, 17%, and 6%
16	34% of 65 patients achieved 1 $\log_{10}$ decline of <400 copies/mL		Baseline RNA ($p = 0.005$); phenotypic resistance to EFV ($p = 0.006$) ABC ($p = 0.006$) predictive of viral load response
24	71% < 500 copies/mL at week 24; 59% < 50 copies/mL at week 24	141	Higher baseline HIV RNA predictive of failure at week 24 ($p = 0.05$)
24	52% ≤ 500 copies/mL at weeks 20 and 24 (ITT)	>200	
24	-1.4 median $\log_{10}$ copies/mL decline at week 4		L90M mutation in 9/13 patients with viral rebound
32 (median)	80% < 500 copies/mL	165	CNS symptoms/diarrhea observed
20	30% across arms HIV RNA < 500 copies/mL at week 16; no difference between NFV and RTV arms ($p = 0.51$); DLV vs. ADF arms had superior VL suppression ($p = 0.003$)	19	No difference between NFV and RTV as 2nd PI with SQVsgc; ADF/DLV no better than DLV alone
12–24	30% < 50 copies/mL		L90M associated with treatment failure
36	78% < 400 copies/mL	104	Diarrhea in 20%

achieved suppression of HIV RNA < 400 copies/mL at week 16, whereas only 4 (19%) of 21 subjects with baseline isolates susceptible to one or none of the drugs attained viral load suppression.

These findings suggested that baseline genotypic and phenotypic assay results might be useful in predicting virologic failure to an alternative regimen. In patients who had a lower baseline viral load and who were NNRTI-naive, superior suppression of viral load occurred.

B.   Dual PI Salvage Therapy

1.   RTV/SQV-based Salvage Regimens

RTV/SQV for NFV Failure.   Tebas et al. (54) evaluated the efficacy of a second PI regimen featuring RTV/SQV in 26 patients who had failed (two consecutive HIV RNA levels > 5000 copies/mL) their initial PI regimen while receiving NFV therapy (Table 3). The mean HIV RNA and median CD4 count were 46,674 copies/mL and 222 cells/mm^3, respectively; median duration of NFV exposure was 48 weeks. Patients were switched to RTV 400 mg /SQV 400 mg plus d4T/3TC twice daily; two patients discontinued the study at 3 weeks. Seventeen of 24 (71%) of the assessable study patients achieved HIV RNA levels < 500 copies/mL that were sustained at week 24. Ten patients (59%) also demonstrated HIV RNA < 50 copies/mL at week 24. Before the switch, the most frequent baseline genotypic mutations observed in these patients were D30N, N88D, and M36I. The L90M mutation was identified in only 5 of 18 patients. Patients with higher plasma viral load (HIV RNA > 30,000 copies/mL) before the switch experienced more virologic failures (HIV RNA > 500 copies/mL) at week 24 than patients with baseline HIV RNA < 30,000 copies/mL ($p = 0.05$). In this study, the presence of L90M was not associated with an increased likelihood of failure after initiating RTV/SQV dual PI therapy ($p = 0.39$); the presence of D30N, N88D, and M36I mutations were also not predictive of short-term virologic response. These study results suggest that dual RTV/SQV-based alternative therapy confers at least short-term suppression of viral load in patients with virologic failure on an NFV-containing regimen.

Zolopa et al. (62) recently reported the week 24 results of a multicenter, retrospective, cohort study that enrolled 97 patients who had failed NFV-based therapy and then switched to RTV/SQV combination therapy plus NRTIs and/or NNRTIs (Table 3). Inclusion criteria stipulated that NFV was the initial PI agent and that patients sustained a virologic rebound (HIV RNA > 0.6 log$_{10}$ copies/mL) after having a confirmed 1 log$_{10}$ decline in plasma HIV RNA. Nine of 97 patients were excluded from study entry. NRTIs and NNRTIs were not restricted; the NNRTI–naive cohort was analyzed separately.

The median baseline HIV RNA and CD4 count for patients were 33,000 copies/mL and 259 cells/mm^3, respectively. Background features pertaining to group I (71 NNRTI-experienced patients) and group II (17 NNRTI-naive patients) included average number of prior NRTIs (two and three), proportion of patients that had received more than three NRTIs (50% and 59%), prior NNRTI use (16% and 0), and duration of NFV exposure (11 and 8 months). Before the switch, 50% of isolates had the NFV-associated D30N resistance mutation; six patients had L90M. By ITT analysis, 52% of group I patients had HIV RNA < 500 copies/mL at week 20 and sustained a median CD4 cell increase > 200 cells/mm^3 with CD4 count of 353 cells/mm^3 observed at week 24 ($p < 0.01$). Baseline predictors for virologic response at 24 weeks included CD4 count at the time of the switch ($p = 0.006$), baseline viral load ($p = 0.002$), and new NRTI ($p = 0.03$). The presence of the D30N mutation was not significant. Fifty-two percent (ITT) of group II patients achieved HIV RNA < 500 copies/mL at week 24. Ten (67%) of 15 group II patients in whom D30N mutation was present achieved HIV RNA < 500 copies/mL at week 24. The addition of an NNRTI agent in group II patients increased the viral load response to 70–85%. The L90M mutation was identified in six patients; four of these patients responded to RTV/SQV (HIV RNA < 500 copies/mL) at week 24. This study confirmed that dual RTV/SQV-based alternative therapy for NFV failure affords substantial virologic activity through week 24 and suggests that the presence of the NFV-associated D30N genotypic mutation does not have a negative impact on response to subsequent PI-based therapy.

RTV/SQV for IDV or RTV Failure. Deeks et al. (63) evaluated the virologic activity of RTV/SQV dual PI therapy in 18 patients who had failed (plasma HIV RNA > 1500 copies/mL after 16 weeks of continuous therapy) a prior IDV- or RTV-containing regimen (Table 3). Baseline viral load and CD4 count before the switch were 4.41 log$_{10}$ copies/mL (branched DNA) and 172 cells/mm^3, respectively; median duration of RTV or IDV before the switch was 8.3 months. All patients switched to RTV (400 mg) plus SQV (400 mg) twice daily in combination with two NRTIs; 12 of 18 patients revised their nucleoside analogue therapy at the time of the switch. Fourteen of 18 patients completed 24 weeks of therapy; 4 patients discontinued salvage therapy after 12 weeks because of intolerance or lack of viral response. Plasma HIV RNA levels declined a median of 1.4 log$_{10}$ after 4 weeks of RTV/SQV + NRTIs therapy. A >0.5 log$_{10}$ decrease in plasma viral load was observed in only four patients.

The V82A protease mutation associated with IDV resistance was identified in 8 of 10 patients before the switch to SQV/RTV therapy. In patients who experienced viral rebound on RTV/SQV therapy, the L90M mutation was detected in 9 of 13 isolates; additional mutations at amino acids 48, 48, and 54 were also identified. Dual RTV/SQV-based salvage PI therapy for patients with confirmed virologic failure on NFV-containing regimens conferred a modest but short-term reduction in viral load. The L90M mutation may have resulted in cross resistance to both RTV and SQV, thereby attenuating the viral load response after switching to dual RTV/SQV therapy. The emergence of mutations, namely the L90M mutation, was associated with viral rebound on RTV/SQV monotherapy.

NFV/SQV and Efavirenz (EFZ) for PI Failure. Duval et al. (64) presented the results of a recently conducted study evaluating a salvage-based regimen featuring NFV (750 mg t.i.d.) plus SQV (600 mg t.i.d.) and EFZ (600 mg/day) in combination with NRTIs in 10 HIV-infected patients who had failed prior PI/NRTI(s) therapy (Table 3). One ($n = 3$) or two to three ($n = 7$) new NRTIs were added at the time of the switch. Mean duration of prior PI exposure was 23 months; baseline viral load and CD4 count at the time of the switch were 5.1 $\log_{10}$ copies/mL and 122 cells/mm^3, respectively. All patients were NFV, SQV, and EFZ naive. Mean follow-up was 8.4 months. At last follow-up, 8 of 10 patients had achieved HIV RNA below the limit of detection and had sustained a mean CD4 cell increase of 165 cells/mm^3. Most patients achieved viral suppression below limit of detection. This salvage regimen was well tolerated with only mild and transient neurologic events and diarrhea observed. These results of this small study suggest that NFV/SQV and EFV may confer short-term viral suppression in selected patients failing their initial PI-containing regimen. Longer follow-up will be essential to evaluate the durability of response.

SQV sgc/RTV or SQV sgc/NFV for IDV Failure. ACTG 359 was a randomized clinical trial (65) that evaluated the efficacy and safety of dual PI (SQV sgc/RTV vs. SQV/NFV) therapy in combination with adefovir and/or delavirdine in patients who had confirmed virologic failure (HIV RNA 2000–200,000 copies/mL) while on an IDV-containing regimen for at least 6 months (Table 3). Two hundred seventy-seven HIV-infected patients with median duration of 14 months IDV exposure whose baseline HIV RNA and CD4 count were 31,476 copies/mL and 229 cells/mm^3, respectively, were randomized to one of six treatment arms: (A) SQV 400 mg twice daily + RTV 400 mg twice daily + delavirdine (DLV) 600 mg twice daily; (B) SQV 400 mg twice daily + RTV 400 mg twice daily + ADF 120 mg once daily; (C) SQV 400 mg twice daily + RTV 400 mg twice daily + DLV 600 mg twice daily + ADF 120 mg once daily; (D) SQV 800 mg three times daily + NFV 750 mg three times daily + DLV 600 mg twice daily; (E) SQV 800 mg three times daily + NFV 750 mg three times daily + ADF 120 mg once daily; and (F) SQV 800 mg three times daily + NFV 750 mg three times daily + DLV 600 mg twice daily + ADF 120 mg once daily.

PIs were administered in an open-label fashion; DLV and ADF were blinded (placebo controlled). L-Carnitine, 500 mg once daily, was given to prevent or diminish ADF-related side effects. Analyses used a factorial design to evaluate the efficacy of a second PI (RTV vs. NFV) and the efficacy of DLV versus ADF versus DLV plus ADF.

The proportion of patients with HIV RNA < 500 copies/mL at week 16 was only 30% (77 of 254 patients): 33% in arm A, 20% in B, 31% in C, 47% in D, 16% in E, and 38% in F. There was no significant difference between the RTV and NFV arms ($p = 0.51$). The addition of DLV conferred superior viral load suppression compared with the use of ADF ($p = 0.003$). The addition of ADF to dual PI regimens containing DLV (arms C and F) provided no greater viral load suppression ($p = 0.47$ in the DLV vs. DLV + ADF arms). Median CD4 cell count increase was +19 cells/mm^3 above baseline among the six treatment arms. During the first 20 weeks, 17% of patients experienced grade 3–4 clinical adverse events, and laboratory abnormalities were observed in 37% of patients. Three cases of nephroxicity were reported in the ADF-containing arms. There was no significant difference between using dual PI-based regimen of SQV/RTV or SQV/NFV in this study population of IDV-experienced NNRTI-naive patients. The addition of DLV provided better HIV RNA suppression than ADF and the combination of DLV/ADF was not better than DLV alone.

Of note, a substudy comprised of 42 patients from ACTG 359 that evaluated pharmacokinetic interactions (66) demonstrated that ADF decreased the area under the curve for DLV plasma levels. From prior studies, DLV is known to inhibit the cytochrome P450 pathway and thereby achieves increased levels of PI agents; the decreased DLV levels due to the addition of ADF may have contributed to decreased SQV plasma concentrations with resultant diminished potency in the DLV + ADF combination arms.

RTV/IDV for PI Failure. RTV/IDV regimens are being intensively evaluated for salvage therapy because this dual PI combination provides markedly enhanced IDV trough concentrations, allows for a b.i.d. dosing schedule, and permits IDV administration with food (Table 3).

The efficacy and safety of IDV (400 mg)/RTV (400 mg) twice daily in combination with d4T/3TC was evaluated in a study conducted by Workman et al. (67) that enrolled 24 HIV-infected patients who were assigned to two treatment groups (A and B). Group A consisted of 12 patients who had been on a stable regimen of RTV/SQV + d4T/3TC for >6 months and who had maintained HIV RNA levels < 400 copies/mL for more than 6 months with stable CD4 counts. Group B featured 12 treatment-naive patients with mean baseline viral load of 65,316 copies/mL (Amplicor assay) who were assigned IDV/RTV + d4T/3TC.

All group A patients maintained HIV RNA < 400 copies/mL up to 36 weeks; 9 of 12 patients sustained substantial CD4 increases after switching therapy. In group B, 10 patients completed at least 12 weeks of ART and all 10 patients achieved HIV RNA < 400 copies/mL. The dual PI combination was well tolerated; mild diarrhea resolved in three group B patients without dose interruption; no nephrolithiasis was reported.

Another recent study reported by O'Brien et al. (68) evaluated IDV/RTV dual PI therapy in 20 treatment-experienced HIV-infected patients with mean prior PI exposure of 15 months. The first phase of this study initially evaluated IDV 800 mg twice daily in combination with RTV 100 mg twice daily taken with food plus two to three NRTIs; in the second phase of the study, the RTV dose was increased to 200 mg twice daily. Twenty patients with baseline HIV RNA and CD4 count of 286,504 copies/mL and 196 cells/mm^3, respectively, were assessable. The IDV trough concentrations obtained in patients after at least 1 month of therapy on the IDV/RTV 800-mg/100-mg dose ($n = 10$) were markedly lower than those observed on the IDV/RTV 800-mg/200-mg dose ($n = 14$). Six of 20 patients achieved HIV RNA < 50 copies/mL at 3–6 months; 4 patients had partial response with HIV RNA decrease of ≥ 1.0 log$_{10}$, and 10 patients were nonresponders. Six of 20 patients developed nephrolithiasis; 3 patients with renal stones required discontinuation from the study. Most patients had numerous genotypic protease resistance mutations observed at baseline; the most frequent mutations occurred at positions 48, 82, 84, and 90. A diminished treatment response was seen in patients with the L90M mutation at baseline. Longer-term follow-up is required to assess durability of response and evaluate the adverse event profile of this dual PI combination.

2. Investigational PI Agents for Salvage Therapy

ABT-378, a novel investigational PI agent that has been coformulated with low-dose ritonavir (ABT-378/r) which functions as a pharmacokinetic enhancer, exhibits a high therapeutic index by achieving trough concentrations that are 30-fold higher than the EC$_{50}$ of wild-type HIV isolates at steady state (69) (Table 3). The high plasma trough concentrations observed with

ABT-378 may serve both as a barrier to the emergence of viral resistance and may make this agent a potentially useful component of salvage therapy.

The M97-765 trial (69) recently evaluated the efficacy and safety of ABT 378/r (400 mg/100 mg vs. 400 mg/200 mg b.i.d.) in salvage combination therapy for 70 PI-experienced patients with virologic failure. Patients had screening HIV RNA levels between 10^3 and 10^5 copies/mL, were receiving stable ART regimens containing one PI and two NRTIs for ≥ 3 months, were naive to at least one NRTI agent, were NNRTI naive, and had not received prior dual PI therapy (Table 3). All patients were assigned ABT/r in combination with nevirapine and at least one new NRTI upon study entry. The baseline median plasma viral load and median CD4 count for these 70 patients were 4.0 $\log_{10}$ copies/mL and 349 cells/mm^3, respectively. Forty-four percent, 36%, 13%, 6%, and 1% of the study patients had received IDV, NFV, SQV, RTV, and amprenavir, respectively, as the single PI agent at the time of virologic failure; 87%, 56%, and 47% of patients had received prior 3TC, d4T, and ZDV, respectively. In phenotypic susceptibility assays obtained on 55 of 70 baseline isolates, 64% demonstrated at least fourfold loss in susceptibility to the previous PI and 33% had at least fourfold loss in susceptibility to at least three PIs. At week 36, 78% and 67% of patients, by on treatment and ITT analyses, respectively, achieved suppression of viral load to <400 copies/mL. The mean CD4 count change from baseline at week 36 was +104 cells/mm^3. The study drug regimen was well tolerated with 14 of 70 (20%) patients experiencing diarrhea as the most frequent adverse clinical symptom; elevated triglycerides and cholesterol were the most frequently observed laboratory abnormalities, and each occurred in 17 of 70 (24%) patients. These preliminary results suggest that ABT-378/r in combination with an NNRTI and new nucleoside analogues may be effective salvage therapy in PI-experienced patients.

VI. ROLE OF INTENSIFICATION STRATEGIES

The role of intensification therapy is currently being explored as a strategic approach in two distinct settings: as a means to prolong the durability of viral load suppression in an already effective regimen and as adjunctive therapy to improve the efficacy of a partially suppressive regimen in which substantial decreases in HIV RNA levels have been achieved but the viral load remains above the limit of detection. For patients who have developed viral rebound on combination therapy, the current treatment guidelines (70) advocate changing at least two and, if feasible, all the drugs in the partially suppressive regimen to attain HIV RNA levels below the level of detection.

Predictors of improved virologic responses observed with subsequent alternative combination therapy in treatment-experienced patients have included switching therapy when HIV RNA levels are relatively low, changing the failing regimen before the accumulation of multiple resistance mutations, and providing a revised regimen that confers adequate potency.

Viral rebounds sustained by patients receiving PI-containing triple combination regimens in several clinical trials were further characterized by gene sequencing in which resistance mutations were noted only in the reverse transcriptase gene and not in the protease gene (71–73). The Trilege trial (71) demonstrated that viral replication was less durably suppressed in ZDV/3TC and ZDV/IDV maintenance arms after a 3-month induction with triple therapy (ZDV/3TC/IDV) compared with continuation of triple therapy. At the time of virologic rebound during the maintenance phase, the M184 mutation was detected in 6 of 8 patients on triple therapy and in 25 of 25 patients on ZDV/3TC maintenance; neither ZDV- nor IDV-associated genotypic resistance mutations were detected at the time of virologic failure except in the protease gene in one patient.

The ACTG 343 (72, 73) trial evaluated an induction maintenance strategy in treatment-naive HIV-infected patients who received triple combination therapy (ZDV/3TC/IDV) for 6 months, followed by randomization to three maintenance arms (ZDV/3TC/IDV montherapy or ZDV/3TC/IDV). Viral rebound (HIV RNA > 500 copies/mL) was observed in 23%, 23%, and 4% of patients in the IDV, ZDV/3TC, and IDV/ZDV/3TC arms, respectively. Further characterization of ACTG 343 viral rebounds was conducted in 26 patients; patients developed viral rebound at a median of 23 weeks with HIV RNA > 10^3 copies/mL. All the IDV monotherapy isolates retained phenotypic susceptibility to IDV; genotypic resistance analyses confirmed no IDV-associated genotypic resistance mutations in the protease gene. In the 17 patients in the ZDV/3TC/IDV arm with viral rebound, no phenotypic IDV resistance was detected, and in genotypic analyses, one isolate had the M46L protease mutation detected. Fourteen (82%) of 17 isolates in the ZDV/3TC//IDV arm possessed the M184V mutation in the RT gene.

The preserved wild-type protease sequences identified in patients experiencing viral rebound on PI-containing triple therapy in these two clinical trials suggest that the PI agent does not have to be automatically replaced when revising a partially suppressive regimen. These data, furthermore, provide a rationale for performing drug resistance testing in the setting of viral rebound and for consideration of intensification with the addition of a single new agent to the existing regimen.

Several clinical trials have been designed to examine the utility of singly adding selected antiretroviral agents with once- or twice-daily dosing schedules, such as ABC or ADF, to background therapy as an intensification strategy in patients with early viral rebound.

The CNA3002 trial (74) recently evaluated the efficacy of an intensification approach that added ABC to stable background ART (≥ 12 weeks) in 185 HIV-infected patients with HIV RNA levels ≥ 400 to $\leq 50,000$ copies/mL and no prior history of CD4 count ≤ 100 cells/mm^3. Patients were randomized to receive ABC 300 mg b.i.d. or ABC placebo in combination with stable background therapy. Randomization was stratified by duration of prior NRTI therapy and 3TC experience; after week 16, patients were allowed to receive open-label ABC and revised background therapy if HIV RNA was >400 copies/mL. Baseline median plasma viral load and CD4 counts were 3.68 log$_{10}$ copies/mL (ABC arm) versus 3.52 log$_{10}$ copies/mL (placebo arm) and 408 cells/mm^3 (ABC arm) versus 410 cells/mm^3 (placebo arm), respectively.

At week 48, 25% (23/92) of patients in the ABC arm compared with 6% (6/93) of patients in the placebo arm achieved HIV RNA < 400 copies/mL ($p < 0.001$; ITT analysis). A subgroup analysis was performed. In the ABC arm, 41% (19/46) of patients with baseline HIV RNA < 5000 copies/mL achieved HIV RNA < 400 copies/mL compared with 9% (4/44) of patients with baseline HIV RNA > 5000 copies/mL. In the placebo arm, 7% (4/55) of patients and 5% (2/38) of patients with baseline HIV RNA levels of <5000 and >5000 copies/mL, respectively, achieved HIV RNA < 400 copies/mL. These results suggest that intensification strategies using the addition of a single new agent to the existing regimen are more likely to be effective if initiated in patients with low level (<5000 copies/mL) virologic failure.

VII. PREDICTORS OF TREATMENT RESPONSE

A number of studies have evaluated whether HIV disease stage, baseline CD4 cell count, baseline viral load, or the presence of baseline genotypic mutations and phenotypic resistance to selected components of a combination regimen were useful predictors of subsequent treatment response. The accurate determination of predictors of response may facilitate devising salvage regimens that exhibit greater likelihood of attaining effective viral suppression and confer more durable responses in treatment-experienced patients.

A. Baseline CD4 Cell Count, Plasma HIV RNA, and Virologic Response

1. Initial Single PI-Containing Regimen

Predictors of viral response were evaluated in 243 HIV-infected patients with baseline median CD4 count and median viral loads of 230 cells/mm^3 and

4.5 $\log_{10}$ copies/mL, respectively, who initiated their first PI-containing regimen and were followed for 32 weeks (75). Most patients were treatment naive ($n = 180$; 74%), and almost half of the patients started two new drugs concurrently with the PI agent; the PI agents included RTV, IDV, and SQV hgc. At week 24, 52.8% of the patients achieved HIV RNA levels < 400 copies/mL. In a multivariate analysis, patients with higher baseline viral load were less likely to achieve suppression of plasma HIV RNA below 400 copies/mL (relative hazard [RH] 0.50; 95% CI, 0.35–0.70; $p < 0.0001$). Those patients who started more new drugs when initiating PI-based therapy, however, were significantly more likely to achieve a plasma viral load below the limit of detection (RH per new drug, 1.54; 95%CI, 1.01–2.11; $p = 0.048$). Time to event analyses showed that among those 111 patients who had attained HIV RNA levels < 400 copies/mL at week 24, 15.5% of patients experienced viral rebound within 24 weeks after the initial undetectable viral load. A higher CD4 count was associated with a lower risk of viral rebound (RH, 0.73; 95% CI, 0.53–1.00; $p = 0.049$) as was treatment with IDV versus other PI agents (RH, 0.17; 95% CI, 0.03–0.86; $p = 0.033$). This study also suggested that treatment-experienced patients could achieve favorable treatment response rates (i.e., proportion with undetectable viral load) comparable with treatment-naive patients, provided that the number of new drugs added to the PI-based regimen was the same.

A retrospective analysis of week 48 viral load (<400 and <50 copies/mL) results derived from a multicenter randomized trial featuring combination ART with NFV plus ZDV and 3TC evaluated baseline variables as early predictors of virologic response (76). In this study, baseline viral load, change in HIV RNA levels over the first 4 weeks of treatment, the 2-hour post-dose NFV levels, and the time to achieve HIV RNA <400 and <50 copies/mL, respectively, were the best predictors of determining treatment response and durability of response. Patients who had lowest HIV RNA nadir (<50 copies/mL) experienced significantly more durable responses compared with patients with nadir HIV RNA levels between 50 and 400 copies/mL. These early predictors identify patients who, shortly after initiation of combination therapy, are determined to be at substantial risk of treatment failure and who would potentially benefit from early interventions, such as intensification strategies or revised combination therapy.

A prospective nonrandomized trial (77) assessed the long-term efficacy of PI-based therapy and evaluated factors associated with virologic response in a cohort of 400 HIV-infected nucleoside experienced patients whose baseline median viral load and CD4 count were 4.6 $\log_{10}$ copies/mL and 86 cells/mm^3, respectively. Of the 400 patients starting initial PI-containing therapy (RTV 26%; SQV 28%; or IDV 46%), 91% had received nucleoside analogues for a median of 28 months. At least one new NRTI was added simultaneously to the PI regimen in 66% of 365 pretreated patients; 335 patients have completed 1 year of follow-up. Long-term virologic efficacy was defined as an HIV RNA level < 200 copies/mL after 12 months of therapy. At 1 year, 45% and 59% of 335 assessable patients had achieved viral load below 200 copies/mL and CD4 cell count increase > 100 cells/mm^3, respectively. In logistic regression analyses, treatment failure was associated with higher baseline plasma viral load (relative risk [RR], 2.10; $p < 0.01$), prior ART (RR, 2.07; $p < 0.01$), and use of SQV (RR, 1.55; $p = 0.03$). A decline in HIV RNA level of more than 1 $\log_{10}$ copies/mL within the first 3 months of therapy was strongly correlated with treatment response (RR, 0.65; $p < 0.01$). There was no strict correlation between virologic and immunologic efficacy. These results suggest that baseline viral load and the decline in HIV RNA levels observed at 3 months are highly predictive of the virologic response at 1 year and indicate that more potent combination therapy is required in pretreated patients to achieve durable viral load suppression.

An observational study of 558 patients participating in the Frankfurt HIV Clinic Cohort who had achieved viral load suppression < 500 copies/mL while receiving HAART was undertaken to investigate the association between CD4 cell count (baseline, updated during follow-up, and change from baseline) and durability of viral load suppression (78). At 24 weeks, the estimate of viral rebound (HIV RNA > 500 copies/mL) was 42.5% patients and at 84 weeks was 64.3% patients. In a Cox proportional model that adjusted for number of new drugs started and time to HIV RNA < 500 copies/mL, the risk of viral rebound was associated with baseline CD4 count ($p = 0.001$), change from baseline ($p = 0.003$), and with the updated CD4 cell count ($p = 0.001$). The risk of viral rebound was independently associated with baseline and change from baseline CD4 count. The achieved CD4 cell count emerged as the most useful predictor of viral rebound (RH 5.4 for an updated CD4 count < 20 vs. >500 cells/mm^3; $p = 0.0001$). Lower baseline CD4 counts conferred an increased risk for viral rebound, but the risk was diminished in patients who sustain a substantial rise in CD4 counts on combination therapy.

2. Virologic Response to Second PI-containing Regimens

Virologic responses after the introduction of a second PI-containing regimen were evaluated in 942 patients with virologic failure (HIV RNA > 1000 copies/mL) on initial PI-based therapy who were enrolled in the longitudinal EuroSIDA study (79). Predictors of viral load response and progression to new AIDS-defining event were examined. Patients had received the following PI agents as the initial PI: RTV (20%), SQV (44%), or IDV (36%).

The baseline median viral load and CD4 count before initiating second PI therapy were 4.56 $\log_{10}$ copies/mL and 160 cells/mm^3, respectively. The second regimen was introduced at least 16 weeks after stopping the first PI; the second PI agents used in the new regimen included RTV (16%), SQV (8%), IDV (45%), or NFV (31%). Fifty-four percent of patients did not add new NRTIs; 35% added at least one new NRTI. At 6 and 9 months after starting the second regimen, patients achieved a median rise in CD4 cell count of 45 and of 75 cells/mm^3, respectively. The median decline in viral load observed at 6 and 12 months was 0.8 $\log_{10}$ copies/mL for each time point; 40% of patients achieved HIV RNA < 400 copies/mL at 24 weeks. Patients whose viral load at baseline was between 5000 and 10,000 copies/mL had a greater likelihood of achieving viral suppression compared with patients whose viral load was >50,000 copies/mL at baseline ($p < 0.0001$). The strongest independent predictors of response were CD4 cell count (RH of response 1.27 per twofold higher; $p < 0.0001$) and viral load (RH 0.60 per 1 $\log_{10}$ copies/mL higher; $p < 0.001$) at baseline. There were 146 treatment failures among 320 patients (51%) and 71 cases of AIDS/deaths. At the time of treatment failure, the median CD4 count and viral load were 50 cells/mm^3 and 4.8 $\log_{10}$ copies/mL, respectively. Thus, the overall response to second PI-containing regimens is generally poor, with high failure rates. Identifying factors contributing to the inadequate treatment response, such as potential cross-resistance and poor adherence, may further explain the high failure rates observed.

A retrospective study determined the rate of virologic failure in an unselected cohort of 198 HIV-infected patients with baseline median plasma HIV RNA and CD4 counts of 4.7 $\log_{10}$ copies/mL and 99 cells/mm^3, respectively, who were receiving PI-based combination therapy (45); 53 patients (23%) had prior PI experience, and a total of 226 treatment episodes featuring PI agents were evaluated (RTV, 47; IDV, 96; and SQV, 83). Treatment failure was defined as <1.0 $\log_{10}$ copies/mL reduction in plasma HIV RNA at 6 months. The overall rate of treatment failure was unexpectedly high at 44% (SQV, 64%; RTV, 38%; and IDV, 30%). In a multivariate model, the RR for virologic failure was lower for patients with higher baseline CD4 counts (RR, 0.997 for each CD4 cell count increase; $p = 0.012$). In pretreated patients, the use of one or two drugs (RR, 2.64; $p < 0.05$) and more than two prior drugs (RR, 2.97; $p < 0.05$) were associated with higher rates of treatment failure. The use of SQV was associated with higher risk of virologic failure (RR, 4.62; $p = 0.001$) compared with IDV use. In this unselected cohort of patients, a higher rate (44%) of virologic failure was reported than in randomized clinical trials. Low baseline CD4 count, pretreatment with antiretrovrial therapy, and use of SQV versus IDV were significant predictors predictors of virologic failure.

3. Dual PI-Based Regimens

Baseline predictors of treatment response and the efficacy of dual PI-based combination therapy using high-dose SQV hgc (800 mg twice daily) plus RTV (400 mg twice daily) were evaluated in a retrospective cohort study featuring 58 HIV-infected patients with baseline median plasma viral load and CD4 count of 4.0 $\log_{10}$ copies/mL and 256 cells/mm^3, respectively, who were failing their first PI-containing regimens (80). Patients achieved a median reduction in plasma HIV RNA > 0.5 $\log_{10}$ copies/mL at 1 year and sustained a median rise in CD4 count of $+89$ cells/mm^3. Overall, 53% of patients achieved HIV RNA levels below 200 copies/mL at 6 months. Patients with higher baseline viral load (RH, 0.46 per $\log_{10}$ higher; 95% CI, 0.29–0.74; $p = 0.0015$) were less likely to attain suppression of HIV RNA < 200 copies/mL; 76% of patients with baseline viral loads < 5000 copies/mL achieved suppression of viral load at 6 months compared with only 30% of patients with baseline HIV RNA levels > 5000 copies/mL. All six patients with two or more major PI resistance mutations experienced virologic failure at 6 months. A switch to dual RTV/SQV combination-based therapy at lower viral loads and the absence of PI-associated resistance mutations at the time of the switch were associated with improved and more durable treatment response to salvage PI therapy.

B. Advanced HIV Disease and Treatment Response to PI-Containing Therapy

An observational study (81) to assess the efficacy of HAART was undertaken in 250 heavily pretreated HIV-infected patients with baseline median viral load and CD4 count ranges of 6498–93,625 copies/mL and 22–209 cells/mm^3, respectively, who had a median duration of NRTI therapy of 26 months. Treatment failure was defined as the occurrence of a new or recurrent AIDS-defining event, death, or any definitive treatment discontinuation. PI-based therapy was initiated among the 250 patients as follows: 153 with IDV, 55 with RTV, and 43 with SQV. During a median follow-up of 8 months, 75 patients (30%) experienced treatment failure attributed to an AIDS-defining event or death ($n = 24$), lack of efficacy ($n = 24$), or severe intolerance ($n = 27$). Of the AIDS-defining events, 20 were new and 6 were recurrent; 9 deaths were reported. CD4 cell counts were above 200 cells/mm^3 at the time of the AIDS diagnosis in only two patients. The SQV-containing regimens correlated independently with treatment failure (RR, 2.46; 95% CI, 1.20–5.03; vs. IDV). Severe immunodepression and AIDS at baseline were predictive of treatment failure.

None of the SQV patients, 12 (7.8%) of the IDV patients, and 15 (27.3%) of the RTV-treated patients were deemed noncompliant; low compliance partially determined the treatment response in RTV-treated patients. The IDV-containing arm demonstrated superior viral load suppression with 68.4% of patients achieving HIV RNA < 500 copies/mL after 6 months; patients treated with IDV or RTV sustained a 10-fold rise in CD4 counts. HAART conferred effective treatment response in 70% of patients with advanced HIV disease stage. A prior AIDS diagnosis and poor adherence to PI-based therapy were predictive of treatment failure.

C. Genotypic and Phenotypic Resistance as Predictors of Treatment Response

1. Virologic Response to NFV Salvage Therapy

The Swiss HIV Cohort study examined the prognostic significance of drug associated genotypic mutations in the protease and reverse transcriptase genes on virologic response to NFV-based salvage therapy (82). Sixty-two patients who had experienced virologic failure (HIV RNA > 1000 copies/mL after >3 months) while receiving HAART and whose baseline median plasma HIV RNA and CD4 count were 5.16 $\log_{10}$ copies/mL and 113 cells/mm^3, respectively, were switched to NFV plus other ARTs. Patients had been previously exposed to reverse transcriptase inhibitors (RTIs) and PIs for a median duration of 35.6 and 12.2 months, respectively. Virologic response was evaluated after 4–12 weeks of NFV-based therapy. A median decline in plasma viral load of 0.38 $\log_{10}$ copies/mL was demonstrated; 32% of patients achieved > 1 $\log_{10}$ decrease. At baseline, 90% of patients had reverse transcriptase inhibitor resistance mutations identified; a median number of four mutations per patient was shown (range, 0–7). Primary and secondary PI mutations were detected in 69% and 89% of patients, respectively. A median of four PI resistance mutations per patient was detected (range, 0–9). Viral load response to NFV-based salvage therapy was associated with number of RTIs, primary and secondary PI resistance mutations, and history of PI use (duration and number) by univariate analysis. Clinical HIV disease stage, baseline viral load, and CD4 count were not associated with treatment response. The number of reverse transcriptase inhibitor plus PI resistance mutations was the only independent predictor of virologic response after adjusting for all variables. These data suggest that the best predictor for virologic response to

NFV-containing therapy in extensively treated HIV-infected patients with advanced disease is the number of baseline reverse transcriptase inhibitor plus PI genotypic mutations associated with drug resistance.

2. Predictors of Response to ABC

Baseline predictors of virologic response (defined as achieving HIV RNA < 400 copies/mL) were examined in 136 ART-experienced patients who intensified their stable background therapy with the addition of ABC (83). The duration of prior ART was significantly associated with treatment response ($p = 0.022$); the number of prior ARTs was not predictive. Baseline HIV RNA was strongly associated with treatment response ($p = 0.0001$), whereas baseline CD4 was not correlated with response. Four genotypic profiles were defined: wild-type virus (11%), M184V mutation *alone* (30%), one to two NRTI mutations excluding M184V alone (24%), and at least three NRTI mutations. Subjects with wild-type genotype exhibited a 53% response; M184V *alone* had a 66% response; one to two NRTI mutations had 33% response; and at least three NRTI mutations had a 17% response. Logistic regression analyses demonstrated that wild-type virus was significantly associated with virologic response compared to virus with at least three NRTI mutations (odds ratio 12.5; 95% CI, 2.5–61.0; $p = 0.002$). M184V *alone* virus was also significantly more likely to achieve HIV RNA < 400 copies/mL than virus with at least three NRTI mutations ($p = 0.002$); no significant differences in response were detected between M184V *alone* and wild-type. The risk of virologic failure (HIV RNA > 400 copies/mL) generally increased with the number of baseline NRTI-associated mutations; no significant increased risk of failure was demonstrated between wild-type and M184V *alone*.

3. Phenotypic Resistance to PIs and Treatment Response

The efficacy and safety of a salvage regimen featuring RTV 100 mg twice daily/SQV 1000 mg twice daily in combination with EFV plus recycled nucleoside analogues was evaluated in an open-label trial that enrolled 32 SQV- and EFV-naive patients who had HIV RNA levels > 1000 copies/mL while receiving a triple RTV or IDV-based combination therapy (84, 85). Median baseline plasma HIV RNA and CD4 counts were 4.31 $\log_{10}$ copies/mL and 258 cells/mm^3, respectively. At week 36, 67% of patients achieved plasma viral load below 500 copies/mL; the HIV RNA level declined by a median of -1.27 $\log_{10}$ copies/mL and CD4 count increased by a median of $+68$ cells/mm^3. Patients whose viral isolates demonstrated phenotypic resistance to SQV at baseline sustained a median decrease in HIV RNA of 0.82 $\log_{10}$ copies/mL at week 36 compared with a 1.52 $\log_{10}$ copies/mL plasma viral load decline in patients whose isolates remained susceptible to SQV ($p = 0.01$). Forty-two percent of patients with SQV phenotypic resistance achieved HIV RNA < 500 copies/mL at week 36 compared with 84% of patients whose isolates demonstrated phenotypic susceptibility to SQV ($p = 0.02$); however, genotypic resistance to SQV did not predict virologic failure. These data indicated that a salvage regimen featuring dual PI RTV/SQV therapy in combination with EFV was effective for most patients experiencing virologic failure on an initial PI-containing regimen and afforded viral load suppression in 67% of patients at week 36. These results suggested that phenotypic resistance may be a more useful predictor of treatment response than the identification of baseline genotypic resistance mutations.

4. Differences in Phenotypic Susceptibility to PIs after Failing Initial PI-Containing Regimen

Differences in phenotypic susceptibility to PI agents were recently examined in patients who had experienced treatment failure (HIV RNA > 400 copies/mL) while receiving an initial PI-based regimen (86). Baseline PI susceptibility (Virologic PhenoSense^{TM} assay) was assessed in an ongoing clinical trial evaluating the utility of phenotypic resistance assays; susceptibility was expressed as the fold change (FC) in 50% inhibitory concentration (IC_{50}) from control and >2.5 FC was considered resistant for this study. Eighty-two patients (median duration of NRTIs, 34 months; median duration of PIs, 15 months) whose baseline median viral load and CD4 count were 4.1 log_{10} copies/mL and 281 cells/mm^3, respectively, were evaluated. Thirteen patients who were PI naive had baseline isolates fully susceptible to PIs. The PI-experienced patients had received NFV ($n = 44$), IDV ($n = 16$), SQV ($n = 5$), RTV ($n = 3$), or APV ($n = 1$). In PI-experienced patients, the mean baseline PI FC by phenotypic assay was significantly different between IDV, NFV, RTV, APV, and SQV (4.9, 20, 7.0, 2.1, and 3.1, respectively; $p < 0.001$). A high proportion of patients failing a PI-based regimen in this study did not have evidence of phenotypic resistance to the current PI agent; most viral isolates except those from patients receiving NFV exhibited low-level phenotypic resistance to the current PI. The proportion of patients who still exhibited drug-susceptible virus (<2.5 FC) was 83% (APV), 84% (SQV), 71% (RTV), 68% (IDV), and NFV (26%).

Prior NFV therapy was associated with infrequent cross-resistance compared with patients with other prior PI exposure: APV (97% vs. 36%; $p = 0.006$), IDV (16% vs. 60%; $p < 0.001$), and RTV (14% vs. 56%; $p < 0.001$). Logistic regression models were performed to predict individual PI resistance based on baseline values (CD4 count, HIV RNA, prior therapy, and AIDS diagnosis). In the best model (NFV; $p = 0.0001$), the correct prediction of resistance was obtained for 81% of cases; 11% (2/18) of patients predicted to be NFV-sensitive were actually resistant, whereas 22% (14/64) deemed NFV resistant were actually determined to be sensitive. In this heavily pre-treated patient population characterized by predominant NFV exposure, viral isolates detained from patients failing NFV therapy frequently demonstrated high-level phenotypic resistance to NFV but generally retained full pheno-typic susceptibility (FC < 2.5) to APV and SQV. The use of NFV as the initial PI agent was associated with less phenotypic cross-resistance in con-trast to that observed with other PI agents, such as IDV, when selected as the first PI-containing regimen. These data indicate that phenotypic susceptibil-ity testing may identify potential PI components of a current failing regimen to which the viral isolate remains sensitive and may therefore preserve fu-ture treatment options by retaining these PI agents that could have continued antiviral activity.

VIII.   ROLE OF GENOTYPIC AND PHENOTYPIC RESISTANCE ASSAYS IN DEVISING SALVAGE THERAPY

The development of treatment failure in patients receiving potent triple combi-nation therapy has frequently been linked to the emergence of drug resistance. The selection of potent salvage therapy in treatment-experienced patients with confirmed virologic failure is limited by fewer available ART agents to which the patient is naive and is hampered by potential cross resistance to selected agents and uncertainty about which, if any, components of the current reg-imen are likely to remain effective. Drug resistance testing (44, 87, 88) of HIV-1 isolates in advance of devising salvage therapy may therefore prove useful in management of treatment failure by guiding the selection of drugs to which the virus remains susceptible and by identifying major genotypic resistance mutations that may preclude introducing a given drug.

Several pilot studies exploring the utility of genotypic and phenotypic re-sistance testing have provided encouraging preliminary results with respect to treatment outcomes. Larger scale trials are warranted to provide clinical validation and to further define the role of resistance testing in clinical prac-tice.

Drug resistance can be evaluated by both genotypic and phenotypic assays (33, 34, 44). Genotyping (44) determines the nucleotide sequence of the specific genes encoding viral proteins such as the reverse transcriptase and protease genes. Any change in genotype from a reference wild-type sequence is reported as a change in the amino acid at a specific codon of the protein (Table 4). Drug susceptibility can be inferred from the genotype. A limitation of the genotypic assay is that it may not detect minority virus subpopulations.

Phenotypic susceptibility assays (44) measure the amount of drug required to inhibit viral replication *in vitro*; phenotypic resistance is based on the ability of the virus to grow in the presence of a given drug compared with a wild-type control virus. Susceptibility *in vitro* is expressed as the IC_{50} or IC_{90}, which refers to the drug concentration required to inhibit viral replication by 50% or 90%, respectively. Phenotypic assays also may fail to detect minor drug-resistant viral species that may contribute to drug failure or transmission of resistant virus.

A. Genotypic Resistance Testing

The VIRADAPT study, a randomized, open, prospective trial (89), evaluated whether the use of genotypic resistance testing in patients failing ART combination therapy would have an impact on the virologic outcome of alternative regimens. One hundred eight patients whose baseline viral load and CD4 count were 4.7 $\log_{10}$ copies/mL and 214 cells/mm^3, respectively, were

Table 4 Major Antiretroviral Genotypic Resistance Mutations

Antiretroviral class	Agent	Primary codon mutation(s)
Nucleoside analogues	Zidovudine (ZDV)	M41L, K70R, T215Y/F
	Didanosine (ddI)	L74V
	Zalcitabine (ddC)	T69D
	Lamivudine (3TC)	M184V
	Abacavir	M184V
	Multinucleoside resistance	Q151M, T69SSS
Nonnucleoside analogues	Nevirapine	K103N, Y181C
	Delavirdine	K103N, Y181C
	Efavirenz	K103N
Protease inhibitors	Saquinavir	G48V, L90M
	Ritonavir	V82A/F/T, 184V, L90M A71V/T, M46I/L
	Indinavir	V82A/F/T; M46I/L
	Nelfinavir	D30N
	Amprenavir	I50V

enrolled. Patients were randomly assigned standard care (control, $n = 43$) or treatment according to the resistance mutations in the protease and reverse transcriptase genes (genotypic group, $n = 65$); the major endpoint was change in plasma viral load. At 3 months, the mean change in plasma HIV RNA was -1.04 $\log_{10}$ copies/mL in the genotypic group compared with -0.46 $\log_{10}$ copies/mL in the control group ($p = 0.01$). At 6 months, the decrease in HIV RNA was -1.15 and -0.67 $\log_{10}$ copies/mL in the genotypic and control groups, respectively ($p = 0.05$). At 3 months, 29% (19/65) of patients in the genotypic group achieved plasma HIV RNA < 200 copies/mL compared with 14% (6/43) of patients in the control group ($p = 0.017$); at 6 months, 32% (21/65) and 14% (6/43) of patients, respectively, had viral suppression < 200 copies/mL ($p = 0.048$).

In extended follow-up, patients in the control group were offered open-label genotype treatment at 6 months (90). In the original genotypic group, the mean decline in plasma viral load was -1.15 and -1.1 $\log_{10}$ copies/mL at 9 and 12 months, respectively. In the control group, 69% (30/43) of patients switched to genotype treatment. In the switched to genotype group, the mean plasma viral load decline was -0.85 and -0.89 $\log_{10}$ copies/mL at 9 and 12 months, respectively. In the open-label genotype group, 14% and 25.7% of patients at 9 and 12 months, respectively, achieved HIV RNA levels < 200 copies/mL. This follow-up phase confirmed the virologic benefit of switching to open-label genotypic testing after 6 months of standard clinical practice. This study determined that genotypic resistance testing in the setting of treatment failure had a favorable impact on virologic outcome of alternative therapy and demonstrated that combination regimens based on genotypic testing could confer durable treatment responses for up to 1 year.

In a related multicenter randomized trial, the CPCRA 046 pilot study evaluated the short-term effects of providing genotypic antiretroviral testing (GART) for the management of 153 HIV-infected patients with treatment failure (viral load rebound after ≥16 weeks of triple therapy) on a PI-containing regimen (91). There were no differences in the number or type of prior PI agents used between the two study groups. Genotyping by Applied Biosystems, Inc. (ABI) sequencing was performed on all patients, followed by randomization to either GART arm or no-GART arm. Genotypic interpretation and suggested therapy were provided to clinicians of patients in the the GART arm. The median baseline viral load and CD4 count of the enrolled study patients were 28,085 copies/mL and 230 cells/mm^3, respectively. Of the 153 patients, specific PI failure was as follows: 82 IDV, 51 NFV, 11 RTV, and 9 SQV. Seventy-three percent of the viral isolates had at least one reverse transcriptase major mutation and at least one major protease mutation. The primary endpoint of the study was defined as the change in viral load from baseline to the average of the week 4 and week 8 measurements. The GART arm sustained a -1.19 $\log_{10}$ copies/mL decline in HIV RNA compared with a -0.61 $\log_{10}$ copies/mL decrease observed in the no-GART arm ($p = 0.00001$). The average difference between treatment groups at 12 weeks was -0.44 $\log_{10}$ copies/mL ($p = 0.003$). The viral load response within each arm correlated with the number of active drugs administered in the alternative regimen. The effect of GART was consistent across all baseline subgroups defined by CD4 counts, baseline viral load, number of prior PIs, and genotypic profile. These results indicated that genotypic resistance testing that directed selection of alternative therapy afforded superior short-term viral load suppression compared with standard clinical care in patients failing triple-drug PI-containing treatment. The benefit of genotypic resistance testing on virologic response was similar in patients failing either an initial PI regimen or having multiple PI exposures.

The impact of drug resistance mutations in viral isolates from patients failing PI-containing regimens on subsequent virologic response to salvage therapy was further examined in the GART study (92). In this analysis, the GART and no-GART groups were combined, and only baseline genotypic mutations with $\geq 5\%$ frequency were evaluated: T69D, M184V, and T215Y/F in reverse transcriptase; and D30N, M46I/L, V82A/F/T, and L90M in the protease gene. A multiple regression analysis was undertaken of the viral load response to the next salvage regimen associated with the presence/absence of each mutation, adjusted for baseline CD4 and HIV RNA, with/without the inclusion of prior drug exposure. In multivariate analyses of reverse transcriptase mutations, the T69D mutation adversely influenced virologic response (change in viral load, $+0.55$ $\log_{10}$ copies/mL; $p = 0.02$) that persisted after adjusting for NRTI exposure history ($p = 0.04$). The presence of T215Y/F and M184V mutations that were detected in most patients did not significantly affect treatment outcome. The D30N mutation exhibited a positive effect on virologic response (change in viral load, -0.41 $\log_{10}$ copies/mL; $p = 0.04$) in multivariate analyses of PI mutations, whereas the L90M mutation conferred a negative impact on virologic response (change in viral load, $+0.31$ $\log_{10}$ copies/mL). The M46I/L, V82A/F/T, and 184V mutations did not significantly affect treatment response to salvage therapy. These data indicated that specific drug mutations in viral isolates obtained at the time of virologic failure on PI-containing regimens were associated with the short-term virologic responses observed after commencing salvage therapy.

A prospective trial evaluating the utility of baseline resistance testing was conducted by Moyle et al. (93) in which genotypic resistance assay results (Vircogen sequencing) were provided in real time (<1 month) for treatment-experienced patients experiencing viral rebound (HIV RNA > 1000 copies/mL) before switching to alternative therapy. Fifty-two HIV-infected patients with baseline median viral load and CD4 count of 4.31 $\log_{10}$ copies/mL and 185 cells/mm^3, respectively, were enrolled. All patients were NRTI experienced; 42 (81%) were PI experienced and 25 (48%) NNRTI experienced, with 15 (29%) exposed to all three classes. Patients were switched to regimens featuring either an NNRTI ($n = 22$), PI ($n = 18$), both NNRTI plus PI ($n = 10$), or NRTI only ($n = 2$). The proportion of patients who received zero, one, two, or three to four drugs to which they were naive were 85%, 27%, 27%, and 38%, respectively. The plasma viral load declined by a median of -1.6 $\log_{10}$ copies/mL and CD4 count increased by a median of $+29$ cells/mm^3 after a median follow-up of 14 weeks. Factors that were associated with treatment response in all patients were a higher baseline CD4 count ($p = 0.04$) and the number of key NNRTI mutations (defined as Y181C and K103N; $p = 0.02$) present at the time of the switch. The number of key NNRTI genotypic mutations were highly predictive of treatment response independent of prior NNRTI exposure. When the analysis was restricted to only those patients who had switched to an NNRTI-containing regimens ($n = 32$), the number of key NNRTI mutations was still associated with treatment response. When the analysis was then restricted to those patients starting a PI-containing regimen ($n = 28$), the number of key PI mutations instead of the number of NNRTI mutations was associated with treatment response. These preliminary results indicate that baseline genotypic resistance mutations influence short-term virologic response and support a role for resistance testing in devising salvage therapy for treatment-experienced patients with viral rebound.

B. Phenotypic Susceptibility Testing as Predictor of Treatment Response

The potential correlation between sustained viral suppression and baseline phenotypic drug susceptibility testing was examined in a cohort study of treatment-experienced HIV-infected patients with viral rebound (HIV RNA > 5000 copies/mL) who were initiating a new salvage therapy (94). Other clinical variables, including regimen selection by prior drug history alone, were also assessed for impact on treatment response. Plasma samples obtained at baseline were tested retrospectively for phenotypic drug susceptibility (ViroLogic PhenoSense^{TM} assay), and complete verified ART history for each patient was reviewed. Two different definitions of drug susceptibility were used: $IC_{50} \leq 2.5$ or $IC_{50} \leq 4.0$ times the drug-sensitive reference IC_{50}. Successful viral suppression was defined as $\geq 0.5 \log_{10}$ copies/mL reduction from baseline plasma viral load at all follow-up visits. Cox proportional hazard analyses were used to assess correlations between study variables and time to virologic failure. Seventy-one patients whose median HIV RNA and CD4 count were 70,644 copies/mL and 142 cells/mm^3, respectively, were enrolled. The median number of prior ART regimens used was 5; 72% of patients were PI experienced and 90% of patients were NNRTI naive. The median duration of follow-up was 15 months. A significant association by univariate proportional hazards analyses was noted between time to virologic failure and (1) the number of drugs in a new regimen to which the baseline viral isolate was susceptible (<2.5 cutoff value; RR 0.67 per susceptible drug in the new regimen; 95% CI, 0.52–0.86); (2) the number of drugs not previously used in a prior regimen (ART history; RR 0.75 per new drug in the regimen; 95% CI, 0.57–0.99); and (3) history of prior PI use (RR 2.12; 95% CI, 1.08–4.16). The baseline viral load, baseline CD4 count, number of previous regimens, PI use in a new regimen, and number of drugs in the new regimens were not significantly associated with time to virologic failure. Multivariate analyses demonstrated that the number of drugs in a new regimen to which the baseline viral isolate was susceptible (using a susceptibility cutoff value of ≤ 2.5 or ≤ 4.0) emerged as the best independent predictor of time to virologic failure (RR 0.59 per susceptible drug in the regimen; 95% CI, 0.46–0.77). Patients who received at least three drugs to which the virus was sensitive in the new regimen experienced a significantly longer time to virologic failure compared with patients who only received less than two drugs to which the virus was susceptible ($p < 0.001$). ART history did not provide additional predictive value when added to the model. These results indicated that sustained viral suppression in treatment-experienced patients with viral rebound is optimally predicted by phenotypic susceptibility to drugs in the new regimen. Although ART history alone was a significant predictor of virologic suppression, it was significantly less predictive compared with phenotypic susceptibility.

These data support a role for phenotypic testing when devising salvage therapy in treatment-experienced patients whose subsequent drug treatment options are increasingly limited. Further refinement in the interpretation and standardization of phenotypic assays is warranted with respect to developing uniform and reproducible cutoff values to define susceptibility.

A prospective study recently evaluated the role of baseline phenotypic drug susceptibility testing in 76 consecutive patients who initiated dual PI therapy with RTV/SQV either alone or in combination with other ART agents (95). Resistance to 10 different drugs was assessed by both phenotype (Virco Antiviogram) and genotype (Vircogen). Resistance inferred from viral genotype was similar to measured phenotypic resistance to both RTV and SQV ($p < 0.01$). Baseline phenotypic drug resistance predicted poor virologic response to dual PI (RTV/SQV)-based regimen; patients were at least four times less likely to achieve a 0.5 $\log_{10}$ decrease in HIV RNA levels if their viral isolates were deemed resistant to SQV or RTV. Patients resistant to both drugs never attained HIV RNA levels $< 10,000$ copies/mL. Patients whose isolates were resistant to either drug sustained median decrease in viral load of 0.05 $\log_{10}$ copies/mL or less, compared with >0.8 $\log_{10}$ copies/mL decline observed in patients with sensitive virus. These data suggest that baseline phenotypic resistance testing may be useful in identifying patients who are less likely to respond to this dual PI combination because even a fourfold reduction in susceptibility to either PI agent was associated with a marginal virologic response.

C. Role of Resistance Testing in Newly HIV-Infected Patients with Resistance Mutations

Although the frequency of transmission of drug resistant strains to newly HIV-infected patients is currently not well defined, therapeutic options for treatment-naive patients may be severely compromised in patients harboring baseline isolates resistant to several classes of antiretroviral drugs. Transmission to newly infected individuals of HIV-1 variants containing multiple mutations that conferred resistance to both PIs and reverse transcriptase inhibitors has been documented (96).

Yerly et al. (97) reported on the frequency of transmission of drug-resistant HIV-1 variants to 82 consecutive individuals with documented primary infection referred to the Geneva AIDS Center between January 1996 and July 1998. ZDV-resistance baseline genotypic mutations were detected in 7 (9%) of 82 patients. Genotypic mutations associated with resistance to other RTIs were identified in two patients. Primary resistance mutations associated with PI agents (V82A, L90M) were detected in 3 (4%) of 70 patients; 2 of these patients also had reverse transcriptase mutations. Diminished sensitivity to three of four PIs was documented in three patients; the virus isolate from one patient harbored 12 mutations that conferred resistance to multiple NRTIs and PIs.

The prevalence of HIV-1 drug resistance mutations in isolates obtained from 80 newly infected individuals (95% homosexual males) identified in the New York metropolitan area (81%) and Los Angeles (14%) was determined by Boden et al. (98). Baseline plasma samples were collected between July 1995 and April 1999; plasma was tested by direct sequencing of three reverse transcriptase-polymerase chain reaction (RT-PCR) reactions. Drug-associated resistance mutations were identified for ZDV (7.5%), 3TC (5.0%), NNRTIs (7.5%), and PIs (2.5%). Multidrug-resistant virus was identified in three (3.8%) patients. Extensive protease gene polymorphism was seen at residues 63 (60.0%), 93 (35%), 10 (17.5%), and 36 (5.0%). Phenotypic testing was performed on 38 samples: Concordance between genotypic and phenotypic data was 100% for resistant genotypes and 87.8% for nonresistant genotypes. The overall prevalence of resistant genotypes to any antiretroviral agent was 17.5%; the prevalence increased to 22.5% for virus with either genotypic or phenotypic resistance.

These studies confirm that baseline resistance testing may warrant an expanded role, especially in endemic areas with extensively treated HIV-infected individuals and increased potential for transmission of drug resistant HIV variants in the management of newly infected individuals with primary HIV-infection before selecting initial antiretroviral combination therapy.

IX. STRUCTURED TREATMENT INTERRUPTIONS

In selected patients who have experienced recurrent virologic failure after receiving multiple combination regimens and for whom there are no readily available new ART agents for salvage therapy, short-term structured treatment interruptions have been investigated in several small pilot trials. The exact scientific rationale for using this strategy is not yet well defined, but it is proposed that the increased viral replication resulting from such ART drug interruptions may potentiate and enhance HIV-specific CD4 and CD8 associated immune responses, thereby limiting viral replication. Treatment interruptions, in effect, remove ongoing selective drug pressure and consequently may permit circulating drug resistant virus to revert to wild-type. Reintroducing ART combination therapy at a later time point (weeks to months post-treatment interruption), which is directed presumably at exclusively wild-type virus, may afford sustained viral suppression. The major obstacle confronting this treatment strategy is that achieving potent suppression of residual resistant virus (which may persist indefinitely at low levels in lymphoreticular compartments or may exist in an integrated provirus form in a reservoir of resting CD4 cells) may not be feasible with the scheduled reintroduction of ART.

Miller et al. (99) investigated the impact of a structured treatment interruption before initiating mega-HAART (using at least six drugs in combination) salvage therapy on treatment response in 94 patients who had virologic failure on PI-containing regimens. CD4 cell count changes and viral load responses were analyzed in 50 patients during treatment interruptions in addition to evaluating changes in viral susceptibility and response to subsequent salvage therapy. At a median follow-up of 12 months mega-HAART therapy afforded a maximum viral load decline of 2.7 $\log_{10}$ copies/mL. Baseline drug susceptibility was associated with virologic response (HIV RNA < 500 copies/mL). Sixty-seven percent of responders had viral populations that were sensitive to at least four drugs in the salvage regimen; 70% of patients failing (never achieving HIV RNA < 500 copies/mL) mega-HAART therapy had viral populations that were sensitive to a maximum of three drugs in the regimen. The responders all experienced a shift to wild-type virus during the prior structured treatment interruption. During the treatment interruption, viral load increased by a median of 0.71 $\log_{10}$ copies/mL and CD4 cell counts decreased by a median of 89 cells/mm^3. Resistance analyses before and after the drug holidays were available for a subset of patients ($n = 39$). A shift to wild-type was observed in 26 of 39 patients. Mega-HAART salvage therapy (three to eight drugs in combination) resulted in a median viral load decrease of 2.9 $\log_{10}$ copies/mL at week 8 for the 26 patients who experienced a shift to wild-type compare with a 0.78 $\log_{10}$ copies/mL decrease in patients (13/39) without a shift to wild-type after treatment interruption. Nineteen of 24 patients with a shift to wild type achieved viral load suppression (HIV RNA < 500 copies/mL) within 24 weeks of resuming salvage treatment compared with 1 of 9 patients in whom a shift to wild-type did not occur.

These data suggest that treatment interruptions in selected patients with virologic failure may allow the predominant virus to shift to wild-type and thereby confer more potent viral suppression upon resuming alternative salvage therapy. CD4 cell counts need to be followed with frequent monitoring because CD4 count declines have been uniformly observed in patients undergoing treatment interruption that may render some patients at increased risk for opportunistic infections. Identifying patients with treatment failure who will derive clinical benefit and improved virologic responses after treatment interruption is not yet defined nor has the optimal duration of treatment interruption been determined.

The treatment strategy of drug interruption merits larger scale controlled clinical trials to better assess whether it enhances durable virologic response in patients failing multiple regimens.

X. MULTIDRUG RESCUE REGIMENS

The optimal approach to managing virologic failure in patients who have developed resistance to all three classes of ART agents or who have experienced recurrent viral rebound on sequential combination regimens has not yet been defined. Multidrug rescue therapy (MDRT) has been investigated in small pilot trials as an alternative approach to managing treatment failure.

The underlying premise of this approach is that although virus may exhibit resistance to several drugs concurrently, each virion is unlikely to be simultaneously resistant to six to nine drugs administered as part of a mega-HAART regimen or MDRT.

Montaner et al. (100, 101) recently reported the results derived from two such patient cohorts treated with MDRT. The initial study evaluated a cohort of 82 failure patients with median baseline viral load and CD4 count of 50,000 copies/mL and 185 cells/mm^3, respectively, who received MDRT that consisted of up to four NRTIs, two PIs, two NNRTIs, and hydroxyurea (up to nine drugs) (100). Median prior ART exposure was seven drugs for 45 months. In an ITT analysis, 56% ($n = 82$), 46% ($n = 80$), 33% ($n = 78$), 23% ($n = 74$), and 16% ($n = 570$) of patients achieved viral load < 400 copies/mL on one, two, three, four, and five consecutive occasions. Of 44 patients, 45% remained suppressed with HIV RNA < 400 copies/mL through median follow-up of 30 weeks. Phenotypic analyses at baseline were available for 60 patients; multivariate analyses demonstrated that sensitivity to three or more drugs in the multidrug rescue regimen ($p = 0.088$) and a low baseline plasma viral load ($p = 0.005$) were predictive of a more favorable virologic outcome.

The second cohort of 67 patients with median baseline HIV RNA and CD4 count of 52,000 copies/mL and 210 cells/mm^3, respectively, who experienced prior virologic failure were enrolled into the MDRT observational trial between June 1998 and December 1998 (101). Median prior ART exposure was seven drugs for 32 months. MDRT regimens consisted of up to nine drugs in combination similar to those featured in the initial cohort. On an ITT analysis, 63% ($n = 67$), 50% ($n = 58$), and 34% ($n = 38$) of patients achieved HIV RNA < 400 copies/mL in one, two, and three consecutive determinations, respectively. Overall, 16% of patients experienced severe adverse events while receiving this MDRT regimen, and 34% of patients had the regimen revised due to side effects. Sixty percent of patients in the second cohort achieved viral load < 400 copies/mL compared with 35% of patients attaining virologic response in the earlier cohort. This observed difference in virologic outcome may in part be due to the fact that more NNRTI agents and a greater number of active drugs were introduced in the MDRT regimens in the second cohort.

A. Dual PI (RTV/IDV) Therapy plus EFV and ddI/Hydroxyurea

Youle et al. (102) evaluated multidrug salvage therapy in 63 patients with virologic failure (>50,000 copies/mL) that developed while receiving a PI-containing regimen for >6 months. The multidrug combination (five to seven drugs) regimen featured a backbone of hydroxyurea, ddI, RTV, and IDV initiated after a median treatment interruption of 8 weeks. Baseline median viral load and CD4 count were 4.8 $\log_{10}$ copies/mL and 128 cells/mm^3, respectively. During the study, 36 subjects revised the regimen largely due to central nervous system toxicity; 13 permanently discontinued study treatment. At week 28, patients sustained a median decrease in plasma viral load of 3.08 $\log_{10}$ copies/mL and had a median rise in CD4 cell count of 120 cells/mm^3. Ninety-one and a half percent of patients who completed week 28 achieved HIV RNA < 400 copies/mL. Lower baseline viral load and longer duration of treatment interruption before multidrug salvage therapy were associated with improved virologic response; patients were 40% less likely to achieve viral suppression with each $\log_{10}$ higher baseline HIV RNA and 15% more likely for every month of treatment break before baseline. These results suggest that salvage will be more effective if started at lower viral load levels and that treatment interruption enhances the short-term virologic response to multidrug salvage therapy.

B. Achieving Viral Load Suppression < 20 copies/mL on Mega-HAART

An open-label observational study evaluated complex mega-HAART regimens in 35 extensively ART-treated patients (mean ART experience of 73 months; mean of nine drugs) with virologic failure (103). Genotyping was available for 21 of 35 patients before initiating mega-HAART. Complex regimens of six to eight drugs, including two or three NRTIs, one NNRTI, two PIs, and hydroxyurea, were administered for 15 months; no patient was lost to follow-up and one patient discontinued due to toxicity. Of the remaining 34 patients, 23 (68%) achieved HIV RNA < 500 copies/mL and 23 (68%) had at least two consecutive determinations of viral loads < 20 copies/mL; 13 (38%) patients have had viral loads < 20–40 copies/mL for more than 6 months. Patients generally tolerated these complex regimens that typically featured every 12 hour dosing schedules. These data indicate that complex multidrug regimens based on genotyping results can achieve impressive suppression of viral load in selected patients for up to >6 months.

XI. CONCLUSIONS

Salvage therapy strategies are rapidly evolving in response to more effective alternative regimens with the recent availability of new antiretroviral drugs that exhibit inherently more potent activity and improved formulations that have allowed more compact dosing schedules. There is, however, an increased recognition within the clinical arena that treatment failure rates on triple-drug PI-containing regimens have been frequently underreported such that a substantial number of extensively treated patients is emerging for whom therapeutic options remain severely limited. Renewed efforts at identifying such patients are underway to better define the reasons for failure and to develop prospective larger scale trials for evaluating different salvage strategies, including structured treatment interruptions and MDRT.

Clinical trial data from several pivotal studies have yielded further insights about devising salvage therapy with regard to predictors of response, the timing of when to switch to alternative therapy, and the optimal role of genotypic and phenotypic resistance testing. The role of intensification is also being explored in patients with early and low level viral rebound with a number of promising ART agents.

At present, clinical trial results suggest that multiple NRTI-exposed individuals with virologic failure may benefit from a salvage regimen of an NNRTI in combination with a new PI or dual PIs. The optimal sequencing of NRTI components and classes of ARTs in a failing regimen is not yet defined, but agents that exhibit uniform cross-resistance, such as the NNRTIs, should not be reintroduced in a salvage regimen unless resistance testing confirms susceptibility. Similarly, RTV should not be substituted in salvage regimen as the sole PI agent for a patient currently failing IDV due to the broad cross-resistance between these agents due to the V82A/F/T genotypic mutation.

Patients with treatment failure have an improved virologic response if salvage therapy is introduced at a lower viral load. There is accumulating evidence that baseline genotypic resistance testing, such as that derived from the GART and VIRADAPPT trials, and phenoptyic susceptibility testing, such as that recently conducted in a clinical cohort reported by Saag et al. (94), have a favorable impact on the magnitude and durability of viral load suppression in salvage-based therapies.

Many aspects of the management of treatment failure remain unanswered, but advances in key areas such as those outlined above are anticipated to translate into more effective therapeutic strategies in the future.

REFERENCES

1. Ho DD, Neumann AU, Perelson AS, ChenW, Leonard JM, Markowitz M. Rapid turnover of plasma virions and CD4 lymphocytes in HIV-1 infection. Nature 1995; 373:117–122.

2. Wei X, Ghosh SK, Taylor ME, Johnson VA, Emini EA, Deutsch P, Lifson JD, Bonhoerrer S, Nowak MA, Hahn BH, et al. Viral dynamics in human immunodeficiency virus type 1 infection. Nature 1995; 373:117–122.

3. Perelson AS, NeumannAU, Markowitz M, Leonard JM, Ho DD. HIV-1 dynamics *in vivo*: virion clearance rate, infected cell life-span, and viral generation time. Science 1996; 271:1582–1586.

4. Coffin JM. HIV population dynamics in vivo: implications for genetic variation, pathogenesis, and therapy. Science 1995; 267:483–489.

5. Pantaleo G, Graziosi C, Demarest J, Butini L, Montroni M, Fox CH, Orenstein JM, Kotler DP, Fauci AS. HIV infection is active and progressive in lymphoid tissue during the clinically latent stages of disease. Nature 1995; 362:355–358.

6. Havlir D, Richman D. Viral dynamics of HIV: implications for drug development and therapeutic strategies. Ann Intern Med 1996; 124:984–994.

7. Mellors JW, Rinaldo CR Jr, Gupta P, White RM, Todd JA, Kingsley LA. Prognosis in HIV-1 infection predicted by the quantity of virus in plasma. Science 1996; 272:1167–1170.

8. Coombs RW, Welles SL, Hooper C, Reichelderfer PS, D'Aquila RT, Japour AJ, Johnson VA, Kuritzkes DR, Richman DD, Kwok S, Todd J, Jackson JB, DeGruttola V, Crumpacker CS, Kahn J. Association of plasma human immunodeficiency virus type-1 RNA with risk of clinical progression in patients with advanced infection. J Infect Dis 1996; 174:704–712.

9. O'Brien WA, Hartigan PM, Martin D,Esinhart J, Hill A, Benoit S, Rubin M, Simberkoff MS, Hamilton JD. Changes in plasma HIV-1 RNA and CD4+ lymphocyte counts and the risk of progression to AIDS. N Engl J Med 1996; 334:426–431.

10. Welles SL, Jackson JB,Yen-Leiberman B, Demeter L, Japour AJ, Smeaton LM, Johnson VA, Kuritzkes DR, D'Aquila RT, Reichelderfer PA, Richman DD, Reichman R, Fischl M, Dolin R, Coombs RW, Kahn JO, McLaren C, Todd J, Kwok S, Crumpacker CS. Prognostic value of plasma human immunodeficiency virus (HIV-1) RNA levels in patients with advanced HIV-1 disease and with little or no prior zidovudine therapy. J Infect Dis 1996; 174:696–703.

11. Mellors JW, Kingsley LA, Rinaldo CR Jr, Todd JA, Hoo BS, Kokka RP, Gupta P. Quantitation of HIV-1 RNA in plasma predicts outcome after seroconversion. Ann Intern Med 1995; 122:573–579.

12. Phillips AN, Eron JJ, Bartlett JA, Rubin M, Johnson J, Price S, Self P, Hill AM. HIV-1 RNA levels and the development of clinical disease. AIDS 1996; 10:859–865.

13. Perelson AS, Essunger P, Cao Y, Vesannen M, Hurley A, Saksela K, Markowitz M, Ho DD. Decay characteristics of HIV-1 infected compartments during combination therapy. Nature 1997; 387:188–191.

14. Chun TW, Carruth L, Finzi D, Shen X, Di Giuseppe JA, Taylor H, Hermankova M, Chadwick K, Margolick J, Quinn TC, Kuo YH, Brookmeyer R, Zeiger MA, Barditch-Crovo P, Silicano RF. Quantitation of latent tissue reservoirs and total body viral load in HIV-1 infection. Nature 1997; 387:183–188.

15. Mellors JW, Munoz A, Giorgi JV, Margolick JB, Tassoni CJ, Gupta P, Kingsley LA, Todd JA, Saah AJ, Detels R, Phair JP, Rinaldo CR Jr. Plasma viral load and CD4+ lymphocytes as prognostic markers of HIV-1 infection. Ann Intern Med 1997; 126:946–954.

16. Carpenter CC, Fischl MA, Hammer SM, Hirsch MS, Jacobsen DM, Katzenstein DA, Montaner JSG, Richman DD, Saag MS, Schooley RT, Thompson MA, Vella S, Yeni PG, Volberding PA. Antiretroviral therapy for HIV infection in 1998: updated recommendations of the international AIDS Society—USA Panel. JAMA 1998; 280:78–86.

17. Centers for Disease Control and Prevention. Report of the NIH panel to define pronciples of therapy of HIV infection and guidelines for the use of antiretroviral agents in HIV adults and adolescents. MMWR Morb Mortal Wkly Rep 1998; 47 (RR-5):43–82.

18. Gulick RM, Mellors JW, Havlir D, Eron J, Gonzalez C, McMahon D, Richman DD, Valentine FT, Jonas L, Meibohm A, Emini E, Chodakewitz JA. Treatment with indinavir, zidovudine, and lamivudine in adults with human immunodeficiency virus infection and prior antiretroviral therapy. N Engl J Med 1997; 337:734–739.

19. Hammer SH, Squires KE, Hughes MD, Grimes JM, Demeter LM, Currier JS, Eron JJ, Feinberg JE, Balfour HH, Deyton LR, Chodakewitz JA, Fischl MA. A controlled trial of two nucleoside analogues plus indinavir in persons with human immunodeficiency virus infection and CD4 cell counts of 200 per cubic millimeter or less. N Engl J Med 1997; 337:725–733.

20. Montaner JSG, Reiss P, Cooper D, Vella S, Harris M, Conway B, Wainberg MA, Smith D, Robinson P, Hall D, Myers M, Lange JA. A randomized, double-blind trial comparing combinations of nevirapine, didanosine, and zidovudine for HIV-infected patients. JAMA 1998; 279:930–937.

21. Palella FJ, Delaney KM, Moorman AC, Loveless MO, Fuher J, Satten GA, Aschman DJ, Holmberg SD. Declining morbidity and mortality among patients with advanced human immunodeficiency virus infection. N Engl J Med 1998; 338:853–860.

22. Hogg RS, Heath KV, Yip B, Craib KJP, O' Shaugnessy MV, Schecter MT, Montaner JSG. Improved survival among HIV-infected individuals following initiation of antiretroviral therapy. JAMA 1998; 279:450–454.

23. Brodt HR, Kamps BS, Gute P, Knupp B, Staszewski S, Helm EB. Changing incidence of AIDS-defining illnesses in the era of antiretroviral combination therapy. AIDS 1997; 11:1731–1738.

24. Mocroft A, Vella S, Benfield TL, Chiesi A, Miller V, Gargalianos P, d'Arminio Monforte A, Yust I, Bruun JN, Phillips AN, Lundgren JD. Changing patterns of mortality across Europe in patients infected with HIV-1. Lancet 1998; 352:1725–1730.

25. Gulick RM, Mellors JW, Havlir D, Eron JJ, Gonzalez C, McMahon D, Jonas L, Meibohm, A, Holder D, Schlief WA, Condra JH, Emini E, Isaacs R, Chodakewitz JA, Richman DD. Simultaneous vs sequential initiation of therapy with indinavir, zidovudine, and lamivudine for HIV-1 infection. JAMA 1998; 280: 35–41.

26. Ledergerber B, Egger M, Opravil M, Telenti A, Hirschel B, Battegay M, Vernazza P, Sudre P, Flepp, Furrer H, Francioli P, Weber R. Clinical progression and virologic failure on highly active antiretroviral therapy in HIV-1 patients: a prospective cohort study. Lancet 1999; 353:863–868.

27. Hirsch M, Steibigel R, Staszewski S, Mellors J, Scerpella E, Hirschel B, Lange J, Squires K, Rawlins S, Meibohm A. A randomized, controlled trial of indinavir, zidovudine, and lamivudine in adults with advanced human immunodeficiency virus type 1 infection and prior antiretroviral therapy. J Infect Dis 1999: 180:659–665.

28. Singh N, Squier C, Wagener M, Nguyen MH, Yu VL. Determinants of compliance with antiretroviral therapy in patients with human immunodeficiency virus: prospective assessment with implications for enhancing compliance. AIDS Care 1996; 8:261–269.

29. Duong M, Piroth L, Forte F, Peytavin G, Benatru I, Rouaud O, Buisson M, Grappin M, Chavanet P, Portier H. Serum protease inhibitor level as marker of adherence to HAART: correlation with self-reported adherence and with HIV RNA. In: Program and abstracts of the 39th Interscience Conference on Antimicrobial Agents and Chemotherapy, September 26–29, 1999, San Francisco, CA. Abstract No. 2069.

30. Breilh D, Pellegrin I, Deneyrolles M, Birac V, Mercie P, Neau D, Masquelier B, Saux M, Fleury H, Pellegrin J. Impact of individual pharmacokinetic parameters and drug resistance mutations on virologic response to ritonavir-saquinavir containing regimens. In: Program and abstracts of the 39th Interscience Conference on Antimicrobial Agents and Chemotherapy, September 26–29, 1999, San Francisco, CA. Abstract No. 2192.

31. Merry C, Barry MG, Mulcahy F, Ryan M, Heavey J, Tija JF, Gibbons SE, Breckenridge AM, Back DJ. Saquinavir pharmacokinetics alone and in combination with ritonavir in HIV-infected patients. AIDS 1997; 11:F29–F33.

32. Sommadossi JP, Zhou XJ, Moore J, Havlir D, Friedland G, Tierney C, Smeaton L, Fox L, Richman D, Pollard R. Impairment of stavudine (d4T) phosphorylation in patients receiving a combination of zidovudine (ZDV) and d4T (ACTG

290). In: Program and abstracts of the 5th Conference on Retroviruses and Opportunistic Infections, February 1–5, 1998, Chicago, IL. Abstract No. 3.

33. Larder B, Kemp SD. Multiple mutations in HIV-1 reverse transcriptase confer high-level resistance to zidovudine (AZT). Science 1989; 246:1155–1158.

34. Richman DD. Drug resistance and its implications in the management of HIV infection. Antiviral Ther 1997; 2(suppl 4):41–58.

35. D'Aquila RT, Johnson VA, Welles SL, Japour AJ, Kuritzkes DR, DeGruttola V, Reichelderfer PS, Coombs RW, Crumpacker CS, Kahn JO, et al. Zidovudine resistance and HIV-1 disease progression during antiretroviral therapy. Ann Intern Med 1995; 122:401–408.

36. St Clair MH, Martin JL, Tudor-Williams G, Bach MC, Vavro CL, King DM, Kellam P, Kemp SD, Larder BA. Resistance to ddI and sensitivity to AZT induced by a mutation in HIV-1 reverse transcriptase. Science 1991; 253:1557–1559.

37. Larder B, Kemp SD, Harrigan PR. Potential mechanism of sustained antiretroviral efficacy of AZT-3TC combination therapy. Science 1995; 269:696–699.

38. Tisdale M, Myers RE, Maschera B, Parry NR, Oliver NM, Blair ED. Cross-resistance analysis of human immunodeficiency virus type 1 variants individually selected for resistance to five different protease inhibitors. Antimicrob Agents Chemother 1995; 39:1704–1710.

39. Ives KJ, Jacobsen H, Galpin SA, Garaev MM, Dorrell L, Mous J, Bragmen K, Weber JN. Emergence of resistant variants of HIV in vivo during monotherapy with the proteinase inhibitor saquinavir. J Antimicrob Chemother. 1997; 39:771–779.

40. Molla A, Korneyeva M, Gao Q, Vasavanonda S, Schipper PJ, Mo HM, Markowitz M, Chernavskiy T, Niu P, Lyons N, Hsu A, Granneman GR, Ho DD, Boucher CA, Leonard JM, Norbeck DW, Kempf DJ. Ordered accumulation for mutation in HIV protease confers resistance to ritonavir. Nature Med 1996; 2:760–766.

41. Condra JH, Schleif WA, Blahy OM, Gabryelski LJ, Graham DJ, Quintero JC, Rhodes A, Robbins HL, Roth E, Shivaprakash M, et al. In vivo emergence of HIV-1 variants resistant to multiple protease inhibitors. Nature 1995; 374:569–571.

42. Vasudevachari MB, Zhang YM, Imamichi H, Imamichi T, Falloon J, Salzman NP. Emergence of protease inhibitor resistance mutations in human immunodeficiency virus type 1 isolates from patients and rapid screening procedure for their detection. Antimicrob Agents Chemother 1996; 40:2535–2541.

43. Condra JH, Holder DJ, Schleif WA, Blahy OM, Danovich RM, Gabryelski LJ, Graham DJ, Laird D, quintero JC, Rhodes A, Robbins HL, Roth E, Shivaprakash M, Yang T, Chodakewitz JA, Deutsch PJ, Leavitt RY, Massari FE,

Mellors JW, Squires KE, Steigbigel RT, Teppler H, Emini EA. Genetic correlates of in vivo resistance to indinavir, ahuman immunodeficiecny virus type 1
protease inhibitor. J Virol 1996; 70:8270–8276.

44. Hirsch MS, Conway B, D'Aquila RT, Johnson VA, Brun-Venizet F, Clotet B,
    Demeter L, Hammer SM, Jacobsen DM, Kuritzkes DR, Loveday C, Mellors
    JW, Vella S, Richman DD. Antiretroviral drug resistance testing in adults with
    HIV infection: implications for clinical management. JAMA 1998; 279:1984–
    1991.

45. Fatkenheuer G, Theisen A, Rockstroh J, Grabow T, Wicke C, Becker K,
    Wieland U, Pfister H, Reiser M, Hegener P, Franzen C, Schwenk A, Salzberger
    B. Virological treatment failure of protease inhibitor therapy in an unselected
    cohort of HIV-infected patients. AIDS 1997; 11:F113–F116.

46. Kempf DJ, Rode Ra, Xu Y, Sun E, Heath-Chiozzi ME, Valdes J, Japour AJ,
    Danner S, Boucher C, Molla A, Leonard JM. The duration of viral suppression
    during protease inhibitor therapy for HIV-1 infection is predicted by plasma
    HIV-1 RNA at the nadir. AIDS 1998; 12:F09–F14.

47. Wong JK, Gunthard HF, Havlir DV, Zhang ZQ, HaaseAT, Ignacio CC, Kwok
    S, Emini E, Richman DD. Reduction of HIV-1 in blood and lymph nodes
    following potent antiretroviral therapy and the virologic correlates of treatment
    failure. Proc Natl Acad Sci USA 1997; 94:12574–12579.

48. Raboud JM, Montaner JSG, Conway B, Rae S, Reiss P, Vella S, Cooper D,
    Lange J, Harris M, Wainberg MA, Robinson P, Myers M, Hall D. Suppression
    of plasma viral load below 20 copies/ml is required to achieve a long-term
    response to therapy. AIDS 1998; 12:1619–1624.

49. Natarajan V, Bosche M, Metcalf JA, Ward DJ, Lane HC, Kovacs JA. HIV-1
    replication in patients with plasma virus receiving HAART. Lancet 1999; 353:
    119–120.

50. Ruiz L, van Lunzen J, Arno A, Stellbrink HJ, Schneider C, Rull M, Castella
    E, Ojanguren I, Richman DD, Clotet B, Tenner- Racz K, Racz P. Protease
    inhibitor-containing regimens compared with nucleoside analogues alone in
    the suppression of persistent HIV-1 replication in lymphoid tissue. AIDS 1999;
    13:F1–F8.

51. Furtado MR, Callaway DS, Phair JP, Kuntsman KJ, Stanton JL, Macken CA,
    Perelson AS, Wolinsky SM. Persistence of HIV-1 trascription in peripheral
    blood mononuclear cells in patients receiving potent antiretroviral therapy. N
    Engl J Med 1991; 340:1614–1622.

52. Zhang L, Ramratnam B, Tenner- Racz K, He Y, Vesanen M, Lewin S, Talal
    A, Racz P, Perelson AS, Korber BT, Markowitz M, HoDD, Yong G, Duran M,
    Hurley A, tsay J, Huang YC, Wang CC. Quantifying residual HIV-1 replication
    in patients receiving combination antiretroviral therapy. N Engl J Med 1999;
    340:1605–1613.

53. Deeks SG, Hecht FM, Swanson M, Elbeik t, Loftu R, Cohen PT, Grant RM. HIV RNA and CD4 cell count response to protease inhibitor therapy in an urban AIDs clinic: response to both initial and salvage therapy. AIDS 1998; 13:F35–F44.

54. Tebas P, Patick AK, Kane EM, Klebert MK, Simpson JH, Erice A, Powderly WG, Henry K. Virologic responses to ritonavir-saquinavir containing regimen in patients who had previously failed nelfinavir. AIDS 1999; 13:F23–F28.

55. Kaufmann D, Pantaleo G, Sudre P, Telenti A, for the Swiss Cohort Study. CD4 cell count in HIV-1 infected individuals remaining viraemic with highly active antiretroviral therapy (HAART). Lancet 1998; 351:90.

56. Hammer SM, Yeni P. Antiretroviral therapy: where are we? AIDS 1998; 12(suppl A):S181–S188.

57. Staszewski S, Morales-Ramirez JO, Godofsky EW, Stryker R, Tashima K, Farina DR, Manion DJ, Ruiz NM. Longer time to treatment failure and durability of response with efavirenz+ZDV+3TC: first analysis of full 1266 patient cohort from study 006. In: Program and abstracts of the 39th Interscience Conference on Antimicrobial Agents and Chemotherapy, September 26–29, 1999, San Francisco, CA. Abstract No. 507.

58. Staszewski S, Keiser P, Gathe J, Haas D, Montaner J, Johnson M, Delfraissy JF, Cutrell A, Lafon S, Thorborn D, Pearce G, Spreen W, Tortell S. Comparison of antiviral response with abacavir/combivir to indinavir/combivir in therapy-naive adults at 48 weeks (CNA3005). In: Program and abstracts of the 39th Interscience Conference on Antimicrobial Agents and Chemotherapy, September 26–29, 1999, San Francisco, CA. Abstract No. 505.

59. Para MF, Collier A, Coombs R, Glidden D, Bassett R, Duff F, Leavitt RY, Pettinelli C. ACTG 333: antiviral effects of switching from saquinavir hard gel capsule (SQVhgc) to soft gelatin capsule (SQVsgc) vs switching to indinavir (IDV) after prior saquinavir. In: Program and abstracts of the Infectious Disease Society of America 35th Annual Meeting, September 13–16, 1997, San Francisco, CA. Abstract No 21.

60. Hammer S, Squires K, Degrutttola V, Fischl M, Bassett R, Demeter L, Hertogs K, Larder B. Randomized trial of abacavir (ABC) and nelfinavir (NFV) in combination with efavirenz (EFV) and adefovir dipivoxil (ADV) as salvage therapy in patients with virologic afilure receiving indinavir (IDV). In: Program and abstracts of the 6th Conference on Retroviruses and Opportunistic Infections, January 31–February 4, 1999, Chicago, IL. Abstract No 490.

61. AIT-Khaled M, Rakik A, Thomas D, Tisdale M, Falloon J. HIV-1 baseline genotype/phenotype and virological response following salvage therapy with ziagen (abacavir, ABC), amprenavir (APV), and sustiva (efavirenz, EFV). In: Program and abstracts of the 6th Conference on Retroviruses and Opportunistic Infections, January 31–February 4, 1999, Chicago, IL. Abstract No. 133.

62. Zolopa A, Tebas P, Gallant J, Keiser P, Sension M, Smith P, Gathe J, Flamm J, Hawkins T, Nadler J, Shafer R, Henry K. The efficacy of ritonavir (RTV)/ saquinavir (SQV) antiretroviral therapy (ART) in patients who failed nelfinavir (NFV): a multicenter clinical cohort. In: Program and abstracts of the 39th Interscience Conference on Antimicrobial Agents and Chemotherapy, September 26–29, 1999, San Francisco, CA. Abstract No. 2065.

63. Deeks SG, Grant RM, Beatty GW, Horton C, Detmer J, Eastman S. Activity of a ritonavir plus saquinavir-containing regimen in patients with evidence of indinavir or ritonavir failure. AIDS 1998; 12:F97–F102.

64. Duval X, Le Moing V, Pettavin G, Ecobichon JL, Damond F, Descamps D, Leport C, Vilde JL. Nelfinavir (NFV)-saquinavir (SQV)-efavirenz (EFV) association as part of antiretroviral therapy in protease inhibitor (PI) experienced HIV infected patients (Pts). In: Program and abstracts of the 39th Interscience Conference on Antimicrobial Agents and Chemotherapy, September 26–29, 1999, San Francisco, CA. Abstract No. 2205.

65. Gulick RM, Katzenstein D, Hu J, Fiscus S, Fletcher CV, Haubrich R, Cheng H Lagakos S, Acosta E, Swanstrom R, Mills C, Snyder S, Fischl M, Pettinelli C. Salvage therapy with saquinavir soft gel capsules in combination with ritonavir or nelfinavir and delavirdine, adefovir dipivoxil, or both: ACTG 359. In: Program and abstracts of the 2nd International Workshop on Salvage Therapy for HIV Infection, May 19–21, 1999, Toronto, Canada. Abstract No. 020.

66. Acosta EP, Gulick R, Katzenstein D, Haubrich R, Fischl M, Raasch R, Mills C, Pettinelli C, Remmel RP, Fletcher CV. Pharmacokinetic (PK) evaluation of saquinavir soft gel capsules (SQV/ritonavir (RTV) or SQV/nelfinavir (NFV) in combination with delavirdine (DLV) and/or adefovir dipivoxil (ADV). In: Program and abstracts of the 6th Conference on Retroviruses and Opportunistic Infections, January 31–February 4, 1999, Chicago, IL. Abstract No.365.

67. Workman C, Musson R, Dyer W, Sullivan J. Novel double protease combinations-combining indinavir (IDV) with ritonavir (RTV): results from first study. In: Program and abstracts of the 12th World AIDS Conference, June 28–July 3, 1998, Geneva. Abstract No. 22372.

68. O'Brien WA, Atkinson TA, Han X, Sova M, East J. Combination therapy with indinavir and ritonavir in antiretroviral-experienced patients. In: Program and abstracts of the 39th Interscience on Antimicrobial Agents and Chemotherapy, September 26–29, 1999, San Francisco, CA. Abstract No. 2209.

69. Eron J, King M, Xu Y, Brun S, Real K, Murphy R, Gulick R, Glesby M, Hicks C, Benson C, Thompson M, Thommes J, Kessler H, Deeks S, Wheeler D, White C, Sryker R, Feinberg J, Albrecht M,Pax P, Riddler S, Hsu A, Bertz R, Molla A, Mo H, Kempf D, Japour A, Sun E. ABT-378/ritoanvir (ABT-378/r) suppresses HIV RNA to < 400 copies/mL in 95% of treatment-naive patients and in 78% of PI-experienced patients at 36 weeks. In: Program and abstracts

of the 39th Interscience of Antimicrobial Agents and Chemotherapy, September 26–29, 1999, San Francisco, CA. Abstract No. LB-20.

70. Feinberg MB, Carpenter C, Fauci AS, Stanley SK, Cohen O, Bartlett JG, Kaplan JE, Abrutyn E. Report of the NIH Panel to define principles of therapy of HIV infection. Ann Intern Med 1998; 12:157–1078.

71. Descamps D, Pettavin G, Calvez V, Flandre P, Meiffredy V, Raffi F, Pialoux G, Aboulker JP, Brun-Vezinet F. Virologic failure, resistance, and plasma drug measurements in induction maintenance therapy trial (Anrs 072, Trilege). In: Program and abstracts of the 6th Conference on Retroviruses and Opportunistic Infections, January 31–February 4, 1999, Chicago, IL. Abstract No. 493.

72. Havlir DV, Marschner IC, Hirsch MS, Collier AC, Tebas P, Bassett RL, Ioannidis JPA, Holohan MK, Leavitt R, Boone G, Richman DD. Mainteance antiretroviral therapies in HIV-infected subjects with undetectable plasma HIV RNA after triple-drug therapy. N Engl J Med 1998; 339:1261–1268.

73. Havlir D, Hellman N, Petropoulos C, Whitcomb JM, Collier AC, Hirsch MS, Tebas P, Sommadossi JP, Richman DD. Drug susceptibility in HIV-infection after viral rebound in patients receiving indinavir-containing regimens. JAMA 2000; 283:229–234.

74. Rockstroh J, Clotet B, Katlama C, Purdon S, Cutrell A, Stone C, Ait-Khaled A. The role of abacavir (ABC, 1592) in antiretroviral therapy-experienced patients: preliminary 48 weeks results from a randomized double-blind trial. In: Program and abstracts of the 39th Interscience Conference on Antimicrobial Agents and Chemotherapy, September 26–29, 1999, San Francisco, CA. Abstract No. 1974.

75. Mocroft A, Gill JM, Davidson W, Phillips AN. Predictors of a viral response and subsequent virological treatment failure in patients with HIV starting a protease inhibitor. AIDS 1998; 12:2161–2167.

76. Powderly WG, Saag MS, Chapman S, Yu G, Quart B, Clendeninn NJ. Predictors of optimal virological response to potent antiretrovial therapy. AIDS 1999; 13:1873–1880.

77. Casado JL, Perez-Elias MJ, Antela A, Sabido R, Martibelda P, Drinda F, Blazquez J, Quereda C. Predictors of long-term response to protease inhibitor therapy in a cohort of HIV-infected patients. AIDS 1998; 12:131–134.

78. Miller V, Staszewski S, Sabin C, Rottman C, Lepri Cozzi A, Hill A, Phillips AN. CD4 lymphocyte count as a predictor of the duration of HAART-induced suppression of HIV-1 virus load. In: Program and abstracts of the 2nd International Workshop on Salvage Therapy for HIV Infection, May 19–21, 1999, Toronto, Canada. Abstract No. 010.

79. Phillips A, Mocroft A, Gatell JM, Van Lunzen J, Lazzarin A, Lundgren J. Virological and clinical response to second line protease inhibitor-containing regimens. In: Program and abstracts of the 39th interscience Conference on An-

timicrobial Agents and Chemotherapy, September 26–29, 1999, San Francisco, CA. Abstract No. 2066.

80. Paredes R, Puig T, Arno A, Negredo E, Balague M, Bonjoch A, Tural C, Sirera G, Veny A, Romeu J, Ruiz L, Clotet B. High-dose saquinavir plus ritonavir-containing HAART salvage therapy: long term efficacy in protease inhibitor-experienced patients and predictors of virological response. In: Program and abstracts of the 2nd International Workshop on Salvage Therapy for HIV Infection, May 19–21, 1999, Toronto, Canada. Abstract No. 007.

81. D'Arminio Montforte A, Testa L, Adorni F, Chiesa E, Bibi T, Moscatelli GC, Abeli C, Rusconi S, Sollima S, Balotta C, Musicco M, Galli M, Moroni M. Clinical outcome and predictive factors of failure of highly active antiretroviral therapy in antiretroviral-experienced patients in advanced stages of HIV-1 infection. AIDS 1998; 12:1631–1637.

82. Lorenzi P, Opravil M, Hirschel B Chave JP, Furrer HJ, Sax H, Perneger TV, Perin L, Kaiser L, Yerly S. Impact of drug resistance mutations on vriologic response to salvage therapy. Swiss HIV Cohort Study. AIDS 1999; 13:F17–F21.

83. Lanier ER, Scott J, Steel H, Hetherington S, Ait-Khaled M, Pearce G, Spreen W, Lafon S. Multivariate analysis of response to abacavir: comparison of prior antiretroviral therapy, baseline HIV RNA, CD4 count and viral resistance. Antiviral Ther 1999; 4(suppl 1):56. Abstract No. 82.

84. Piketty C, Race E, Castiel P, Belec L, Peytavin G, Si-Mohammed A, Gonzalez-Canali G, Weiss L, Clavel F, Kazatchkine MD. Efficacy of a five-drug combination including ritonavir, saquinavir, and efavirenz in patients who failed on a conventional triple-drug regimen: phenotypic resistance to protease inhibitors predicts outcome of therapy. AIDS 1999; 13:F71–F77.

85. Picketty C, Race E, Castiel P, Belec L, Peytavin G, Si-Mohamed A, Gonzalez-Canali G, Weiss L, Clavel F, Kazatchkine MD. Phenotypic resistance to protease inhibitors predicts outcome of a five drug combination including ritonavir, saquinavir, and efavirenz in patients who failed on HAART. In: Program and abstracts of the 39th Interscience Conference on Antimicrobial Agents and Chemotherapy, September 26–29, 1999, San Francisco, CA. Abstract No. 2068.

86. Haubrich R, Kemper C, Witt M, Keiser P, Dube M, Forthal D, Currier J, Hwang J, Richman D, Hellman N, Heilek G, Lie Y, McCutchan JA. Differences in protease inhibitor (PI) phenotypic susceptibility after failure of the first PI-containing regimen. In: Program and abstracts of the 39th Interscience Conference on Antimicrobial Agents and Chemotherapy, September 26–29, 1999, San Francisco, CA. Abstract No. 1167.

87. Rodriguez-Rosado, R, Briones C, Soriano V. Introduction of HIV drug resistance testing in clinical practice. AIDS 1999; 13:1007–1014.

88. Erickson JW, Gulnik SV, Markowitz M. Protease inhibitors: resistance, cross-resistance, fitness and the choice of initial and salvage therapies. AIDS 1999; 13(suppl A):S189–S204.

89. Durant J, Clevenbergh P, Halfon P, Delgiudice P, Porsin S, Simonet P, Montagne N, Boucher CAB, Schapiro JM, Dellamonica P. Drug-resistance genotyping in HIV-1 therapy: the VIRADAPT randomised trial. Lancet 1999; 353:2195–2199.

90. Clevenbergh P, Durant J, Halfon P, del Giudice P, Simonet P, Montagne N, Schapiro JM, Boucher CAB, Dellamonica P. Persisting long-term benefit of antiretroviral genotypic guided treatment for HIV-infected patients failing HAART: the VIRADAPT study, week 48 follow-up. Antiviral Ther 1999; 4(suppl 1):42. Abstract No. 60.

91. Baxter JD, Mayers DL, Wentworth DN, Neaton JD, Merigan TC. Final results of CPCRA 046: a pilot study of antiretroviral management based on genotypic antiretroviral resistance testing (GART) in patients failing antiretroviral therapy. Antiviral Ther 1999; 4(suppl 1):43. Abstract No. 61.

92. Mayers DL, Baxter JD, Wentworth DN, Neaton JN, Merigan TC. The impact of drug resistance mutations in plasma virus of patients failing on protease inhibitor-containing HAART regimens on subsequent vriological response to the next HAART regimen: results of CRCRA 046 (GART). Antiviral Ther 1999; 4(suppl 1):51. Abstract No. 74.

93. Moyle G, Iverson JA, Basar A, Sabin CA, Gazzard BG. Predictors of virological response to salvage regimens in treatment-experienced patients. Antiviral Ther 1999; 4(suppl 1):53. Abstract No. 78.

94. Call S, Westfall A, Cloud G, Johnson V, Raper J, Stewart K, Hellman N, Saag M. Predictive value of HIV phenotypic susceptibility testing in a clinical cohort. In: Program and abstracts of the 39th Interscience Confernce on Antimicrobial Agents and Chemotherapy, September 26–29, 1999, San Francisco, CA. Abstract No. LB-17.

95. Harrigan PR, Hertogs K, Verbiest W, Pauwels R, Larder B, Kemp S, Bloor S, Yip B, Hogg R, Alexander C, Montaner JSG. Baseline HIV drug resistance profile predicts response to ritonavir-saquinavir protease inhibitor therapy in a community setting. AIDS 1999; 13:1863–1871.

96. Hecht FM, Grant RM, Petropoulos CJ, Dillon B, Chesney MA, Hellman NS, Bandrapalli NI, Branson B, Kahn JO. Sexual transmission of an HIV-1 variant resistant to multiple reverse-transcriptase and protease inhibitors. N Engl J Med 1998; 339:307–311.

97. Yerly S, Kaiser L, Race E, Bru J-P, Clavel F, Perrin L. Transmission of antiretroviral-drug resistant HIV-1 variants. Lancet 1999; 354:729–733.

98. Boden D, Hurley A, Zhamg L, Cao Y, Guo Y, Farthing C, Limoli K, Parkin N, Markowitz M. Prevalence of HIV-1 drug resistance mutations in 80 newly infected individuals. Antiviral Ther 1999; 4(suppl 1):85. Abstract No. 120.

99. Miller V, Rottman C, Hertogs K, Larder BA, Phillips AN, Cozzi-Lepri A, Sturmer M, Gute P, Staszewski S. Mega-HAART, resistance and drug holidays. In: Program and abstracts of the 2nd International Workshop on Salvage Therapy for HIV Infection, May 19–21, 1999, Toronto, Canada. Abstract No. 030.

100. Montaner JSG, Harrigan PR, Jahnke NA, Hogg RS, Ypi B, Harris M, Montessori V, O'Shaughnessy MV. Multidrug rescue therapy for HIV-infected individuals with prior virological failure to multiple regimens: results from an initial cohort. In: Program and abstracts of the 2nd International Workshop on Salvage Therapy for HIV Infection, May 19–21, 1999, Toronto, Canada. Abstract No. 015.

101. Montaner JSG, Harrigan PR, Jahnke NA, Hogg RS, Yip B, Harris M, Montessori V, O'Shaughnessy MV. Multidrug rescue therapy for HIV-infected individuals with prior virological failure to multiple regimens: results from a second cohort. In: Program and abstracts of the 2nd International Workshop on Salvage Therapy for HIV Infection, May 19–21, 1999, Toronto, Canada. Abstract No. 016.

102. Youle M, Mocroft A, Johnson M, Tyrer M, Madge S, Dykhoff A, Drinkwater A. Surrogate marker responses to multidrug combinations comprising hydroxyurea, efavirenz, double protease inhibitors (PI) and nucleoside analogues in PI failures. In: Program and abstracts of the 2nd International Workshop on Salvage Therapy for HIV Infection, May 19–21, 1999, Toronto, Canada. Abstract No. 018.

103. Grossman H, Frechette G, Reyes F. Mega-HAART: complex protective regimens for HAART failure. In: Program and abstracts of the 2nd International Workshop on Salvage Therapy for HIV Infection, May 19–21, 1999, Toronto, Canada. Abstract No. 023.

8

Drug Interactions of Antiretroviral Agents

Bradley W. Kosel and Francesca Aweeka
San Francisco General Hospital, University of California, San Francisco, San Francisco, California

I. OVERVIEW

The pillbox has become an infamous symbol for the complexity of treating human immunodeficiency virus type 1 (HIV-1). This mixture of capsules and tablets includes medications for HIV and prophylaxis for opportunistic infections. Highly active antiretroviral therapy (HAART) is currently the standard of care for HIV-1 and requires minimum administration of three antiretroviral (ARV) medications. Such combination therapy results in mortality rates reduced 4-fold and opportunistic infections decreased 5-fold when compared with response rates with monotherapy (1). Currently, the duration of therapy necessary to optimize response and whether HIV-infected individuals can maintain treatment in the face of medication toxicity and rapidly evolving viral resistance are unclear.

A 1994 report estimated that patients with acquired immunodeficiency syndrome, on average, take over seven medications per month (2). For HIV alone, patients and clinicians must choose from a multitude of ARVs currently available, with each possible combination potentially resulting in unique drug interactions and toxicities. These interactions, if not fully characterized, can have profound effects on the outcome of a patient's therapy and may result in virologic failure, emergence of drug resistance, or unnecessary adverse effects. Efficient understanding and recognition of these interactions can be a valuable tool for clinicians and patients alike.

Extensive efforts have been devoted toward elucidating ARV drug interactions as such information is clearly essential for optimizing patient therapy. Clinical pharmacokinetic studies serve as the basis for quantitating the effect of one or more compounds on the exposure of the affected drug. The most fundamental concept of drug interactions may be the identification of inhibition and/or induction of medication metabolism. Compounds that inhibit metabolism can potentially increase the plasma concentration of concurrently administered medications, whereas induction of metabolism diminishes concentrations of the affected drug(s). In the simplest sense, such interactions may lead to recommendations to decrease and increase the dose of the affected compound, respectively.

The medical literature contains a wealth of information regarding the pharmacokinetic parameters and drug interactions of the ARVs. However, the major dilemma lies in the decisions that must be made clinically on a daily basis. Terminology such as area under the curve (AUC) and minimum concentration (C_{min}) have little value to the patients and physicians who need to interpret this information to make accurate adjustments in ARV dosing. Alterations in these parameters may or may not warrant modified therapy, and additional factors must be considered (e.g., the therapeutic window of the drugs and the magnitude of the interaction). The basis for creating a resource of ARV drug interactions, such as this chapter, is to provide a guide that includes information on ARV interactions but emphasizes how best to manage such interactions clinically.

The phrase, "medication interaction" is usually associated with a negative stigma. However, a large part of HAART uses advantageous interactions for simplifying regimens (reduction of dose or frequency) and improving efficacy. Medication adherence is now recognized as a crucial factor in the battle against HIV. Thus, simplification of regimens for optimizing adherence is a high priority. Rather than dosing three or four times daily, regimens set for once- or twice-daily dosing are most desirable, with simplified regimens clinically used as soon as valid research deems such strategies safe and efficacious (regardless of U.S. Food and Drug Administration [FDA]-approved guidelines).

All three major classes of ARVs and their interactions are discussed throughout this chapter. A section is also devoted to evaluating the interactions involving medications used to treat HIV-associated complications. Most importantly, clinical application is emphasized and dosing recommendations are provided.

II. INTERPRETATION OF DRUG CONCENTRATIONS

The importance of ARV concentrations is discussed briefly to provide a basis for interpreting results of drug interaction studies. Pharmacodynamics is the study of the relationship between drug exposure and clinical response. Which specific measurement of drug exposure (i.e., AUC, trough concentration) is most predictive of response remains unclear. For the protease inhibitors, some work has illustrated the importance of drug plasma AUC and/or trough concentrations in ensuring the desired decline in viral load (3–5) and for preventing viral breakthrough and resistance. Maintaining target plasma measurements is presumed to be key for optimizing nonnucleoside reverse transcriptase inhibitor (NNRTI) use as well, although work for this class of drugs is more limited.

For the nucleoside reverse transcriptase inhibitors (NRTIs), the pharmacologically active form of these compounds is the intracellular triphosphate moiety, thus making the utility of plasma drug concentrations questionable. This is underscored by work demonstrating that plasma concentrations of zidovudine (ZDV) do not correlate linearly and are not predictive of active ZDV–triphosphate levels (6). Thus, higher ZDV plasma concentrations do not necessarily translate into higher intracellular triphosphate concentrations (7).

In general, recommendations to modify dosages in the context of combination therapy are in response to altered plasma measurements for protease inhibitors (PIs) and NNRTIs. For optimizing NRTIs, data on the intracellular disposition of the active triphosphate are best obtained to fully evaluate a potential drug interaction.

III. INTERACTION TYPES

The potential for a multitude of interactions can occur when two or more compounds are introduced into the body. The two prominent categories of interactions, especially for the ARVs, are intracellular and extracellular (usually plasma). Most intracellular interactions involve the NRTIs as their mechanism of action is dependent on the conversion of the parent drug to the triphosphate form inside the cell (8). However, the ability to extract the pharmacokinetic data needed to predict these types of interactions is often arduous and difficult compared with determination of plasma pharmacokinetic (PK) or extracellular interactions. The prediction of clinical outcome and determining appropriate dose adjustments invariably will be difficult once an intracellular interaction has been established.

More straightforward are the extracellular interactions involving the PI and NNRTI classes of ARVs with the need for dosage alterations more easily determined when an interaction has been detected. Most drug metabolism for the PIs and NNRTIs occurs via the cytochrome P450 (CYP450) enzymatic system in the liver and gut, with these compounds acting as both substrate and modifier (inhibitor or inducer) of this system. Thus, as the list of available new ARVs grows, the list of potential drug interactions expands exponentially. Often, the documentation needed to identify and evaluate probable drug interactions is lacking for many of the newer agents. An understanding of the pharmacokinetic and dynamic characteristics of the ARVs can have some value for predicting interactions in unknown situations. Nevertheless, in many cases, unique ARV combinations should be evaluated clinically becauase pharmacokinetic changes are difficult to estimate.

IV. INHIBITOR AND/OR INDUCER

The CYP450 enzymatic system performs two primary biological functions: metabolism of endogenous compounds and detoxification of exogenous compounds. Metabolic reactions are categorized into two distinct phases. Phase I consists of oxidation, reduction, and hydrolysis—all associated with basic polarization (addition of functional groups) of parent compounds forming metabolites that may or may not exhibit loss of pharmacological activity. Phase II involves conjugation of the resulting molecule and combines it with an endogenous substrate forming a water-soluble conjugate that can be excreted in the urine or bile. The most common conjugation occurs with glucuronic acid, resulting in drug inactivation, although exceptions to the rule exist. Most reactions that occur in phase I are mediated by the CYP450 enzyme system.

The system is divided into families of enzymes (e.g., CYP3, CYP2) with similar amino acid sequences and can further be divided into subfamilies (e.g., CYP3A, CYP2D) and finally individual enzymes (e.g., CYP3A4, CYP2D6). The primary enzymes involved in metabolism of the PIs and NNRTIs include CYP3A4, CYP2D6, CYP2C9, and CYP2C19. Understanding which family of enzymes or isozyme substrates each drug affects can help predict which type of interaction may occur (Table 1). All the currently approved PIs exhibit a certain degree of inhibition and/or induction on the CYP450. The most potent isozyme inhibitor is ritonavir (RTV), but it may at the same time also induce

Table 1 Metabolic Characteristics of Antiretrovirals

Drug	Primary metabolism	Inhibitor	Inducer
PI			
Amprenavir	3A4	3A4	
Indinavir	3A4	3A4	
Nelfinavir	3A4, 2C19, 2D6	3A4	Glucuronyl transferase, 3A4?
Ritonavir	3A4,[a] 2D6, 2C9, 2C19, 2A6, 1A2, 2E1		3A, 1A2, 2C9, glucuronyl transferase
Saquinavir	3A4	3A4	
NNRTI			
Delavirdine	3A4	3A4, 2C9, 2C19	
Nevirapine	3A4		3A4
Efavirenz	3A4	3A4, 2C9, 2C19	3A4

[a]Ritonavir inhibition: 3A4 > 2D6 > 2C9 > 2C19 >> 2A6 > 1A2 > 2E1.
Source: Ref. 63.

its own metabolism during the first few weeks of administration. Amprenavir (APV), nelfinavir (NFV), and indinavir (IDV) have moderate inhibitory effects, leaving saquinavir (SQV) the least potent inhibitor. The strong effects of RTV on the P450 isozyme system, specifically CYP3A4 (9), tend to result in the most significant clinical drug interactions. RTV will often be used clinically for the sole purpose of inhibiting this isozyme, dramatically elevating plasma levels of coadministered medications. The quantity of isoforms in the CYP450 system has been shown to vary by 10- to 20-fold (10), and studies indicate this factor contributes to differences in systemic concentrations of PIs, causing an unpredictability for maintaining a certain threshold value of plasma concentrations to achieve optimal antiviral response (3). Individual variability of gut absorption and metabolism and hepatic first-pass effect can lead to widely ranging plasma levels. First-pass effect can greatly reduce the amount of drug delivered to the plasma. Further, the short half-lives of the PIs make them more vulnerable to undesirable effects (e.g., decreased plasma concentrations, increased clearance) caused by drug interactions, predisposing patients to drug failure. Adjusting doses to correct for altered PI metabolism and thus maintaining adequate plasma levels seems to be essential to the longevity of this ARV class use.

The NNRTIs primarily metabolized by the CYP3A4 isozyme family elicit some degree of inhibition and/or induction upon the CYP450 system. Delavirdine (DLV) is a moderate inhibitor of CYP3A4 that includes inhibiting its own metabolism (11). In contrast, nevirapine (NVP) has been labeled a potent inducer of CYP450, including its own induction, leading to a unique starting dosage (12). Efavirenz (EFV), the latest to be approved for use, has a complex dual effect involving induction and inhibition and can affect multiple families of the CYP450 system. Interestingly, these opposing effects are observed when coadministered with drugs of the same class (i.e., PIs). The unpredictability of EFV on the CYP450 creates confusion for optimizing drug dosing of the coadministered ARVs. All three of the NNRTIs have numerous interactions with the PIs, making these combinations a challenge to use in a clinical setting.

In addition to metabolism by the CYP450, the possible impact PIs and NNRTIs may have on glucuronidation of concomitant medications has been considered. The NRTIs have very little effect on the CYP450, are not substrates for CYP450 isozymes, and only ZDV undergoes glucuronidation via hepatic metabolism. No study has definitively demonstrated clinically important interactions between the PIs/NNRTIs and NRTIs.

Unfortunately, metabolism by the CYP450 system is not confined to the ARVs. A multitude of concurrent medications used in the treatment of HIV-1 complications are also substrates of the CYP450 system and can be affected in similar ways (see Sec. VIII).

V. NUCLEOSIDE REVERSE TRANSCRIPTASE INHIBITORS

A. Intracellular Interactions

The investigation of nucleoside analogue intracellular interactions is a priority area of pharmacologic investigation. The currently approved NRTIs are abacavir (ABC), didanosine (ddI), lamivudine (3TC), stavudine (d4T), zalcitibine (ddC), and ZDV. The antiviral effect and clinical efficacy of this class of drugs is dependent on the extent to which these drugs are transformed to their active triphosphate moiety inside the cell. The mechanism of action of the NRTIs is based on competition with endogenous nucleosides (adenine, guanine, cytosine, thymidine, uracil) for incorporation into the reverse transcriptase of HIV-1. Each agent is identified as an "analogue" of the naturally occurring nucleoside, which are divided into the substrates of the purines (e.g., adenosine and guanine) and the pyrimidines (e.g., thymidine, cytosine, uracil). Because there are a limited number of unique endogenous nucleosides, competition involving drugs of the same substrate (ZDV and d4T) that use the same enzyme conversion to the triphosphate form, can occur inside the cell. Intracellular interactions occur within the NRTI class itself and with other nucleoside analogues (e.g., ribavirin [RBV]) used for treatment of various disease states (Table 2).

The use of NRTIs with the PIs is a potent and necessary combination in ARV treatment. Interaction evaluation between NRTIs and the PIs—SQV, RTV, and IDV—resulted in no effect on phosphorylation of nucleoside analogues in vitro (13).

The process of intracellular phosphorylation of the nucleoside analogues involves numerous enzymes that expedite the conversion of the parent drug to the active triphosphate. The pyrimidines analogues (e.g., ZDV, d4T, 3TC, ddC) have a more straightforward pattern of conversion than the purine compounds, with fewer processing steps and less enzymes involved. The thymidine analogues ZDV and d4T are initially converted by the same enzyme, thymidine kinase, to the monophosphate form. Further conversion to the diphosphate and triphosphate forms uses the same enzymes for both drugs. The cytosine analogues ddC and 3TC exhibit similar overlap with monophosphate formation via deoxycytidine kinase and identical enzymes responsible for conversion to the triphosphate. Because the analogues with identical substrates use the same pathways, they can potentially elicit competition for the enzymes responsible for phosphate formation and ultimately decrease conversion of one drug to the active triphosphate, reducing antiviral potency. Conversely, the purine analogues ddI and ABC each have unique patterns

Table 2 Alteration of NRTI Phosphorylation In Vitro

Competing nucleoside analogue	Change in phosphorylation					
	ZDV	3TC	ddC	D4T	ddI	ABC
ZDV		↔	↔	↓	↔	No data
3TC	↔		↓	↔	↔	No data
ddC	↔	↓		↔	↔	No data
d4T	↔	↔	↔		↔	No data
ddI	↔	↔	↔	↔		No data
ABC	↔	↔	No data	No data	No data	
RBV	↓	No data	↓	↓	↑	No data

↑, increase; ↓, decrease; ↔, no change.

of phosphorylation involving multiple enzymes and seem to be linked to additive or synergistic interactions with other medications using nucleosidic mechanisms of action. In fact, the antitumor agent hydroxyurea and the anti-hepatitis C (HCV) drug RBV have both demonstrated in vitro synergistic effects with ddI (14, 15). Unfortunately, there is no clear model to measure in vivo synergy. Although numerous studies of hydroxyurea in combination with ddI have been carried out, the long-term antiviral effects are unknown.

The understanding of the nature of NRTI intracellular interactions has been instrumental in establishing guidelines (16) for optimal combinations of NRTIs and eliminating unnecessary interactions within the class.

B.   Extracellular Interactions

There are few clinically consequential extracellular interactions involving the NRTIs. One reason for this may be the lack of correlation between plasma and intracellular concentrations (6, 17). However, because ZDV is glucuronidated there are some reported interactions to note. Plasma alterations of ZDV have been seen in combination with ddI but with varying results reported. Notable changes in ZDV and 3TC plasma concentrations occurred when ABC was administered in combination to a small number of HIV patients (18). Plasma interactions involving other combinations have been evaluated, producing insignificant results. Moreover, resulting changes in plasma levels may not be predictive of intracellular exposure and thus may have limited effect on antiviral activity.

Another factor to consider is the physical administration of multiple drugs and the importance of gastrointestinal absorption. Specific instructions are provided for each ARV regarding to correct administration with or without food. ddI absorption is enhanced by formulation with an alkaline buffer and must be exclusively taken on an empty stomach, which logically precludes it from coadministration with ARVs requiring food for increased absorption. Most PIs and NNRTIs that are taken with food should be taken at least 1 hour apart from ddI. However, IDV requires administration on an empty stomach and uses an acidic environment in the gut for maximal absorption and is compromised by the antacid formulated ddI. IDV plasma levels are unaffected when ddI is taken 1 hour before IDV despite elevated gastric pH at the time of IDV dosing (19). Coadministration of ddI with DLV and IDV results in AUC decreases of 20 and 86%, respectively. NFV should also be taken at least 1 hour after ddI to provide adequate absorption (20). Manipulation of ARV administration times with consideration for patient's daily activities may be required to eliminate unwanted absorption interactions of these medications.

C. Pharmacokinetic Application

Coadministration of the combination of nucleosides that contain the same pyrimidine analogues (ZDV/d4T, ddC/3TC) should be avoided. In vitro discovery of NRTI antagonism, particularly for the ZDV/d4T combination, has led to confirmation of these results in vivo. The antagonistic effect of ZDV on d4T phosphorylation suggests a much higher affinity of ZDV for thymidine kinase, the enzyme responsible for the conversion of both drugs to their monophosphate (21). Clinically, a reduction in d4T triphosphate formation has been observed in a small number of subjects (22). As expected with the lower thymidine kinase affinity, d4T had no effect on ZDV phosphorylation (23). Although unconfirmed in vivo, antagonism between 3TC and ddC is also attributed to varying enzyme affinity (24), and therefore this combination should be avoided clinically (24, 25). Most of other intracellular interactions for NRTI combinations are of minor importance.

Extracellular interactions were reported in a few cases involving NRTI combinations. ddI and ABC were shown to increase the plasma AUC levels of ZDV by 35 and 24%, respectively (18, 26). Other studies examining the ZDV and ddI combination found no evidence of interaction but did show alteration of the ZDV glucuronide metabolite, which is unlikely to have clinical significance (27). In contrast, ABC decreased the AUC of 3TC by 15% (18). Nonetheless, such moderate changes in NRTI plasma concentrations may have little impact on intracellular phosphorylation and thus have questionable clinical relevance.

PIs have little impact on intracellular activation of nucleoside analogues but have been shown to alter plasma exposure. The AUCs of ZDV and 3TC were decreased by 35 and 10%, respectively, with NFV. RTV reduced the AUC of ZDV by 25% and of ddI by 13% (28). All were deemed to be insignificant in terms of efficacy considering the magnitude of the change and the unknown effects on active triphosphate exposure. Conversely, APV increased ZDV AUC by 31% (29), but clinical significance is unknown, and no adjustment of dosage has been recommended.

D. Clinical Application

The relevance of NRTI intracellular interactions is still being evaluated. In vitro studies demonstrate antagonism (and potentially synergy) for various combinations. However, in vivo analysis is needed to fully understand the ramifications of these results. Unless clinical pharmacological and virological findings prove otherwise, the use of analogues of the same pyrimidine (e.g., thymidine) is not recommended at this time.

For NRTI combinations deemed safe to use, dosage adjustments are not recommended, despite reports of minor changes in plasma pharmacokinetics. However, dosage adjustments and drug selection should be considered in light of potential overlapping toxicities, such as peripheral neuropathy or pancreatitis. In addition, the timing of dose administration relative to concomitant therapies is crucial for patients managed with ddI, as the optimal absorption of NNRTIs and PIs can only be assured if dosed at least 1 hour from the time of ddI dosing. Fortunately, ddI can be dosed once daily, which permits flexibility. In summary, the NRTIs have minimal interactions considered clinically relevant and are therefore the least troublesome ARV class when used as part of combination therapy.

VI. PI COMBINATIONS

The most potent class of ARVs is also associated with the most numerous and clinically significant drug interactions. A 1997 retrospective analysis reported that the probability of one or more drug interactions occurring in patients receiving IDV, SQV, or RTV ranged from 31 to 77% with increased probabilities of 55 to 93% in patients with CD4 counts less than 100 cells/mL, presumably due to an increase in total medications taken in advanced disease state (30). Some of these interactions involving inhibition of drug metabolism are considered advantageous in that they permit simplification of PI regimens (e.g., less frequent dosing), a change paramount to improving adherence. Such interactions, along with improved dosing formulations and the introduction of new compounds with favorable pharmacokinetic profiles, may lead to all PIs being dosed once or twice daily. Drugs with less optimal formulations and poor bioavailability (i.e., SQV) greatly benefit from such interactions, which has led to the commonly prescribed RTV/SQV combination.

Unfortunately, ARV interactions are potentially dangerous clinically, and the concern over enhanced untoward effects or the possibility of metabolic induction has prompted careful consideration of new combinations and how best to optimize dosing. Not all possible PI regimens have been evaluated pharmacokinetically, and such study is warranted before unique drug combinations can be trusted clinically. Hence, new combinations are being studied with great interest and expediency (Fig. 1).

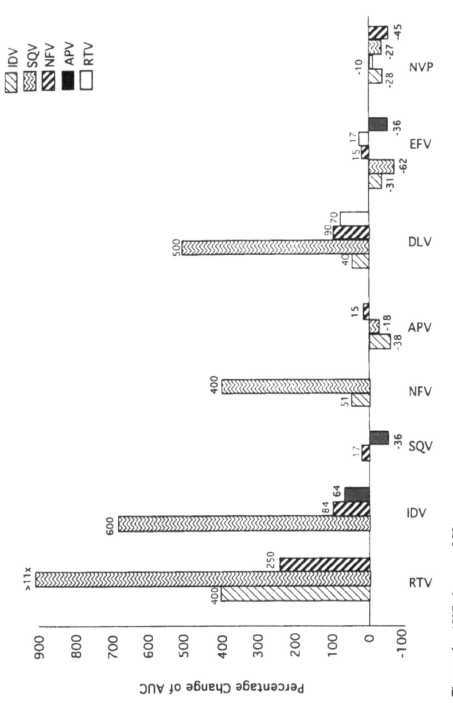

Figure 1   AUC changes of PIs.

A.   Pharmacokinetic Application

Because RTV is the most potent inhibitor of the CYP450, it maintains the most clinically significant interactions. As a strong inhibitor of CYP3A4, it increases plasma concentrations of CYP3A4 substrates such as other PIs or the NNRTIs and thus is combined with other ARVs to improve plasma concentrations, providing either enhanced efficacy, modified dose adjustment, or both. Unfortunately, if adequate dosage adjustments are not used, RTV coadministration can also result in increased adverse effects of the affected drug.

1.   RTV/IDV

One of the most favorable interactions occurs between RTV and IDV. IDV alone requires strict every 8 hour dosing and fasting administration. Single PI dosing with IDV administered twice daily failed in the Merck 069 study, and other alternatives were sought. Less frequent coadministration of IDV with RTV has proven to produce IDV pharmacokinetic exposure similar to IDV alone dosed every 8 hours (31). Another RTV/IDV combination study produced dramatic pharmacokinetic changes in healthy volunteers, increasing the AUC of IDV over 400% using various dosing strategies. RTV kinetics were not altered (32).

2.   RTV/SQV

The combination of RTV with the soft-gel formulation of SQV (Fortovase [FTV]) revealed similar effects in altering the dosing schedule and minimizing pill burden. The reduction of SQV first-pass metabolism by RTV increased the AUC of FTV by >50-fold (33) with minimal effect on RTV levels. Clinically, the combination is favorable as it counteracts the poor oral bioavailability and large pill burden of FTV.

3.   RTV/NFV

NFV plasma exposure is also improved by the coadministration of RTV, elevating the AUC of NFV by 152 to 250% after single-dose administration in two studies (34, 35). There was no effect seen on the PK of RTV in both cases. Precise dosing of this combination is still being considered (see Clinical Application).

4.   FTV/NFV/IDV

Other PIs that enhance the plasma concentrations of FTV include IDV and NFV with the AUC of FTV increased 500 and 392% with IDV and NFV, respectively (34, 36). The AUC of NFV was increased 17% by FTV (37).

Despite these pharmacokinetic improvements, pill burden may be an issue with the NFV and FTV combination as the doses remain large.

PI interactions between IDV and NFV exhibit modest alterations in PK exposure but nonetheless may be clinically advantageous. AUC increases occurred for both IDV (51%) and NFV (84%) when administered together (35). Ideal dosing for this combination is being evaluated (see Clinical Application).

5. APV

APV is the newest PI approved and is characterized by an interesting profile of interactions with other PIs. Although APV is labeled a moderate inhibitor of CYP450, specifically 3A4, it conversely diminishes levels of IDV and FTV to a degree that may prove clinically relevant. The mechanism of these reductions in IDV and FTV plasma exposure is not fully understood.

Coadministration of IDV and APV produced an increase in APV AUC of 64% but decreased the AUC of IDV by 38%. In addition, APV reduced the AUC of FTV by 18%, which is not statistically significant but is undesirable considering the already low bioavailability of FTV. Even modest elevations in dose of either drug would make the pill burden unreasonable. Therefore, combinations of APV with IDV or FTV are not advised at this time.

NFV had no impact on APV AUC but resulted in a significant increase in the minimum concentration of APV of 189% (38). NFV AUC increased slightly by 15% in a separate study in HIV infected patients (39).

B. Clinical Application

Dual PIs are commonly prescribed and often result in adequate antiviral efficacy in naive and heavily pretreated patients (40, 41). However, as the emergence of viral resistance is growing, the need for novel combinations and information that ensures optimum dosing is also increasing. Evaluating potential drug interactions for new regimens and gathering information on exposure-response are two areas of focus for pharmacological investigations.

Improved adherence is a likely result of some combination regimens as the dosing amount and frequency are often reduced. Simplification and reduction of pill burden may be the grandest outcome of the investigation of multiple PI dosing. Already new PIs, like ABT-378, are being developed as a combination formulation to exploit the potent inhibitory properties of RTV.

The use of RTV and IDV together is a promising dual PI combination. In addition to reduced pill burden, RTV allows IDV to be administered with food (less that 32% as fat kcal) (42), making this an attractive regimen to patients. The correct dose of this combination when considering the side effect and resistance profiles is yet to be determined . Evidence of RTV resistance may warrant the use of lower RTV doses of 200 mg b.i.d. with IDV 800 mg b.i.d . This elevates IDV plasma exposure and possibly overcomes phenotypic IDV cross-resistance (if present). The AUC of IDV is greater with the 800/200-mg (IDV/RTV) combination as compared with the 800/400-mg regimen and the 400/400-mg combination (31).

The pharmacokinetics of RTV were altered by IDV more substantially at the lower doses of RTV, but the AUC of RTV 400 mg remained predictably higher than the AUC of RTV 200 mg. Based on pharmacokinetics and reported adverse effects (31), the most favorable combination is the 800/200-mg IDV/RTV regimen, dosed b.i.d. However, the antiviral potency of RTV may be diminished at lower doses, and thus the larger dose of RTV within the 400/400-mg combination may be more desirable in cases where resistance to both drugs is absent. Further, it may be easier to overcome IDV resistance rather than RTV resistance due to the exaggerated increase in IDV plasma concentration (AUC, C_{min}) created by RTV and not vice versa. Future use of phenotypic analysis may help decipher which combination is best for a specific patient, making useful the comparison of predicted plasma concentrations with viral inhibitory concentrations.

RTV and SQV 400/400-mg combination was one of the first dual PI combinations to be used for first-line and salvage therapy and has been widely used in clinical practice (43, 44). One issue of concern is patient tolerance due to increased side effects, mainly gastrointestinal disturbances. However, adherence is likely improved with the reduced pill burden and twice daily dosing.

RTV 400 mg b.i.d. and NFV 500 or 750 mg b.i.d. is currently being evaluated for efficacy (45) with definitive information still lacking. A pharmacokinetic study in HIV-infected individuals revealed marginal differences between the 500- and 750-mg doses of NFV with regard to the impact of RTV on NFV AUC (46). The combination was found to be well tolerated, with diarrhea and nausea the most noticeable adverse effects.

Coadministration of NFV with IDV also allows less frequent administration of IDV based on a single-dose study (35). Furthermore, doses of NFV at 1250 mg b.i.d. and IDV 1000 mg b.i.d. produced similar pharmacokinetic results for IDV compared with monotherapy at standard q8h dosing (47). Administration of the two agents with regard to food intake was not discussed.

Combinations of PIs that appear advantageous pharmacokinetically may have limited clinical utility due to unacceptable adherence requirements associated with excessive pill burden and compounded adverse effects. This is exemplified by the combination of NFV and FTV. Doses of 1250 mg b.i.d. and 1200 mg b.i.d. for the two drugs, respectively, are necessary, which is equivalent to a daily intake of 22 capsules. In addition, this combination is associated with an increased incidence of gastrointestinal side effects.

The safety of the combination of APV and NFV administered twice daily depends on future pharmacokinetic evaluation. One small study used doses of 1250 mg of NFV with 1200 mg APV in combination with EFV and ABC (48). Investigation of APV and NFV disposition in the absence of EFV must be completed to determine safety and tolerability. Alleviation of pill burden in the context of specific combinations is feasible once the 625-mg formulation of NFV, currently under investigation, becomes available.

Many potential PI combinations with APV have not been evaluated pharmacologically or with regard to clinical potency, and suggestions for concurrent use and dosing adjustments are unavailable. Unfortunately, the RTV and APV interaction has not been characterized but has great potential in reducing the number of APV capsules currently prescribed per day (16 capsules/day).

No dosage adjustments have been suggested for the combination of APV with either IDV or FTV. As the reduction of plasma IDV AUC is significant and dosage modification not yet recommended, an alternate combination should be sought to ensure patient safety. APV and FTV should also be avoided because the plasma levels for both are diminished. Moreover, the large pill burden makes this combination an undesirable option for patients regardless of altered pharmacokinetics.

The PI combinations discussed above have been most commonly evaluated for pharmacokinetic alterations and clinical efficacy. In many cases, such study has resulted in recommendations for the best dosage adjustments (Table 3). However, despite strong pharmacokinetic information in controlled clinical studies, clinical monitoring of individual patients may be warranted because between-patient variability in absorption and metabolism is considerable. It remains unclear if therapeutic monitoring of PI drug concentrations is important for ensuring optimum ARV treatment. Current work is underway to evaluate this potential tool and decipher if such "real-time" evaluation is crucial to patient care.

VII. NNRTI AND PI COMBINATIONS

Until recently, the use of NNRTIs as potent initial ARV therapy in a combination drug regimen without a PI was not recommended. However, recent use of EFV as initial therapy (16) (in PI sparing regimens) may increase the efficacy of PIs used in salvage regimens for HIV-infected individuals. The

Table 3   Investigational PI and NNRTI Dosing Regimens

DOSE of → with ↓	Ritonavir 600 mg b.i.d.[a]	Indinavir 800 mg q8h[a]	Saquinavir 1200 mg t.i.d.[a]	Nelfinavir 750 mg t.i.d.[a]	Amprenavir 1200 mg b.i.d.[a]
PI					
Ritonavir		800 mg b.i.d.[b], 600 mg b.i.d.[b], 400 mg b.i.d.[b]	400 mg b.i.d.[b], 1600 mg q.d.[b]	500 mg b.i.d.[b], 750 mg b.i.d.[b]	No data
Indinavir	100 mg b.i.d.[b], 200 mg b.i.d.[b], 400 mg b.i.d.[b]		No data	1250 mg b.i.d.	Avoid
Saquinavir	400 mg b.i.d.[b], 100 mg q.d.[b]	No data		1250 mg b.i.d.	Avoid
Nelfinavir	400 mg b.i.d.	1200 mg b.i.d.	1000 mg b.i.d.[b], 1200 mg b.i.d.[b]		No data
Amprenavir	No data	Avoid	Avoid	No data	
NNRTI					
Delavirdine, 400 mg t.i.d.	Standard	600 mg q8h	800 mg t.i.d.	1250 mg b.i.d. (DLV600 mg b.i.d.)	No data
Nevirapine, 200 mg b.i.d.[a]	Standard	1000 mg q8h	Avoid	1000 mg t.i.d. or standard	Avoid
Efavirenz 600 mg q.d.[a]	600 mg b.i.d. (can → to 500 mg b.i.d.)	1000 mg q8h	Avoid	Standard	Avoid

[a]FDA-approved standard doses, optimal dosing for once daily (q.d.) = every 24 hours (q24h), two times a day (b.i.d.) = every 12 hours (q12h), and three times a day (t.i.d.) = every 8 hours (q8h).
[b]Determination of optimal dosing strategies (i.e., multiple RTV/IDV combinations) is dependent on patient variability and clinical evaluation.
Sources: Refs. 31, 34, 38, 44, 47, 49–55.

increasing popularity of PI-sparing regimens will obviously deviate interactions between the PI and NNRTI classes of drugs. But as the emergence of viral resistance and failure to previous ARV combinations grows, the use of PI/NNRTI combinations may increase as well.

NNRTI and PI-based combination regimens can include one or more drug from each class. The NNRTIs each have unique metabolic characteristics. Although DLV causes inhibition of CYP450, induction of metabolism is a consequence of both NVP and EFV use that invariably reduces the plasma concentrations of affected drugs. Metabolic induction is detrimental to the integrity of PI-containing regimens, and any reduction of plasma levels is undesirable. Interestingly, EFV also inhibits the activity of CYP450 isozymes, making prediction of the resulting effect difficult. Thus, evaluating potential interactions between the NNRTIs and 3A4 substrates is a priority focus for pharmacological investigations. Clinical trials to evaluate new combination regimens may be placed on hold to await definitive pharmacokinetic interaction information.

A. DLV Interactions

DLV is the only NNRTI that is a predictable inhibitor of CYP450 enzymes. The most notable changes include plasma AUC increases of 90, 70, and 500% for NFV, RTV, and SQV hard gel capsule (hgc), respectively (49–51). Data also show an increase in plasma IDV AUC up to 40% with DLV (52). Alternately, the impact on DLV plasma levels in combination with the PIs is minimal except for a 50% decrease seen with NFV (49). As all four DLV/PI combinations result in increased PI plasma exposure, the incidence of adverse effects may also increase and therefore patient monitoring is advised. However, dose adjustments are not recommended for RTV, NFV, and SQV(hgc) when used with DLV, and all are administered at standard doses. Preliminary data indicate the possibility of elevated APV levels due to metabolism inhibition by DLV (48), but further evaluation is needed to confirm the degree of alteration.

B. NVP Interactions

In contrast to DLV, the metabolic induction effects of NVP result in unwanted reductions in PI plasma concentrations, potentially compromising PI antiviral activity. A questionable interaction occurs with NPV and NFV—two studies have reported conflicting results. In one, a decrease in NFV AUC of approximately 50% was observed (53), whereas another reported only an 8% reduction (54). The former results suggest an NFV dosage adjustment; however, the investigators likely failed to consider the autoinductive effects of NFV, which may explain the findings.

Dose adjustment of IDV is potentially required when administered with NVP. Although IDV plasma AUC decreases a moderate 28% (12), the C_{min} of IDV is reduced by almost 50%, which may impact IDV efficacy. Moreover, due to large interpatient variability for IDV pharmacokinetic (3), an increase in IDV dose is advised.

A moderate decrease of 27% is reported for the plasma SQV (hgc) AUC when coadministered with NVP (55). However, no studies have been done assessing the soft gel formulation, which is now exclusively used in clinical practice. No recommendations have been made for combined use of FTV and NVP.

The minimal 10% drop in RTV AUC with NVP is not likely clinically significant considering the adequate absorption of RTV (56). Interestingly, despite knowledge of NVP induction, there is little information regarding the potential effect of this compound on APV. Therefore, avoidance of APV/NVP is warranted with the need for rigorous pharmacokinetic analysis before safe concomitant use.

C. EFV Interactions

The third NNRTI to be licensed, EFV, possesses the ability to promote both inhibition and induction of the CYP isozyme system. The ability of EFV to induce or inhibit metabolism is dependent on which particular PI is being used in combination. Moderate induction of metabolism occurs with three of the five approved PIs with a resulting decrease in their plasma drug exposure. The plasma AUC and maximum concentration of IDV are decreased by 31 and 16%, respectively, with the former of potential clinical significance (57). The AUCs of APV and FTV are diminished by 36 and 62% (57), and thus FTV and EFV coadministration is contraindicated. Additional investigation between EFV and APV is ongoing with the need for specific dosage recommendation before their combined use.

RTV AUC is slightly elevated by 18% and EFV AUC is increased 21% during coadministration, the latter attributed to RTV inhibition of metabolism (58). Of note is the RTV dose of 500 mg used in this study instead of the standard 600 mg. Neither pharmacokinetic alteration requires dosage modification. However, increases in side effects of both drugs may be seen and monitoring of liver function tests is advised. EFV given at 600 mg daily elevated the NFV AUC by 20% while decreasing the M8 metabolite of NFV by 37%, requiring no dose adjustment (59).

Due to the unpredictability of EFV on the metabolism of other ARV medications, caution should be taken in cases where incomplete pharmacokinetic data are available. This agent in particular underscores the need for early and rapid pharmacokinetic study of potential ARV regimens, and new combinations including EFV are rarely used clinically before acquisition of these data.

D.   Clinical Application

The pharmacokinetic effects of the NNRTIs on the disposition of combined PIs are generally significant enough to warrant PI dosage adjustments, but modifications in NNRTI doses are unnecessary.

Dose reductions are recommended for IDV and FTV when coadministered with DLV with the dose of IDV decreased to 600 mg q8h to achieve plasma levels similar to standard 800-mg q8h dosing. Reduction of FTV to 800 mg three times a day (16) is also suggested due to a report of early increases in hepatocellular enzymes in healthy subjects receiving standard doses (51). As formal evaluation of this combination has not been completed, monitoring of transanimase levels is advised. Amplification of toxicities with other PIs may also occur, and appropriate precautions should be taken.

Despite the reported 90% increase in NFV AUC and subsequent 50% decrease in DLV concentrations during combined use, standard doses are recommended with close monitoring for neutropenia (rare side effect of NFV).

Currently, an IDV regimen of 1000 mg q8h is recommended when coadministered with NVP. However the clinical efficacy of this regimen is presently being evaluated, with antiviral and clinical responsiveness being the ultimate determinant of optimum treatment guidelines. To date, small studies have demonstrated no loss of antiviral activity and continued virological control (12, 60), but the lack of clear differences may be attributed to the extensive variability in the magnitude of HIV-1 disease progression. Moreover, pharmacokinetic variability is also associated with variable disease state with decreased plasma concentrations and increased clearance observed in patients with advanced disease (3). In general for IDV, factors such as large interpatient pharmacokinetic variability, present disease state, likelihood of adverse effects, and variable adherence should be considered when selecting specific patient doses.

NVP and FTV coadministration is not advised, despite the lack of data with the soft gel formulation. This is based on results demonstrating reduced SQV levels using the hard gel capsule. Addition of RTV to this combination could eliminate the induction effects of NVP, but no formal investigation has been done.

RTV and IDV require dose modifications when given concurrently with EFV. Adjustment of the IDV dose to 1000 mg q8h is recommended to compensate for EFV induction. One may mitigate the need for two separate dosage formulations (200- and 400-mg capsules) by administering three 333-mg IDV capsules. The already reduced dose of 500 mg of RTV studied for pharmacokinetic analysis with EFV still resulted in mild increases in plasma drug exposure for both agents but attenuated the side effects seen with the 600-mg RTV dose. Thus, intolerance to RTV 600 mg due to increased toxicity (mainly central neurons system) justifies the use of 500 mg b.i.d. of RTV with no loss of antiviral activity.

Neither FTV nor APV as a sole PI should be coadministration with EFV. One unpublished study evaluated the APV/EFV combination with concurrent administration of either low dose RTV (200 mg) or NFV (1250 mg) twice daily that attenuated the reduction of APV caused by EFV. Any further increase of dose with these two PIs administered with EFV would create a very large pill burden, which may not be optimal for successful patient adherence.

The inductive effects of NVP and EFV can cause undesired reduction of PI plasma levels and create confusion in PI dosing. Questions arise when unfamiliar combinations of these drugs are used in cases where therapeutic options are limited. Often, potentially beneficial dosing regimens are not fully validated with rigorous clinical study despite the priority for rapid assessment of unique combinations. In the absence of definitive information, clinical judgement may need to suffice coupled with close patient monitoring and possible drug level determinations. However, whenever possible, alternate drug combinations should be used when optimal dose adjustments cannot be determined.

VIII. MANAGEMENT OF NON-ARV DRUG INTERACTIONS

The era of HAART therapy has greatly reduced the incidence of opportunistic infections and extended survival of HIV-infected individuals (61). However, therapeutic antiviral failure and a growing incidence of other coexisting infections (i.e. chronic hepatitis B and C) has increased the need for multidrug approaches. The proper clinical management of multiple disease states such as opportunistic infections in the context of HIV infection can be very difficult because the decisions and choices of drugs to treat these conditions are limited by drug interactions. This added complexity underscores the need to recognize possible interactions and take the proper precautions, including dose modifications and monitoring to ensure patient safety.

Many coadministered drugs are metabolized by CYP450 enzymes, as are the PIs and NNRTIs, and references are available that categorize which drug is metabolized by which specific isozyme(s) and which compounds are likely to induce or inhibit specific metabolic systems (62, 63). Such knowledge helps predict clinically relevant interactions that may occur when medications are coprescribed. The following section provides drug interaction information for the most commonly used non-ARVs, with a focus on those interactions serious enough that dosage adjustment are necessary or coadministration is strictly contraindicated. It should be noted that many pharmacokinetic evaluations were conducted in healthy volunteers. Nevertheless, these studies provide important information for guiding dosage decisions.

A. Antibiotics

1. Antimycobacterial Agents

Most commonly used for mycobacterium avium complex (MAC) and tuberculosis, the rifamycins are well-defined inducers of the CYP3A4 and generally reduce plasma concentrations of coadministered medications. Rifampin (RFP) is the most potent inducer, decreasing the AUC of the available PIs from 35 to 89% (16). Rifabutin (RBT) has less inducing effect with PI AUC reductions ranging from 14 to 45% (16, 64, 65). Little data are available for rifapentine, but it is described as an intermediate inducer with effects greater than those of RBT (66).

RFP also induces the metabolism of NVP (67) and DLV (68), resulting in a 37 and 96 reduction in AUCs, respectively, but only moderate reduction of EFV AUC (25%). RBT similarly alters the disposition of NVP and DLV; however, only the 80% plasma AUC decrease for DLV is clinically significant, and EFV concentrations remain unchanged (68, 69). The effects of coadministration on RFP PK is negligible. However, in contrast, the plasma levels of RBT are markedly increased when combined with DLV, NFV, RTV, or IDV and decreased when combined with NVP (16%) or EFV (35%) (67, 69).

Concurrent use of RFP with any of the five PIs, DLV, or NVP is contraindicated. The only acceptable concurrent use is with EFV when standard doses of both drugs administered. Potential for use with RTV seems limited due to possible increased liver toxicity and limited pharmacokinetic data. The substitution of RBT for RFP should be made in almost all cases where a rifamycin is needed in the context of concurrent PI and/or NNRTI therapy.

The growing use of RBT for mycobacterial infections in patients with HIV has warranted concern regarding optimum dosing. As the magnitude of the interactions with ARVs are variable, dose adjustments are in turn drug specific, and not all dose modifications have been fully evaluated in HIV-infected individuals. Use of FTV with RBT is contraindicated. RBT dose reduction from 300 mg daily to 150 mg q.d. is suggested when combined with APV, IDV, or NFV. A scheduled 150-mg dose of RBT every other day is necessary when RTV is included in antiviral therapy (as RBT levels can quadruple with standard doses of RTV). Further, RBT toxicities (uveitis, arthralgias, and leukopenia) should be closely monitored while the patient remains on the combination. Dose increases for IDV and NFV to 1000 mg q8h are suggested to offset plasma AUC reductions, but this is not confirmed clinically and clinician judgement for individual patients is advised.

Proper dosing guidelines for RBT when combined with NNRTIs are less concrete. Most clear is the contraindication of RBT with DLV due to the 80% change in DLV exposure. Limited data reported for interaction with NVP reveal slight enhancement of NVP clearance but no need for dose adjustment (70). However, until more extensive evaluation is available for dose recommendations, clinical judgment and monitoring should be applied to cases when the combination is clearly indicated. Reduction of RBT AUC when used with EFV warrants an RBT dose increase to 450 mg daily (16) or 600 mg daily (66).

2. Macrolide/Azalide

The treatment and the prophylaxis of MAC primarily includes a macrolide or azalide antibiotic such as clarithromycin (CLR) or azithromycin (AZM) (71). CLR inhibits CYP 3A4 and therefore alters the pharmacokinetics for many ARVs. In contrast, AZM is primarily eliminated in the gut with no evidence for CYP450 induction or inhibition (72). Despite these data, some precautions are still issued (73).

Dose modifications of CLR are recommended only with RTV and DLV in the presence of renal insufficiency. It is recommended that the CLR dose be reduced by 50% with a creatinine clearance of 30–60 mL/min and by 75% when less than 30 mL/min. Elevation of PI plasma concentrations does occur, but dose changes have not been recommended. Confusion about the potential alteration of the effectiveness of CLR with EFV is due to contrasting pharmacokinetic results, indicating a reduction of parent drug AUC but an increase in metabolite concentrations. Conversely, AZM concentrations are not significantly affected by EFV, suggesting metabolism by CYP3A4 is not the primary route of elimination. Substitution to AZM may be considered when concomitant use with EFV is required. AZM remains the principle alternative for mycobacterium infections if drug interactions are suspected with clarithromycin.

B. Antifungals

Treatment and prophylaxis for *Candida albicans* and other mycotic infections often includes the use of an azole antifungal agent. Included in this class are ketoconazole, itraconazole, and fluconazole (listed in descending order of inhibitory potency of the CYP450 enzyme system). The predicted effect of inhibition upon coadministered medications is increased plasma drug exposure requiring dose reduction of the affected drug. CYP3A4 inhibition is confirmed clinically to be greater with ketoconazole and itraconazole and less with fluconazole (e.g., there is no significant change in IDV and DLV levels with fluconazole). The effect of fluconazole may be more pronounced with either the CYP2C9 or 2C10 subfamily as indicated by interactions with drugs using this subfamily of enzymes (74). Nevertheless, the potential for a fluconazole interaction with a CYP3A4 substrate cannot be ruled out, and further study with ARVs to establish safety is needed. Generally, minimal information is available regarding drug interactions of all the azoles with ARVs, and dose adjustments are only suggested for ketoconazole. Dose reduction of IDV to 600 mg q8h may obviate increased side effects (i.e., nephrolithiasis) due to the 68% increase in IDV plasma levels with ketoconazole coadministration. Elevated plasma concentrations of FTV do not require dose reduction as increased bioavailability is especially beneficial for FTV with less severe side effects seen. Alteration in ketoconazole plasma levels are mediated by RTV, resulting in higher levels and necessity for ketoconazole dose reduction to 100 mg. Avoidance of concurrent administration with NVP should be practiced because subtherapeutic ketoconazole levels may result.

C. Ribavirin

The mechanism of action of the nucleoside analogue RBV has lead to in vitro studies examining the agonism/antagonism in efficacy occurring when used in combination with NRTIs (15, 21, 75, 76). The basis of these interactions occurs at the level of phosphorylation and inhibition of enzymes responsible for active triphosphate formation. RBV has demonstrated variable effects on NRTI triphosphate formation in vitro. Coexposure with RBV has resulted in antagonistic effects upon AZT (76) as well as d4T to a lesser extent (21). Conversely, the effects on the purine analogues of adenosine and guanosine show an additive or even synergistic effect based on a decrease in the EC_{50}

against HIV (15). RBV has also been reported to work synergistically with ddI, an additional purine analogue (75). The most recently approved NRTI, ABC, a purine analogue, may also exhibit enhanced activity in combination with RBV. Although ABC has a unique pattern of phosphorylation, it is still considered a guanosine (purine) analog. In vitro study has not been done with ABC, but synergistic potential could promote its use especially with patient coinfected with hepatitis C.

Of importance presently is the potential antagonism RBV may possess with ZDV and d4T. There is a need to confirm in vitro results in in vivo pharmacology studies. The effect of RBV on ZDV phosphorylation is likely due to RBV-induced increase in deoxythymidine triphosphate (dTTP) levels, resulting in feedback inhibition of thymidine kinase (76). This in turn will diminish the amount of ZDV phosphorylated and limit antiviral activity. The net effect is increased formation of dTTP that directly competes with ZDV–triphosphate for binding to the reverse transcriptase and decreased ZDV–triphosphate concentrations (76, 77). One study reported a three- to fivefold decrease of ZDV–triphosphate when combined with RBV (76). A second study reported total phosphorylation reduced to 25% of the control value ($p < 0.001$) when using RBV concentrations of 20 nM (77). The mechanism is similar for d4T due to the similarities of enzymatic phosphorylation. Inhibition of the thymidine kinase enzyme decreases phosphorylation and ultimately d4T–triphosphate formation.

The activity of the NRTIs is dependent on the ratio of dideoxynucleoside triphosphates (ddNTPs) to endogenous deoxynucleoside triphosphates (dNTPs). Thus, an increase of ZDV–triphosphate/dTTP ratio increases the antiviral activity of the ZDV. Conversely, decreases in levels of ZDV–triphosphate or d4T–triphosphate and increases in dTTP (as suggested above) would shift the ratio to favor endogenous nucleosides. Since intracellular concentration of ZDV–triphosphate is low, any further decrease could impact the antiviral drug potency. No recommendations for concurrent use of RBV with any of the NRTIs are available, but evaluation of antagonistic effects on ZDV and d4T in vivo are underway.

D. Anticonvulsants

Central nervous system involvement by HIV or opportunistic infections (i.e. toxoplasmosis) can result in the occurrence of seizures and may require concomitant use of anticonvulsants (AC). Although the concurrent use of these medications may not be common in the HIV-positive population, they can impose a dramatic effect on the PK of the ARVs and impact the integrity of stable ARV regimens. Anticonvulsants such as phenytoin and carbamazepine have potent inducting effects on CYP3A4 and therefore could reduce PI and NNRTI concentrations. However, this has not yet been evaluated clinically. Uncertainty also exists with regards to the impact the antiretrovirals have on AC efficacy, thus clinical monitoring of AC plasma levels is advised. Substitution of medications such as phenytoin, carbamazepine and phenobarbital with drugs less likely to interact is recommended. Neurontin, widely used as treatment for peripheral neuropathy, possesses antiepileptic properties but is renally eliminated and not metabolized. Lamotrigine and valproic acid are substrates of glucuronyl transferase and have less effect on the CYP450. Dosing of these alternative AC drugs should be titrated based on clinical efficacy and therapeutic monitoring of plasma AC drug levels.

E.   Oral Contraceptives and Lipid-Lowering Agents

Diminished effectiveness of oral contraceptives including ethinyl estradiol and to a lesser extent norethindrone occurs in combination with RTV and NFV due to induction of glucuronyl transferase. Increased plasma AUC concentrations (37%) (57) of ethinyl estradiol are seen with EFV, and the clinical effects are unknown at this time. Avoidance of concurrent use with RTV and NFV is recommended. In the case of EFV, use of barrier contraceptive method is advised in light of the teratogenic effects observed in animals (57). IDV, on the other hand, is not altered in the context of oral contraceptive therapy and therefore its use with oral contraception is acceptable (78).

Hyperlipidemia and other metabolic changes are becoming an increasingly common manifestation of prolonged ARV therapy. Dramatic increases in serum lipids has necessitated the use of lipid-lowering agents in HIV-positive patients on HAART. Primary treatment of hyperlipidemias is often managed with 3-hydroxy-3-methylglutaryl coenzyme A reductase inhibitors, referred to as "statins." All current statins are metabolized by the CYP450, and the potential for drug interaction exists. The Department of Health and Human Services guidelines for ARV use (16) list simvastatin and lovastatin as contraindicated for administration with the four protease inhibitors (APV not listed). Pravastatin may not be as susceptible to these interactive effects due to decreased avidity to CYP3A4 (79). A recent study of HIV-negative subjects demonstrated the interaction potential between the RTV/FTV combination with pravastatin, atorvastatin, and simvastatin (80). Steady-state drug interactions were evaluated using 24 hour AUCs. RTV 400 mg and FTV 400 mg b.i.d. combined with the statins (40-mg dose for all) demonstrated increases in median AUCs of 4.5-fold and 2-fold for atorvastatin and total active atorvastatin (includes atorvastatin plus active metabolites) respectively. Furthermore, a 31.6-fold increase in the AUC of simvastatin was observed. Pravastatin median AUC was decreased by 0.5-fold. Cautious initiation of atorvastatin is advised with potential need for dose reductions. Simvastatin use with RTV should be contraindicated. Pravastatin may require higher doses with RTV coadministration. Clinical monitoring of myopathy and elevated liver function tests is recommended with all PI and statin coadministration. Additionally, use with the NNRTI delavirdine may also increase the risk of myopathy due to expected increases in plasma levels of the statins. Further evaluation of the pharmacokinetic interactions of statins and ARVs is currently underway.

F. Sildenafil

The use of sildenafil (Viagra®) has become a common treatment for erectile dysfunction in HIV-positive men. However, the benign side effects and pharmacodynamic properties of the medication can become severe when combined with inhibitors of the CYP450 (i.e., PIs). Sildenafil is metabolized and acts as a weak inhibitor of the CYP3A4 and CYP2C9 (81). The PIs SQV, RTV, and IDV were shown to elevate the plasma AUC after a single 25-mg dose of sildenafil by 2-fold, 4.4-fold and 11-fold (82, 83). Because elevation of sildenafil plasma AUC is seen with even the weakest inhibitor (SQV) of the CYP450, dose reduction should be considered with initial coadministration. Possible interaction may also take place with DLV due to CYP450 inhibition. Initial starting doses of 12.5 to 25 mg of sildenafil may be advised with concurrent administration of the PIs and/or DLV. Use of sildenafil with RTV should be avoided as extremely high plasma concentrations of sildenafil may cause severe adverse effects.

IX. CONCLUSION

Combination therapy with ARV medication is currently the standard of care for HIV disease. Extensive metabolism of these medications by the CYP450 enzyme system produces a multitude of drug interactions. The ability of the ARVs to perform optimally is dependent on numerous factors, including concomitant drug interactions with the potential to diminish antiviral potency. Clinicians and patients require the knowledge and ability to recognize possible interactions to ensure successful treatment of HIV and its complications.

Utilizing beneficial interactions (dual PIs) is a unique way to minimize the demands of some regimens with the reduction of dose frequency and pill burden, enhancing the quality of life and adherence of many patients, However, untoward interactions are more common, and the magnitude of possible alterations in drug levels and interactions at the level of adverse effects increases as more compounds are introduced clinically. Clinical evaluation and management of interactions is one of the paramount factors for eliminating detrimental outcomes and providing safe effective care to patients.

REFERENCES

1. Palella FJ Jr, Delaney KM, Moorman AC, Loveless MO, Fuhrer J, Satten GA, Aschman DJ, Holmberg SD. Declining morbidity and mortality among patients with advanced human immunodeficiency virus infection. HIV Outpatient Study Investigators [see comments]. N Engl J Med 1998; 338:853–860.

2. Fogelman I, Lim L, Bassett R, Volberding P, Fischl MA, Stanley K, Cotton DJ. Prevalence and patterns of use of concomitant medications among participants in three multicenter human immunodeficiency virus type I clinical trials. AIDS Clinical Trials Group (ACTG). J Acquir Immune Defic Synd 1994; 7:1057–1063.

3. Acosta E, Henry K, Baken L. Indinavir concentrations and antiviral effect. Pharmacotherapy 1999; 19:708–712.

4. Fletcher C, Kakuda T, Anderson P, Henry K, Schacker T, Brundage R. Viral dynamics of concentration-targeted (C) vs. standard-dose (S) therapy with zidovudine (ZDV), lamivudine (3TC), and indinavir (IDV). 39th Interscience Conference on Antimicrobial Agents and Chemotherapy, San Francisco, CA, 1999.

5. Burger D, Hugen P, Prins J, Van De Ende M, Reiss P, Lange J. Pharmacokinetics of an indinavir/ritonavir 800/100 mg BID regimen. 6th Conference on Retroviruses and Opportunistic Infections, Chicago, IL, 1999.

6. Peter K, Gambertoglio JG. Zidovudine phosphorylation after short-term and long-term therapy with zidovudine in patients infected with the human immunodeficiency virus. Clin Pharmacol Ther 1996; 60:168–176.

7. Barry MG, Khoo SH, Veal GJ, Hoggard PG, Gibbons SE, Wilkins EG, Williams O, Breckenridge AM, Back DJ. The effect of zidovudine dose on the formation of intracellular phosphorylated metabolites. AIDS 1996; 10:1361–1367.

8. St. Clair MH, Richards CA, Spector T, Weinhold KJ, Miller WH, Langlois AJ, Furman PA. 3′-Azido-3′-deoxythymidine triphosphate as an inhibitor and substrate of purified human immunodeficiency virus reverse transcriptase. Antimicrob Agents Chemother 1987; 31:1972–1977.

9. Kumar GN, Rodrigues AD, Buko AM, Denissen JF. Cytochrome P450-mediated metabolism of the HIV-1 protease inhibitor ritonavir (ABT-538) in human liver microsomes [published erratum appears in J Pharmacol Exp Ther 1997; 281:1506]. J Pharmacol Exp Ther 1996; 277:423–431.

10. Wrighton SA, VandenBranden M, Ring BJ. The human drug metabolizing cytochromes P450. J Pharmacokinet Biopharmaceut 1996; 24:461–473.

11. Batts D, Freimuth W, Cox S. Open-label escalating multiple-dose study of the safety, tolerance and pharmacokinetics of oral U-90152S (delavirdine, DLV) in HIV infected males and females who are maintained on stable doses of AZT. First National Conference on Human Retroviruses and Related Infections, Washington, DC, 1993.

12. Murphy RL, Sommadossi JP, Lamson M, Hall DB, Myers M, Dusek A. Antiviral effect and pharmacokinetic interaction between nevirapine and indinavir in persons infected with human immunodeficiency virus type 1. J Infect Dis 1999; 179:1116–1123.

13. Hoggard PG, Manion V, Barry MG, Back DJ. Effect of protease inhibitors on nucleoside analogue phosphorylation in vitro. Br J Clin Pharmacol 1998; 45:164–167.

14. Kewn S, Hoggard P. Intracellular activation of $2',3'$-dideoxyinosine and drug interactions in vitro. AIDS Res Human Retrovir 1999; 15:793–802.

15. Baba M, Pauwels R, Balzarini J, Herdewijn P, De Clercq E, Desmyter J. Ribavirin antagonizes inhibitory effects of pyrimidine $2',3'$-dideoxynucleosides but enhances inhibitory effects of purine $2',3'$-dideoxynucleosides on replication of human immunodeficiency virus in vitro. Antimicrob Agents Chemother 1987; 31:1613–1617.

16. Department of Health and Human Services (DHHS). Guidelines for the use of antiretroviral agents in HIV-infected adults and adolescents. 1999.

17. Stretcher BN, Pesce AJ, Frame PT, Stein DS. Pharmacokinetics of zidovudine phosphorylation in peripheral blood mononuclear cells from patients infected with human immunodeficiency virus. Antimicrob Agents Chemother 1994; 38: 1541–1547.

18. Symonds W, McDowell J. The safety and pharmacokinetics of GW 1592U89, zidovudine (ZDV) and lamivudine (3TC) alone and in combination after single-dose administration in HIV-infected patients (abstract P19). AIDS 1996; 10(suppl 2):S23.

19. Mei J, Shelton M, Bartos F, DiFrancesco R, Hewitt R. If taken 1 hour before indinavir (IDV), didanosine (ddI) does not affect IDV exposure, despite persistent buffering effects. 39th Interscience Conference on Antimicrobial Agents and Chemotherapy, San Francisco, CA, 1999.

20. Squibb BM. Videx (didanosine) package insert. 1999 (July).

21. Hoggard PG, Kewn S, Barry MG, Khoo SH, Back DJ. Effects of drugs on $2',3'$-dideoxy-$2',3'$-didehydrothymidine phosphorylation in vitro. Antimicrob Agents Chemother 1997; 41:1231–1236.

22. Sommadossi J, Zhou X, Moore J. Impairment of stavudine phosphorylation in patients receiving a combination of zidovudine and d4T (ACTG 290). Fifth National Conference on Human Retroviruses and Related Infections, Chicago, IL, 1998.

23. Brody S, Aweeka F. Pharmacokinetics of intracellular zidovudine and its phosphorylated anabolites in the absence and presence of stavudine using an in vitro human peripheral blood mononuclear cell (PBMC) model. Int J Antimicrob Agents 1997; 9:131–135.

24. Kewn S, Veal GJ, Hoggard PG, Barry MG, Back DJ. Lamivudine (3TC) phosphorylation and drug interactions in vitro. Biochem Pharmacol 1997; 54:589–595.

25. Veal GJ, Barry MG, Khoo SH, Back DJ. In vitro screening of nucleoside analog combinations for potential use in anti-HIV therapy. AIDS Res Human Retrovir 1997; 13:481–484.

26. Barry M, Howe JL, Ormesher S, Back DJ, Breckenridge AM, Bergin C, Mulcahy F, Beeching N, Nye F. Pharmacokinetics of zidovudine and dideoxyinosine alone and in combination in patients with the acquired immunodeficiency syndrome. Br J Clin Pharmacol 1994; 37:421–426.

27. Sahai J, Gallicano K, Garber G, Pakuts A, Cameron W. Pharmacokinetics of simultaneously administered zidovudine and didanosine in HIV-seropositive male patients. J Acquir Immune Defic Syndr Human Retrovirol 1995; 10:54–60.

28. Flexner C. HIV-protease inhibitors. N Engl J Med 1998; 338:1281–1292.

29. Sadler B, Wald J, Lou Y. The single-dose pharmacokinetics of 141W94, zidovudine, and lamivudine, when administered alone and in two- and three-drug combinations. 6th European Conference on Clinical Aspects and Treatment of HIV-Infection, Hamburg, Germany, 1997.

30. Van Cleef GF, Fisher EJ, Polk RE. Drug interaction potential with inhibitors of HIV protease. Pharmacotherapy 1997; 17:774–778.

31. Saah S, Winchell G. Multiple-dose pharmacokinetics(PK) and tolerability of indinavir(IDV)-ritonavir(RTV) combinations in healthy volunteers (Merck 078). 6th Conference on Retroviruses and Opportunistic Infections, Chicago, IL, 1999.

32. Hsu A, Granneman GR, Cao G, Carothers L, Japour A, El-Shourbagy T, Dennis S, Berg J, Erdman K, Leonard JM. Pharmacokinetic interaction between ritonavir and indinavir in healthy volunteers. Antimicrob Agents Chemother 1998; 42:2784–2791.

33. Hsu A, Granneman GR, Cao G, Carothers L, el-Shourbagy T, Baroldi P, Erdman K, Brown F, Sun E, Leonard JM. Pharmacokinetic interactions between two human immunodeficiency virus protease inhibitors, ritonavir and saquinavir. Clin Pharmacol Ther 1998; 63:453–464.

34. Agouron Pharmaceuticals I. Nelfinavir (Viracept) package insert. 1998: La Jolla, CA.

35. Yuen G, Anderson R, Daniels R. Investigations of nelfinavir mesylate (NFV) pharmacokinetic (PK) interactions with indinavir (IDV) and ritonavir (RTV). Conference on Retroviruses and Opportunistic Infections, Washington, DC, 1997.

36. McCrea J, Buss N. Indinavir-saquinavir single dose pharmacokinetic study. Fourth Conference on Retroviruses and Opportunistic Infections, Washington, DC, 1997.

37. Kravick S, Sahai J, Kerr B. Nelfinavir mesylate (NFV) increases saquinavir-soft gel capsule (SQV-SGC) exposure in HIV+ patients. 4th Conference on Retroviruses and Opportunistic Infections, Washington, DC, 1997.

38. Glaxo-Wellcome Inc. Amprenavir (Agenerase) package insert, 1999.

39. Sadler S, Gillotin C, Chittick G. Pharmacokinetic drug interactions with amprenavir. 12th World AIDS Conference, Geneva, Switzerland, 1998.

40. Deeks S, Grant R, Horton C, Simmonds N. Virologic effect of ritonavir plus saquinavir in subjects who have failed indinavir. Proceedings of the Interscience Conference on Antimicrobial Agents and Chemotherapy, Toronto, Canada, 1997.

41. Batisse D, Salmon-Seron S, Karmochkine M, Ginsburg C. Efficacy and safety of ritonavir and saquinavir in combination in protease inhibitor-experienced patients. Proceedings of the Interscience Conference on Antimicrobial Agents and Chemotherapy, Toronto, Canada, 1997.

42. Hsu A, Granneman G, Molla A. Indinavir can be taken with regular meals when taken with ritonavir. Abstracts of the 12th World Congress on AIDS, Geneva, Switzerland, 1998.

43. Tebas P, Patrick A, Kane E, Klebert M, Simpson J, Atkinson B, Isaacson J, Powderly W, Henry K. 60-Week virologic responses to a ritonavir/saquinavir containing regimen in patients who had previously failed nelfinavir. 6th Conference on Retroviruses and Opportunistic Infections, Chicago, IL, 1999.

44. Cameron DW, Japour AJ, Xu Y, Hsu A, Mellors J, Farthing C, Cohen C, Poretz D, Markowitz M, Follansbee S. Ritonavir and saquinavir combination therapy for the treatment of HIV infection. AIDS 1999; 13:213–224.

45. Gallant J, Raines C, Sun E, Lewis R, Apuzzo L, Deetz C, Fields C, Flexner C. A phase II study if ritonavir-nelfinavir combination therapy: 48-week data. 6th Conference on Retroviruses and Opportunistic Infections, Chicago, IL, 1999.

46. Flexner C, Hsu A, Kerr B, Wong C, Gallant J, Anderson R. Steady-state pharmacokinetic interaction between ritonavir (RTV), nelfinavir (NFV), and the nelfinavir active metabolite M8. 12th World AIDS Conference, Geneva, Switzerland, 1998.

47. Squires K, Riddler S, Havlir D, Kerr B, Yeh K, Lewis R, Hawe L, Zhong L, Deutsch P, Saah A. Co-administration of indinavir (IDV) 1200 mg and nelfi-

navir (NFV) 1250 mg in a twice daily regimen: Preliminary PK activity. 6th Conference on Retroviruses and Opportunistic Infections, Chicago, IL, 1999.

48. Manufacturer Information. Glaxo Wellcome. Personal Communication, October 1999.

49. Cox S, Schneck D, Herman B. Delavirdine (DLV) and nelfinavir (NFV): a pharmacokinetic (PK) drug-drug interaction study in healthy adult volunteers. 6th Conference on Retroviruses and Opportunistic Infections, Chicago, IL, 1999.

50. Morse G, Shelton M, Hewitt R. Ritonavir (RIT) pharmacokinetics (PK) during combination therapy with delavirdine (abstract). 5th Conference of Retroviruses and Opportunistic Infections, Chicago, IL, 1998.

51. Cox S. Evaluation of pharmacokinetic (PK) interaction between saquinavir (SQV) and delavirdine (DLV) in healthy volunteers. 4th Conference on Retroviruses and Opportunistic Infections, Washington, DC, 1997.

52. Ferry JJ, Herman BD, Carel BJ, Carlson GF, Batts DH. Pharmacokinetic drug-drug interaction study of delavirdine and indinavir in healthy volunteers. J Acquir Immune Defic Syndr Human Retrovirol 1998; 18:252–259.

53. Merry C, Barry MG, Mulcahy F, Ryan M, Tjia JF, Halifax KL, Breckenridge AM, Back DJ. The pharmacokinetics of combination therapy with nelfinavir plus nevirapine [see comments]. AIDS 1998; 12:1163–1167.

54. Skowron G, Leoung G, Kerr B, Dusek A, Anderson R, Beebe S, Grosso R. Lack of pharmacokinetic interaction between nelfinavir and nevirapine [editorial; comment]. AIDS 1998; 12:1243–1244.

55. Sahai J, Cameron W, Salgo M. Drug interaction study between saquinavir (SQV) and nevirapine (NVP). 4th Conference on Retroviruses and Opportunistic Infections, Washington, DC, 1997.

56. Lamson M, Gangnier P, Greguski R, Myers M, Leonard J, Lauva I, Hsu A. Effect of nevirapine (NVP) on pharmacokinetics of ritonavir (RTV) in HIV-1 patients. 4th Conference on Retroviruses and Opportunistic Infections, Washington, DC, 1997.

57. Dupont-Merck. Efavirenz (Sustiva) package insert, 1998.

58. Fiske W, Benedek I. Pharmacokinetics of efavirenz (EFV) and ritonavir (RIT) after multiple oral doses in healthy volunteers. 12th World AIDS Conference, Geneva, Switzerland, 1998.

59. Fiske W, Benedek I. Pharmacokinetic interaction between efavirenz (EFV) and nelfinavir mesylate (NFV) in healthy volunteers. 5th Conference on Retroviruses and Opportunistic Infections, Chicago, IL, 1998.

60. Harris M, Durakovic C, Rae S, Raboud J, Fransen S, Shillington A, Conway B, Montaner JS. A pilot study of nevirapine, indinavir, and lamivudine among patients with advanced human immunodeficiency virus disease who have had failure of combination nucleoside therapy. J Infect Dis 1998; 177:1514–1520.

61. Consensus. Report of the NIH Panel to define principles of therapy of HIV infection. MMWR Morb Mortal Wky Rep 1998; 47(RR-5):1–41.

62. Michalets EL. Update: clinically significant cytochrome P-450 drug interactions. Pharmacotherapy 1998; 18:84–112.

63. Tseng AL, Foisy MM. Significant interactions with new antiretrovirals and psychotropic drugs. Ann Pharmacother 1999; 33:461–473.

64. Cato A 3rd, Cavanaugh J, Shi H, Hsu A, Leonard J, Granneman R. The effect of multiple doses of ritonavir on the pharmacokinetics of rifabutin. Clin Pharmacol Ther 1998; 63:414–421.

65. Polk R, Israel D, Patron R. Pharmacokinetic (PK) interaction between 141W94 and rifabutin (RFB) and rifampin (RFP) after multiple-dose administration. 5th Conference on Retroviruses and Opportunistic Infections, Chicago, IL, 1998.

66. Burman WJ, Gallicano K, Peloquin C. Therapeutic implications of drug interactions in the treatment of human immunodeficiency virus-related tuberculosis. Clin Infect Dis 1999; 28:419–429; quiz 430.

67. Roxanne. Nevirapine (Virammune) package insert, 1997.

68. Borin MT, Chambers JH, Carel BJ, Freimuth WW, Aksentijevich S, Piergies AA. Pharmacokinetic study of the interaction between rifabutin and delavirdine mesylate in HIV-1 infected patients. Antiviral Res 1997; 35:53–63.

69. Benedeck I, Fiske W. Pharmacokinetic interaction between multiple doses of efavirenz and rifabutinin healthy volunteers [abstract]. Clin Infect Dis 1998; 27:1008.

70. Maldonado S, Lamson M, Gigliotti M, Pav J, Robinson P. Pharmacokinetic (PK) interaction between nevirapine (NVP) and rifabutin (RFB). 39th Interscience Conference on Antimicrobial Agents and Chemotherapy, San Francisco, CA, 1999.

71. Horsburgh C. Epidemiology of mycobacterium avium complex disease. Am J Med 1997; 102:11–15.

72. Schlossberg D. Azithromycin and clarithromycin. Med Clin North Am 1995; 79:803–815.

73. Pfizer Labs. Zithromax (azithromycin) capsule package insert, 1996, New York.

74. Doecke CJ, Veronese ME, Pond SM, Miners JO, Birkett DJ, Sansom LN, McManus ME. Relationship between phenytoin and tolbutamide hydroxylations in human liver microsomes. Br J Clin Pharmacol 1991; 31:125–130.

75. Balzarini J, Lee CK, Herdewijn P, De Clercq E. Mechanism of the potentiating effect of ribavirin on the activity of $2',3'$-dideoxyinosine against human immunodeficiency virus. J Biol Chem 1991; 266:21509–21514.

76. Vogt MW, Hartshorn KL, Furman PA, Chou TC, Fyfe JA, Coleman LA, Crumpacker C, Schooley RT, Hirsch MS. Ribavirin antagonizes the effect of azidothymidine on HIV replication. Science 1987; 235:1376–1379.

77. Hoggard PG, Veal GJ, Wild MJ, Barry MG, Back DJ. Drug interactions with zidovudine phosphorylation in vitro. Antimicrob Agents Chemother 1995; 39:1376–1378.

78. Merck & Co. Crixivan (indinavir) package insert, 1998.

79. Neuvonen PJ, Kantola T, Kivistö KT. Simvastatin but not pravastatin is very susceptible to interaction with the CYP3A4 inhibitor itraconazole. Clin Pharmacol Ther 1998; 63:332–341.

80. Fichtenbaum C, Gerber J, Rosenkranz S, Segal Y, Blaschke T, Aberg J, Royal M, Burning W, Lamb K, Ferguson E, Alston B, Aweeka F. Pharmacokinetic interaction between protease inhibitors and selected HMG-CoA reductase inhibitors. Abstract. 7th Conference on Retroviruses and Opportunistic Infections, San Francisco, CA, January 2000.

81. Goldenberg MM. Safety and efficacy of sildenafil citrate in the treatment of male erectile dysfunction. Clin Ther 1998; 20:1033–1048.

82. Pfizer Labs. Sildenafil (Viagra) package insert. Revised June 1999, New York.

83. Merry C, Barry M, Ryan M, Tjia J, Hennessy M, Eagling V, Mulcahy F, Back D. Interaction of sildenafil and indinavir when co-administered to HIV-positive patients. AIDS 1999; 13:F101–F107.

9

Rationale for Immune-Based Therapies for Human Immunodeficiency Virus Type 1 Infection

Michael M. Lederman and Hernan Valdez
Case Western Reserve University and University Hospitals of Cleveland, Cleveland, Ohio

.

Replication of human immunodeficiency virus type 1 (HIV-1) occurs primarily in CD4+ lymphocytes, in mononuclear phagocytes, and in dendritic cells, all critical to host immune responses. In most infected persons, cell-mediated defenses become progressively and profoundly impaired. As is typical with intracellular pathogens, completion of the HIV-1 propagation cycle depends on efficient interaction with and utilization of numerous host cellular elements. Moreover, it appears that immune activation enhances HIV-1 propagation. Thus, the relationship between HIV-1 and immune function is intimate, complex, and, by most standards, difficult to unravel.

I. RATIONALE FOR IMMUNE-BASED THERAPIES

Although immune deficiency is the hallmark of infection with HIV-1, immune defenses, particularly cytotoxic T-lymphocyte responses, are essential regulators of viral propagation after acquisition of infection (reviewed in Reference 1) and by inference are critical predictors of long-term prognosis (2–4). Nonetheless, progressive depletion of cell-mediated immune responses, as characterized by losses in circulating and lymph node T-lymphocyte populations and functional impairments of the remaining cells, are expected long-term consequences of HIV-1 infection. This immune dysfunction predisposes to the opportunistic infections and neoplasms that define acquired immuno-deficiency virus (AIDS).

Despite profound immune deficiency, HIV-1 infection is also associated with evidence of immune activation such as increased plasma levels of the proinflammatory cytokines tumor necrosis factor alpha (TNF-α) and inter-leukin-6 (IL-6), increased immunoglobulin synthesis, and increased activation antigen expression on CD8+ and CD4+ lymphocytes (5, 6). It is posited that dysregulated immune activation may contribute directly to the morbidity of HIV-1 infection (wasting and autoimmune phenomena) and accelerate HIV-1 propagation.

The introduction of highly active antiretroviral therapy (HAART) regi-mens has dramatically changed the outlook for HIV-1-infected persons (7–9). A decreased incidence of opportunistic infections and decreased mortality have been the consequences of these treatments. Presumably, these benefits are related to a cessation of virus-induced immune deterioration and to some degree of immunological reconstitution. Preliminary data indicate that in the short-term immune reconstitution in subjects with chronic HIV-1 infection is incomplete after HAART. In subjects with chronic infection, HAART in-duces increases in circulating CD4+ lymphocyte numbers and improvements in lymphocyte proliferation in response to prevalent antigens. A consistent finding in these subjects is that HIV-1-specific immune responses are not re-stored after treatment with potent combination therapy (10, 11). In addition, perturbations in the distribution of lymphocyte T-cell-receptor Vβ families (a reflection of the potential diversity of antigen recognition by T lymphocytes) are not corrected or only minimally corrected by HAART, at least in the short term, in HIV-1-infected persons (11). Perhaps more prolonged suppression of viral replication will permit increasing degrees of immune restoration, but the durability of antiviral therapies is limited by the emergence of viral es-cape mutants, and the likelihood of escape is promoted by the unforgiving clinical requirements for strict adherence to suppressive treatment regimens that ensure viral replication is continuously blocked.

During the early stages of HIV-1 infection, a virus reservoir is established in resting memory CD4+ lymphocytes (12). The existence of this cellular reservoir, which has a very prolonged half-life due to its slow turnover, makes the possibility of cure of HIV-1 infection with antiretroviral therapy alone very unlikely. If eradication and cure of HIV-1 infection is a goal, different therapeutic approaches are needed.

Thus, HIV-1 parasitizes immune-competent cells, uses host-cellular ele-ments and immune activation for propagation, and induces progressive life-threatening immune deficiency that is only partly improved as a result of suppressive antiviral therapies. The rationale for treatment trials of host-directed and immune-based therapies for HIV-1 infection can be therefore summarized as follows. Host-directed antiviral therapies may interfere with HIV-1 replication and may be less susceptible to the emergence of viral escape mutation. Treatment with immune-based therapies may enhance immune responses in persons with HIV-related immune deficiency thereby improving the clinical outcome of HIV-1 disease. Because HIV-1 infection is unusual among pathogens in its ability to block the development of effective defenses to clear or control infection, therapies designed to induce host defenses against HIV-1 itself or to target long-lived reservoirs of infection may help to control or resolve HIV-1 replication. Well-designed trials of host-directed or immune-based therapies will not only test the utility of a treatment intervention but can also provide an opportunity to test critical hypotheses of HIV-1 disease pathogenesis.

II. HOST-DIRECTED THERAPIES

Host-directed therapies may interfere with HIV-1 replication and may be less susceptible to the emergence of viral escape mutation. A rate-limiting factor in successful antiviral treatment strategies is the predictable emergence of viral escape mutations as a consequence of continuous, high-level viral replication, and an error-prone reverse transcriptase. Because host elements are used for every phase of viral replication, targeting host–virus interactions may prove a reasonable therapeutic strategy to block viral replication. Mutational escape from these interventions is less likely, since the target elements are encoded in host genes. On the other hand, immunological toxicities of host-directed therapies are predictable, but the redundancy of host-immune defenses may permit targeting of these elements without dose-limiting toxicity.

Several potential targets for host-directed antiviral treatment strategies include host nuclear factors that enhance HIV-1 transcription (13); cellular cofactors for Tat, the transcriptional regulatory protein that mediates high level expression of HIV-1 genes (14–16); cellular chaperones for assembly of viral proteins (17) ; enzymes responsible for the generation of dinucleotide triphosphates needed to assemble proviral DNAs (18); and the chemokine receptors that serve as coreceptors for cell entry of both macrophage-tropic HIV-1 and lymphocytotropic HIV-1 isolates (19, 20).

Of these, targeting chemokine coreceptors may prove a particularly interesting strategy. Persons homozygous for a 32-bp deletion in the chemokine receptor gene that results in a failure of surface CCR-5 expression have been found to have significant resistance to acquisition of HIV-1 infection in vivo (21). This resistance is mirrored in cellular resistance to HIV-1 isolates that are macrophage-tropic in vitro (22). Most importantly, these persons, although relatively resistant to HIV-1 in vivo, are otherwise healthy and not immune impaired. Thus, targeting of the CCR-5 receptor may block viral replication without deleterious effects on the host. The potential utility of this approach is underscored by the clinical observations that persons who are homozygous for this allele tend to have lower plasma HIV-1 RNA levels (23), a more benign clinical outcome of HIV-1 infection (24), and a greater likelihood of durable response to antiretroviral therapies (25). Amino-terminus modification of the beta-chemokine RANTES can result in a molecule with limited agonist activity (26) and the ability to block HIV-1 replication in vitro (27, 28) and in animal models (29). These large molecules may work in part through down-modulation of surface CCR-5, thereby limiting virus access to critical coreceptors. Detailed study of these agents may help in the design of smaller molecules that are more convenient as therapeutics.

Although the foregoing approach may prove useful, additional coreceptors may be used for HIV-1 entry (30), and introduction of a selection pressure against macrophage-tropic CCR-5-dependent HIV-1 isolates may facilitate emergence of CXCR4-dependent syncitium-inducing strains that are associated with a more accelerated disease course (31). These considerations underscore the importance of carefully designed preclinical and clinical studies to ensure that treatment strategies targeting host elements are developed in a rational and safe manner. In this regard, host targeted agents that are active against CXCR4-dependent strains, such as AMD-3100, T-22, and T-134, have been identified (32, 33), and at least one of these agents, AMD-3100, is in human trials.

A. Hydroxyurea

HIV-1 replication depends on adequate intracellular levels of deoxynucleotide triphosphates (dNTP) (34). Hydroxyurea inhibits ribonucleotide reductase, the rate-limiting step for dNTP synthesis, creating a competitive advantage for the incorporation of nucleoside reverse transcriptase inhibitors. Because hydroxyurea depletes deoxyadenosine triphosphates to a greater extent than deoxythymidine triphosphate, the combination of hydroxyurea with didanosine appears to be more potent than the combination of hydroxyurea with zidovudine (35). Hydroxyurea does not reduce the prevalence of HIV-1 isolates genotypically resistant to didanosine (36), but by decreasing intracellular dNTP, hydroxyurea places didanosine at a favorable competitive position with respect to cellular dNTP and may restore the antiviral activity of didanosine. In vitro, HIV-1 isolates resistant to didanosine are more sensitive in the presence of hydroxyurea (37). Finally, because hydroxyurea inhibits S-phase of the cell cycle (38), it may reduce the availability of target cells for HIV-1 infection.

Recent trials of hydroxyurea have shown that this drug can potentiate the antiviral activity of didanosine in vivo. Montaner et al. (39) gave hydroxyurea to patients receiving didanosine (ddI) monotherapy. After 4 weeks of therapy, a 0.6 $\log_{10}$ decrease in plasma HIV-1 RNA levels was noted with no increase in CD4+ cell counts.

Rutschmann et al. (40) randomized 144 patients with a mean baseline plasma HIV-1 RNA level of 4.53 $\log_{10}$ and 370 CD4+ cells/μL to receive ddI, d4T (stavudine), plus hydroxyurea or placebo. After 12 weeks of therapy, the mean decrease in plasma HIV-1 RNA level was 1.7 and 2.3 $\log_{10}$, and 8% and 19% of patients had fewer than 20 copies/mL in the placebo and hydroxyurea arms, respectively. Despite greater decreases in viral load, patients randomized to hydroxyurea had an increase of 28 CD4+ cells/μL, compared with 38 CD4+ cells/μL in the group randomized to placebo. Patients receiving hydroxyurea experienced more neutropenia and thrombocytopenia, and they tended to have an increased occurrence of diarrhea and neuropathy.

Vila et al. (41) treated 25 ddI-naive patients with more than 200 CD4+ cells/μL and a median viral load of 29,000 copies/mL with ddI and hydroxyurea. After 1 year of therapy, 50% of patients had plasma HIV-1 RNA levels below 200 copies/mL, their CD4+ cell counts had increased from 525 to 601 cells/μL, and eight patients studied had very low levels of HIV-1 RNA in lymph nodes (41). After 1 year of treatment, two of these patients had no detectable HIV-1 RNA in lymph nodes and stopped therapy. These two patients had started therapy within 1 year of acquiring HIV-1 infection and had very low baseline HIV-1 RNA levels (676 and 1120 copies/mL). After 1 year of follow-up without resuming therapy, these patients had not experienced viral rebound in plasma, maintained normal CD4+ cell counts, and had very low levels of proviral DNA in lymph nodes (42). It is not known whether hydroxyurea had any role in preventing viral rebound in these unusual patients.

Recently, Lori et al. (43, 44) reported the immunological status of selected patients who were treated with hydroxyurea-containing regimens for 13–30 months. These patients experienced an increase in the percentage of naive CD4+ and CD8+, a decrease in the percentage of activated CD8+ lymphocytes, and an increase in CD8+ lymphocytes expressing CD28. Surprisingly about half of the hydroxyurea-treated patients showed lymphocyte proliferative responses after stimulation with HIV-1 p24 antigen. Because no baseline lymphocyte proliferation data were available for these patients, it is hard to know whether these HIV-1-specific responses are related to treatment.

More than 200 patients who had had excellent control of HIV-1 replication while receiving therapy with zidovudine, lamivudine, and indinavir were randomized to continue that regimen or to switch to ddI, d4T, and indinavir or ddI, d4T, indinavir, and hydroxyurea. The combined primary endpoint of the study was loss of viral suppression and drug toxicity necessitating discontinuation of treatment. After 24 weeks of follow-up, patients in the hydroxyurea-containing arm experienced a significantly increased occurrence of primary endpoints (mainly treatment-limiting toxicities), with two fatalities due to pancreatitis (ACTG 5025 summary). Thus, the long-term safety and efficacy of hydroxyurea in patients with advanced HIV-1 disease and the place of hydroxyurea in the treatment of HIV-1 disease remain to be determined. The antiviral activity of hydroxyurea when used in combination with ddI must be balanced against the effects that this agent may have on blunting the rise in CD4+ T cells, which may mediate the immunological benefits of viral suppression.

B.   Mycophenolate Mofetil

Other compounds also may interfere with synthesis of cellular nucleotides needed for HIV-1 replication (45). Mycophenolate mofetil is the prodrug of mycophenolic acid (MA); MA reversibly inhibits inosine monophosphate dehydrogenase, limiting the de novo synthesis of guanosine nucleotides. Because monocytes and lymphocytes are dependent on de novo synthesis of purines, MA is a relatively selective inhibitor of lymphocyte and monocyte proliferation (46). Although in vitro MA can directly inhibit HIV-1 replication at concentrations that are clinically achievable (45), MA also potentiates the antiviral activity of abacavir, a guanosine analogue (47), and this activity of MA provides a rationale for additional investigation.

Margolis et al. (47) confirmed that MA can inhibit HIV-1 replication in vitro at clinically achievable concentrations. Furthermore, synergy was demonstrated between abacavir and MA. Moreover this combination is active in vitro against lymphocyte and macrophage tropic strains of HIV-1, even in the presence of a M184V mutation that confers partial resistance to abacavir. These authors also showed that although MA had an additive effect with cytosine and adenosine analogues, MA had antagonistic antiviral activity when combined with thymidine analogues such as stavudine and zidovudine.

Carefully designed clinical trials are needed to confirm the in vivo antiviral activity of this combination, to identify the optimal MA dose, and to determine the activity of MA against viruses with mutations that confer resistance to nucleoside analogues. In addition, the immunological effects and safety of MA, an agent associated with the development of Kaposi's sarcoma, cytomegalovirus and other viral infections, and fungal infections in transplant recipients (48, 49) must be evaluated carefully.

III.   CYTOKINES AND GROWTH FACTORS

Cytokine dysregulation may play an important role in HIV-1 disease pathogenesis. Cytokine profiles are altered early in HIV-1 infection (50). Expression of T-helper cytokines is decreased during the course of HIV-1 disease (51–53), and this decrease may contribute to the functional impairment in immune responses seen in HIV-1 disease. Administration of T-helper cytokines is undergoing study in the hope that these agents may help correct these abnormalities. T-helper cytokines and growth factors are also undergoing evaluation because of additional effects of these agents on cellular homeostasis and perhaps on HIV-1 replication.

A.   Interleukin-2

IL-2 broadly enhances immune responsiveness; it induces T-cell proliferation, enhances cell-mediated cytotoxicity, and also enhances antigen presentation through increasing cell-surface human leukocyte-associated antigen DR (HLA-DR) expression. In vitro, IL-2 partly corrects the impaired lymphocyte natural killer (NK) cell activity and impaired CD8+-lymphocyte cytotoxicity in patients with AIDS (54) and the increased tendency of lymphocytes to undergo apoptosis (55) seen in HIV-1 disease. In addition, IL-2 enhances CD8+-lymphocyte-mediated nonlytic suppression of HIV-1 replication (56). This IL-2 effect may not be mediated by chemokines because IL-2 administration does not increase beta chemokine production by peripheral blood mononuclear cells (PBMC) of HIV-1-infected patients (57).

IL-2 production and phytohemagglutinin (PHA)-stimulated IL-2 receptor expression on CD4+ lymphocytes are decreased in patients with untreated HIV-1 disease (51, 53, 58, 59). Although the abnormalities in IL-2 receptor expression, in IL-2 production, and in response to IL-2 tend to decrease, they do not normalize after administration of suppressive antiretroviral therapies (59, 60).

Trials of low doses of IL-2 (36,000 to 500,000 U) administered subcutaneously daily or twice daily to HIV-infected patients with CD4+ counts greater than 200 cells/μL resulted in increases in lymphocyte-proliferative responses, NK cell number and activity, and enhanced delayed-type hypersensitivity responses. At higher doses, modest but transient increases in CD4+ cell counts were also seen (61–63).

Higher doses of IL-2 (6 to 18 MU daily) have been given intravenously in 5-day cycles every 8 weeks to HIV-infected patients with CD4+ cell counts greater than 200 cells/μL (64, 65). In these trials, more than half of the patients experienced a substantial polyclonal increase in circulating CD4+ cells. This was associated with transient bursts in circulating HIV-1 RNA levels. The increase in CD4+ cells appears to be greater in patients with lower plasma HIV-1 RNA levels at the time of initiation of IL-2 (66). When similar IL-2 doses were given to patients with fewer than 200 CD4+ cells/μL, a smaller proportion of patients experienced an increase in CD4+ cells, the increases in p24 antigen levels appeared to be more sustained, and more patients experienced adverse reactions (64). Conceivably in patients with more advanced disease and poorly controlled HIV-1 replication, the blunted CD4+ T-cell increase reflects both the effects of heightened HIV-1 replication and a diminished ability of IL-2 to induce cellular expansion.

Subcutaneous administration of IL-2 twice daily for 5 days every 8 weeks in doses up to 15 MU/day was also shown to provide significant increases in circulating CD4+ lymphocyte numbers (67, 68). Patients treated with nucleoside analogues with a mean baseline CD4+ count of 384 cells/μL experienced a mean increase of greater than 500 cells/μL and 70% of patients had an 80% increase in CD4+ cells after seven cycles. These increases were similar to those obtained using intravenous IL-2 (68, 69). As in the continuous intravenous infusion trials, plasma HIV-1 RNA levels increased transiently during the period of IL-2 administration.

After the first cycle of administration of IL-2, the increase in CD4+ cells is mainly constituted of memory CD4+ cells, but subsequently there is an increase in naive CD4+ cells (68, 69). The proportion of CD4+ cells expressing CD25 and the proportion of CD4+ cells expressing CD28 also increase after administration of IL-2 (68). CD8+ memory and naive lymphocyte numbers do not increase after IL-2 administration, but the proportion of CD8+ lymphocytes that coexpress CD28 increases and the proportion that coexpress the activation markers CD38 and HLA-DR decrease (64, 68). These changes suggest that IL-2 administration causes an increase in CD4+ cells with a more functional phenotype. The mechanisms that underlie the decrease in activation phenotype of CD8+ T cells is not well understood.

Administration of 6 to 18 MU of IL-2 daily for 5 days every 6 to 8 weeks to HIV-1-infected patients has shown to cause an increase in PHA-stimulated IL-2, IL-4, and interferon-γ production (70); to increase lymphocyte proliferative responses to tetanus toxoid (69); and to increase the size of delayed-type hypersensitivity skin test responses to recall antigens (66).

Fever, rash, capillary leak, and increased serum transaminases are common toxicities of high-dose IL-2 administration. As plasma levels of TNF-α rise during IL-2 infusions, this clinical syndrome and the transient increases in viral load have been attributed to induction of TNF-α expression by IL-2. However, neither thalidomide nor chimeric murine-human monoclonal anti-TNF-α antibodies prevented the clinical toxicities or transient increases in plasma HIV-1 RNA levels seen during IL-2 infusions (71).

As is the case with other immune-based therapies (72), patients with fewer CD4+ cell counts, those who would benefit the most from an IL-2-induced increase in CD4+ cell number and function, are the least likely to respond. Furthermore, as mentioned above, patients with lower CD4+ cell counts tend to experience more sustained increases in HIV-1 replication and an increased frequency of side effects after IL-2 administration.

Will adequate control of viral replication with HAART allow for safe and effective use of IL-2 in patients with low CD4+ cell counts? Recently, Arno et al. (73) reported the results of a small study performed among persons with advanced HIV-1 disease. Thirteen patients with a mean CD4+ cell count of 68 cell/μL initiated treatment with a protease inhibitor-containing regimen. After a mean of 11 months on therapy, the mean CD4+ cell counts had increased to 165/μL and plasma HIV-1 RNA levels were below the limit of detection. The patients then initiated IL-2—3 to 6 MU subcutaneously daily for 5 days every 4 weeks—and a comparable group of 12 controls who remained on antiretrovirals alone was also followed. After 24 weeks, CD4+ cell counts had significantly increased in the IL-2-treated group only (105 vs. 30 cells/μL). Thus, it appears that patients with advanced HIV-1 disease also can experience an increase in circulating CD4+ T cells from IL-2 therapy after viral replication is well controlled.

The clinical significance of the increases in circulating CD4+ T-lymphocyte numbers seen after IL-2 administration remains to be determined. Despite often dramatic increases in circulating CD4+ T-lymphocyte counts, prolonged therapy with IL-2 did not correct the perturbed T-cell receptor Vβ repertoire seen in HIV-1 disease (74), and the increase in delayed-type hypersensitivity responses was mainly due to the increase in diameter of preexistent responses and not to development of new responses (66). A clinical endpoint trial may be needed to establish the clinical significance of the CD4+ cell increases seen after IL-2 infusions. The design of such trial is challenging, because persons with lower CD4+ cell counts who are at greatest risk of opportunistic infection are less likely to experience an increase in CD4+ T-cell counts in response to IL-2 unless they are also treated with a regimen that effectively controls viral replication. Patients with controlled viral replication and CD4+ lymphocyte increases are at very low risk for developing opportunistic infections (75). Therefore, clinical trial strategies to explore the clinical benefit of IL-2 administration may require either very large numbers of patients or may need to focus on unique populations such as patients with advanced disease who do not experience CD4+ T-cell increases on antiretroviral therapies or populations at high risk for opportunistic infections that tend to occur with higher CD4+ T-cell counts such as, for example, persons at high risk for tuberculosis.

The early establishment of a viral reservoir in resting memory cells renders the possibility of eradicating HIV-1 with antiretroviral therapy unlikely (12, 76). This pool of cells is long lived and decays very slowly, with a mean half-life estimated to range between 6 and 43.9 months (77–79); it is not surprising therefore that after stopping suppressive antiretroviral therapies, viral rebound is observed in almost all instances. It has been proposed that activation of these cells with agents such as IL-2 while patients are receiving antiretroviral therapy may lead to induction of HIV-1 expression without subsequent infection of new cells. In this model, decay of this reservoir would be the cytolytic consequence of viral activation.

Chun et al. (80) examined retrospectively the frequency of latently infected memory cells in 12 HIV-1-infected patients who had received potent antiretroviral therapy and 14 patients who had received IL-2 (median of 10 cycles) in addition to potent antiretroviral therapy. The two groups were comparable in baseline characteristics. Patients receiving IL-2 had fewer infectious units per million cells than patients receiving antiretrovirals alone. In three patients in the IL-2 group, no virus could be isolated even when the cell input was as high as 330 million resting CD4+ cells. Two of these three patients had excisional lymph node biopsies and no replication-competent virus could be isolated. Nevertheless, proviral DNA could be identified in every patient (80), and after stopping antiviral therapy these two patients experienced viral rebound in plasma (81).

The significance of these findings remains to be determined. First, the apparent decrease in the frequency of culturable virus must be confirmed in a controlled randomized trial. If IL-2 administration is associated with a decrease in the frequency of latently infected cells, then the mechanism for this must be established. Is this related to enhancement of HIV-specific host defenses or to the induction of HIV-1 expression from these cells even though they do not express detectable IL-2 receptors? Clearly, in this small group, decreases in the size of the reservoir were insufficient to prevent viral rebound after suppressive antiviral therapies were withdrawn.

B. Granulocyte-Macrophage Colony-Stimulating Factor (GM-CSF)

GM-CSF is a growth factor that has been used to treat neutropenia due to HIV-1 or its therapy (82–86). In addition to increasing leukocyte numbers, GM-CSF also exerts quantitative and qualitative changes in lymphocytes and antigen-presenting cells (APC) that may be useful in the setting of HIV-1 infection (87). GM-CSF augments IL-2-induced proliferation and the effects of IL-2 on lymphokine-activated killer cell function. Furthermore, although T lymphocytes do not express GM-CSF receptors, GM-CSF, but not G-CSF, accelerates the reconstitution of CD4+ lymphocytes after autologous bone marrow transplantation (88). In APC, GM-CSF induces the expression of class I and class II molecules that may enhance antigen presentation. GM-CSF also decreases in vitro the expression of the chemokine receptor CCR-5, the major coreceptor for M-tropic HIV-1 entry into cells (89, 90), and may enhance the antiviral effect of zidovudine by increasing intracellular concentrations of zidovudine triphosphate (91). For these reasons, there has been a long-standing interest in the use of GM-CSF for the treatment of HIV-1 infection.

In vitro studies have shown enhancement, inhibition, or no effect of GM-CSF on HIV-1 replication (92–95). Differences in culture condition, differentiation stage, and cell type (monocyte vs. macrophage) may account for these different results. In vivo, GM-CSF administration was associated with a greater than 200% increase in serum p24 antigen levels in HIV-1-infected patients receiving chemotherapy but no antivirals for non-Hodgkin's lymphoma, whereas there was no increase in serum p24 antigen levels in patients only receiving chemotherapy (85). Other studies using insensitive techniques to quantitate viral load (e.g., p24 antigen or viral culture) have shown either no change (82–84, 96) or a trend to a decrease in HIV-1 levels (86). More recently, using polymerase chain reaction (PCR)-based assays to measure plasma HIV-1 RNA levels, Scadden et al. (97) showed that administration of GM-CSF to patients with advanced HIV-1 disease receiving zidovudine is not associated with increases in plasma HIV-1 RNA levels. There was a trend toward increased intracellular levels of phosphorylated zidovudine after GM-CSF administration.

As has also been seen in autologous bone marrow transplantation, patients with HIV-1 infection receiving GM-CSF may also experience CD4+

cell rises (82). Bernstein et al. (98) treated 13 HIV-1-infected patients on a stable antiviral regimen with 5 μg/kg of GM-CSF for 3 months. Plasma HIV-1 RNA levels did not change significantly, but 7 of 11 patients completing therapy experienced increases in CD4+ cell counts. Brites et al. (99) administered GM-CSF 125 μg/M^2 twice weekly or placebo for 6 months to 105 HIV-1-infected patients with fewer than 300 CD4+ cells/μL on nucleoside analogue therapy. After 6 months, a nonsignificant increase in CD4+ cells and a significant progressive decrease in plasma HIV-1 RNA levels was noted in GM-CSF-treated patients (-0.5 log$_{10}$ compared to -0.01 log$_{10}$ in the placebo arm). More recently, Skowron et al. (100) reported results of a study where 20 HIV-1-infected patients receiving a protease inhibitor-containing regimen were randomized to receive either GM-CSF 250 μg or placebo subcutaneously thrice weekly for 8 weeks. There was a trend toward greater HIV-1 RNA reductions and CD4+ cell increases in GM-CSF-treated subject. Finally, Angel et al. (101) presented a study wherein 309 HIV-1 infected subjects with fewer than 100 CD4+ cells/μL while receiving a stable antiretroviral regimen were randomized to receive either placebo or GM-CSF 250 μg subcutaneously thrice weekly for 24 weeks. Patients receiving GM-CSF experienced a significant rise in CD4+ cells compared with placebo recipients. Furthermore, among patients who started the trial with plasma HIV-1 RNA levels below the limit of detection (<400 copies/mL), 83% of GM-CSF recipients but only 54% of placebo recipients maintained control of viral replication.

Although these preliminary results are encouraging, many questions remain. First, the effects of GM-CSF administration on CD4+ T-cell numbers and HIV-1 replication must be confirmed. If GM-CSF increases the numbers of circulating CD4+ T-cell counts, is this through enhancing bone marrow release of progenitors for T-cell maturation or through other mechanisms? If HIV-1 replication is decreased, is this related to an effect of GM-CSF on CCR-5 expression? If GM-CSF downregulates CCR-5 expression in vivo, does this occur by induction of chemokine production and indirectly down-regulating CCR5 or does GM-CSF directly down-modulate CCR5 production (89, 102). The absence of recognized receptors for GM-CSF on T cells suggests an indirect mechanism would be more likely.

IV. ENHANCEMENT OF HIV-1-SPECIFIC IMMUNE RESPONSES

Strong HIV-1-specific immune responses correlate with a less aggressive course of disease. T-helper-cell proliferative responses to HIV-1 antigens,

HIV-1 specific cytotoxic T lymphocyte (CTL) responses, and neutralizing antibody levels to HIV-1 antigens are all higher in subjects with slowly progressive disease than in subjects with rapidly progressive illness (103–106). Are these relationships causal? The decrease in plasma HIV-1 RNA levels after acute HIV-1 infection is temporally associated with the appearance of HIV-1-specific CTL responses (2, 107). Patients with higher frequencies of HIV-1-specific memory CTL have lower viral loads and experience a slower CD4+ cell decline than patients with lower frequencies of these cells (108). Infused ex vivo expanded HIV-1-specific CTL accumulate in lymph nodes (the main site of HIV-1 replication) and cause a transient decrease in the number of productively infected CD4+ cells (109). In the simian immunodeficiency virus (SIV)-infected macaque, depletion of CD8+ cells results in marked increases in viremia; when SIV-specific CD8+ cells reappear, viremia is again suppressed (110).

HIV-1-specific CD4+ T-cell proliferative responses are absent in most HIV-1-infected individuals, even at a stage when these patients are able to respond to other recall antigens (111). HIV-1-specific proliferative responses are more often detected in long-term nonprogressors who have very low viral loads, and the magnitude of the HIV-1-specific proliferative response correlates inversely with plasma HIV-1 levels (106, 112, 113). Furthermore, the magnitude of HIV-1-specific helper cell responses correlates positively with the frequency of HIV-gag-specific CTL precursors (114).

The failure to restore HIV-1-specific CD4+ T-cell responses after HAART administration to persons with established HIV-1 infection (10, 11) is puzzling. In contrast, administration of HAART soon after acute HIV-1 infection permits the development of strong CD4+ T-cell responses to HIV antigens (106, 115). Therefore, either HIV-1-reactive CD4+ T cells are depleted during periods of uncontrolled HIV-1 replication or somehow are rendered anergic. Low frequencies of HIV-reactive CD4+ T lymphocytes have been detected in chronically infected persons using short-term assays, but the frequency of these cells may fall with duration of HAART administration (116). CD4+ T cells may be required to maintain cytolytic activities of CD8+ T cells as suggested in animal models of viral infection (117), and administration of HAART results in a decrease in the frequency of HIV-1-specific CD8+ T cells (118). Thus, treatment with antiretroviral therapies in chronic infection does not appear to result in the development of host immune responses to HIV-1 that may permit control of HIV-1 replication. Rather, host immune responses to HIV-1 may diminish as HIV-1 replication is decreased. A key question is whether induction of HIV-1-specific responses will provide HIV-1-infected persons the means to control HIV-1 replication in the absence of antiretroviral therapies.

Host immune responses are critical for control of viral infection. In this regard, HIV-1 may be unique among viral pathogens in that infection and depletion of CD4+ T cells may interfere with the ability of the immune system to control infection. Because treatment with potent antiretroviral agents during acute HIV-1 infection preserves HIV-1-specific responses (106, 115), it is likely that HIV-1-specific helper cell responses are generated during the early stages of infection and if viral replication is not controlled, these CD4+ lymphocytes are eliminated by a direct HIV-1 cytopathic effect or by activation-induced cell death. Alternatively, HIV-1-specific CD4+ lymphocytes may be rendered anergic. Proposed mechanisms for this are presented in Figure 1. In this model, naive CD4+ T cells with T-cell receptors (TCR) capable of recognizing HIV-1-derived peptides accumulate at sites of HIV-1 replication and are activated to proliferate and release cytokines by recog-

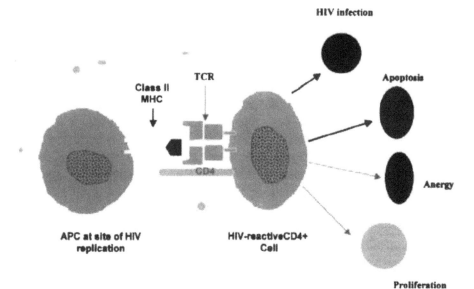

Figure 1   During uncontrolled HIV-1 replication, CD4+ lymphocytes with receptors capable of recognizing HIV-1 antigens accumulate in the lymph nodes, the sites of HIV-1 replication. Once activated, these lymphocytes are more susceptible to viral infection and cytolytic death; activated lymphocytes are also susceptible to death through apoptosis. Inappropriate triggering of the T-cell receptor in the absence of coreceptor activation may lead to anergy. Finally, some CD4+ lymphocytes may proliferate normally. The balance among these four possible outcomes may determine the course of disease. APC, antigen-presenting cell; MHC, major histocompatibility complex molecule; TCR, T-cell receptor.

nition and binding of HIV-1-derived peptides presented in the context of class II major histocompatibility complex (MHC) molecules. As these cells are activated by TCR stimulation, several possible outcomes can result. The benign and "normal" outcome of TCR stimulation that is seen in the absence of HIV-1 infection is the appropriate activation and proliferation of antigen-reactive cells and the development of a memory response. As activated CD4+ T cells are targets for productive HIV-1 replication, these cells may become infected and die as a result of virus-induced cytolysis (119). The lymphoid tissues in untreated HIV-1 disease are also characterized by high level immune activation (120, 121). T-cell activation in this setting also may result in the induction of activation-induced apoptosis (122) and cell death. Finally, dysregulated TCR triggering such as may be seen in the absence of appropriate coreceptor (e.g., CD28) stimulation also may induce a hyporesponsive state or anergy that may render HIV-1-reactive cells incapable of appropriate immune responsiveness (123). How these potential outcomes of antigen-induced activation are balanced in acute HIV-1 infection may determine the outcome of disease. Thus, antiretroviral therapies applied early after acquisition of infection may help to preserve HIV-1-specific CD4+ T-cell responses by decreasing the magnitude of HIV-1 replication and resultant inappropriate immune activation Whether preservation of these responses will affect control of HIV-1 replication remains to be determined.

As noted above, patients with chronic HIV-1 infection do not restore HIV-1-specific proliferative responses after treatment with HAART, although responses to other prevalent recall antigens tend to improve (10, 11). Although viral antigen is still present in lymph nodes of subjects with HIV-1 infection and plasma HIV-1 RNA levels below the limit of detection (124), it appears that for maintenance or regeneration of HIV-1-specific responses either the amount of antigen is insufficient and/or HIV-1-reactive CD4+ cells have been depleted or rendered anergic or the setting in which HIV-1 antigens are provided is inimical to the development of appropriate immune responses.

Two different approaches are being taken in an attempt to generate HIV-1-specific immune responses: scheduled treatment interruptions and therapeutic immunization.

A. Scheduled Treatment Interruptions

The rationale for scheduled treatment interruptions is based on the hypothesis that exposure to HIV-1 antigens may be required to develop or sustain an HIV-1-specific immune response. Thus, brief treatment interruptions that are expected to permit some degree of HIV-1 replication may result in the development or enhancement of HIV-1-specific immune defenses as HIV-1 antigens are exposed to immune-competent cells. Several critical issues must be addressed by these studies. First, is treatment interruption safe? Second, does treatment interruption result in increases in HIV-1-specific immune responses? Third, are these responses durable? Fourth, will these responses enhance control of HIV-1 replication?

After stopping combination antiviral therapy, most HIV-1-infected subjects experience viral rebound within 1 to 3 weeks (125, 126). Because HAART is associated with an apparent decline in HIV-1-specific immune responses, it is reasoned that brief interruptions of HAART after control of HIV-1 replication may expose the immune system to enough antigen to reelicit immune responses. Ten antiviral-naive subjects with a mean baseline CD4+ cell count of 414 were treated with zidovudine, lamivudine, and indinavir for 28 days. When treatment was stopped for 28 days, patients experienced virologic rebound; treatment resumption allowed regain in control of viral replication (127). Furthermore, no protease or reverse transcriptase mutations associated with resistance were observed, suggesting that at least a single therapy interruption in this small group of patients was safe.

Ortiz et al. (128) reported five subjects who started antiretroviral therapy shortly after acquiring HIV-1 infection and one who started therapy during chronic infection. After stopping antiretroviral therapy, three subjects failed to contain viral replication. The remaining three patients did not experience viral rebound or regained control of viral replication after a brief rebound. The patients who were able to control HIV-1 replication once therapy was withdrawn had or developed broad and strong HIV-1-specific CTL responses. Another group reported two subjects who started HAART during seroconversion and then interrupted treatment. After the first treatment interruption and upon reinstitution of HAART, these patients regained control of viral replication and HIV-1-specific CD4+ and CD8+ responses increased. After the second course of structured treatment interruption, these patients evidenced partial control of viral replication (129).

These preliminary results are intriguing, but many questions remain. Will scheduled treatment interruption permit sufficient control of HIV-1 replication without antiviral therapy? How many cycles of therapy interruption and resumption will be needed to achieve this? How much HIV-1 replication is enough to induce a helper cell response without destroying it? Can HIV-1-specific immune responses also be generated or boosted in subjects with chronic infection? Finally, how applicable will these approaches be in the clinic setting? Well-designed carefully controlled studies are needed to resolve these key issues.

B. Therapeutic Immunization

Enhancement of HIV-1-specific immune responses through immunization has been a strategy for the treatment of HIV-1 infection since before the availability of HAART (130). In these earlier studies, although some degree of immune responsiveness to immunization could be demonstrated, there was no evidence that the development of these HIV-1 specific immune responses could affect the clinical course of disease or could result in enhanced control of HIV-1 replication (131, 132). Interest in therapeutic immunization for HIV-1 infection has been rekindled after the realization that HIV-1-specific responses are not restored in subjects with chronic HIV-1 infection even after prolonged successful control of viral replication and that CD4+-dependent responses to HIV-1 can be generated after administration of potent antiretroviral therapy shortly after acquisition of infection.

Administration of envelope-based vaccines, such as recombinant gp160, has resulted in the generation of HIV-1-specific proliferative responses in HIV-1-infected patients with relatively preserved immune systems (CD4+ lymphocyte counts over 300 cells/μL) (133, 134). These augmented responses did not result in plasma viral load decreases. When patients with more advanced immunodeficiency and fewer CD4+ cell counts were immunized with rgp120, no significant improvement in HIV-1-specific proliferative responses was obtained (135).

A large placebo-controlled trial of rgp160 administered to HIV-1-infected subjects who were either untreated with more than 500 CD4+ cells/μL or had between 200 and 500 CD4+ cells/μL while taking nucleoside analogues was published recently (132). Although vaccine recipients developed increased proliferative responses directed against gp160, there was no difference between the groups in the rate of decline of CD4+ cells, in plasma HIV-1 RNA levels or proviral DNA levels or time to an AIDS-defining event. Another randomized, double-blind, placebo-controlled study using rgp160 enrolled more than 800 subjects with HIV-1 infection stratified by CD4+ cell counts (>400 cells/μL and 200 to 400 cells/μL) and had a clinical endpoint of mortality or a new AIDS-defining opportunistic infection. Antiviral therapy was allowed but HAART was not available at the time the trial was conducted. Recipients of rgp160, but not placebo recipients, developed proliferative responses to gp160. Interestingly, fewer patients in the immunized group reached a CD4+ endpoint (CD4+ cell count decrease of 30%). There was, however, no effect of immunization on the primary clinical endpoint of death or a new AIDS-defining condition. The clinical results of this study maybe somewhat confounded by a study design that permitted rgp160 immunization of patients who reached a CD4+ cell endpoint (131).

Inactivated, gp120-depleted HIV-1 in incomplete Freund's adjuvant (Remune) has also been used for therapeutic immunization. In subjects with relatively preserved immune systems (CD4+ cell counts usually over 300 cells/ μL), Remune has been shown to increase HIV-1-specific lymphocyte proliferative responses, to increase lymphocyte production of interferon gamma and RANTES after stimulation with HIV-1 antigens, to increase HIV-1-specific antibody responses, and to induce an HIV-1-specific delayed-type hypersensitivity response (136–138). The results of a clinical endpoint trial of Remune versus placebo were presented recently. In this study, more than 2500 patients with CD4+ T-cell counts between 300 and 550 were randomized to receive Remune or placebo in addition to their current antiretroviral therapies. Although 34 to 45% of the patients receiving Remune and fewer than 1% of the patients receiving placebo developed HIV-1-specific proliferative responses, the rate of clinical progression and the changes in plasma HIV-1 RNA levels were the same in both groups (139). Conceivably, patients with uncontrolled HIV-1 replication are unlikely to develop responses to immunization (140, 141) and are more likely to develop clinical endpoints (9) than patients with well-controlled HIV-1 replication. Alternatively, immunization with Remune failed to support HIV-specific CD8+ cell responses despite inducing CD4+ cell responses.

Because inactivated vaccines are not expected to elicit strong MHC class I restricted CTL responses, other strategies have been tested to induce or expand HIV-1-specific CTLs, the direct mediators of antiviral activity. Canarypox virus is a large avian DNA virus that can infect human cells but cannot complete a replication cycle. Recombinant canarypox expressing gp160 has been used in a double-blind trial in untreated HIV-1-infected patients who had over 500 CD4+ cells/μL (142). Immunization with gp160 expressing canarypox did not induce an increase in either gp160 antibody concentrations or CTL responses, but patients receiving the canarypox HIV-1 immunogen and patients receiving the canarypox rabies vaccine experienced nonspecific increases in lymphocyte proliferative responses to p24 and gp160. Two groups have conducted small trial using naked DNA vaccines expressing HIV-1 antigens (143, 144). Both found small increases in HIV-1-specific CTL, proliferative, and antibody responses in a minority of immunized subjects.

Thus, immunization trials in persons with HIV-1 infection and ongoing HIV-1 replication have shown only modest immunogenicity and no clear evidence that HIV-1 replication is affected by the induction of these responses. This is not particularly surprising, as there is limited precedent that immunization strategies are effective in the control of infectious diseases (as opposed to their prevention). On the other hand, HIV-1 is a unique pathogen in that HIV-

1-reactive CD4+ T cells are likely directly targeted in the course of HIV-1 replication and the diminution of detectable CD4+ T-cell responses to HIV-1 may determine the failure of host defenses to control HIV-1 replication. Thus, strategies designed to enhance HIV-1 specific CD4+ T-cell responses during uncontrolled HIV-1 replication may be counterbalanced by virus-induced cytopathic effects or other mechanisms that cripple the induction or preservation of CD4+ T-cell responses to HIV-1 antigens. A key question is whether immunization or other reexposures to HIV-1 antigens after HIV-1 replication is controlled with antiviral therapies will permit the establishment and survival of CD4+ T-cell helper responses sufficient to support the survival of brisk CTL responses and endogenous control of HIV-1 replication.

Valentine et al. (145) have reported the results of a study wherein HIV-1-infected subjects who had more than 400 CD4+ cells/μL were vaccinated with either Remune or incomplete Freund's adjuvant shortly after initiating HAART. Subjects receiving Remune had a 0.7-$\log_{10}$ increase in stimulation index to HIV-1 antigens after immunization. After 32 weeks of follow-up, 94% of patients in the group that received Remune had plasma viral loads below 40 copies/mL, compared with 75% of patients in the group who received the adjuvant (not statistically significant) (145).

The magnitude of the CD4+ T-cell response to immunization in this study is encouraging yet raises many questions. Will the patients who start HAART with fewer CD4+ cells also develop a strong response to HIV-1 antigens? Will the induction of a brisk CD4+ T-cell response to HIV-1 proteins also enhance CTL responses? Finally, the key question is whether any immunization strategy will permit a better control of HIV-1 replication through the induction of HIV-1-specific responses. This can be tested by comparing the durability of antiretroviral therapies in immunized and nonimmunized subjects or by examining the control of HIV-1 replication after withdrawal of antiviral therapies.

V. CONCLUSION

Host-directed and immune-based therapies are offering increasing promise to persons with HIV-1 infection. This is in part a consequence of the successes of newer antiretroviral therapies that for the first time have permitted substantive control of HIV-1 replication. Better control of HIV-1 replication and consequent escape from HIV-1-induced immune paralysis has permitted better responses to immunization and to administration of other immune-based therapies. The next few years should determine if the promise of these therapies will be translated into clinical, virological, and immunological benefit.

REFERENCES

1. Lederman M. Role of cytotoxic T lymphocytes in the control of HIV-1 infection and HIV-1 disease progression. Curr Opin Infect Dis 1996; 9:14–18.

2. Borrow P, Lewicki H, Hahn BH, Shaw GM, Oldstone MB. Virus-specific CD8+ cytotoxic T-lymphocyte activity associated with control of viremia in primary human immunodeficiency virus type 1 infection. J Virol 1994; 68:6103–6110.

3. Kaslow RA, Carrington M, Apple R, Park L, Munoz A, Saah AJ, Goedert JJ, Winkler C, O'Brien SJ, Rinaldo C, Detels R, Blattner W, Phair J, Erligh H, Mann DL. Influence of combinations of human major histocompatibility complex genes on the course of HIV-1 infection. Nat Med 1996; 2:405–411.

4. Mellors JW, Rinaldo CR, Jr., Gupta P, White RM, Todd JA, Kingsley LA. Prognosis in HIV-1 infection predicted by the quantity of virus in plasma. Science 1996; 272:1167–1170.

5. Aukrust P, Liabakk NB, Muller F, Lien E, Espevik T, Froland SS. Serum levels of tumor necrosis factor-alpha (TNF alpha) and soluble TNF receptors in human immunodeficiency virus type 1 infection—correlations to clinical, immunologic, and virologic parameters. J Infect Dis 1994; 169:420–424.

6. Giorgi JV, Ho HN, Hirji K, Chou CC, Hultin LE, O'Rourke S, Park L, Margolick JB, Ferbas J, Phair JD. CD8+ lymphocyte activation at human immunodeficiency virus type 1 seroconversion: development of HLA-DR+ CD38+ CD8+ cells is associated with subsequent stable CD4+ cell levels. The Multicenter AIDS Cohort Study Group. J Infect Dis 1994; 170:775–781.

7. Palella FJ Jr, Delaney KM, Moorman AC, et al. Declining morbidity and mortality among patients with advanced human immunodeficiency virus infection. HIV Outpatient Study Investigators. N Engl J Med 1998; 338:853–860.

8. Cameron DW, Heath-Chiozzi M, Danner S, et al. Randomised placebo-controlled trial of ritonavir in advanced HIV-1 disease. The Advanced HIV Disease Ritonavir Study Group. Lancet 1998; 351:543–549.

9. Hammer SM, Squires KE, Hughes MD, et al. A controlled trial of two nucleoside analogues plus indinavir in persons with human immunodeficiency virus infection and CD4 cell counts of 200 per cubic millimeter or less. AIDS Clinical Trials Group 320 Study Team. N Engl J Med 1997; 337:725–733.

10. Li TS, Tubiana R, Katlama C, Calvez V, Ait Mohand H, Autran B. Long-lasting recovery in CD4 T-cell function and viral-load reduction after highly active antiretroviral therapy in advanced HIV-1 disease. Lancet 1998; 351: 1682–1686.

11. Lederman MM, Connick E, Landay A, et al. Immunologic responses associated with 12 weeks of combination antiretroviral therapy consisting of zidovudine, lamivudine, and ritonavir: results of AIDS Clinical Trials Group Protocol 315. J Infect Dis 1998; 178:70–79.

12. Chun TW, Carruth L, Finzi D, et al. Quantification of latent tissue reservoirs and total body viral load in HIV-1 infection. Nature 1997; 387:183–188.

13. Nabel G, Baltimore D. An inducible transcription factor activates expression of human immunodeficiency virus in T cells [published erratum appears in Nature 1990; 344:178]. Nature 1987; 326:711–713.

14. Kashanchi F, Piras G, Radonovich MF, et al. Direct interaction of human TFIID with the HIV-1 transactivator tat. Nature 1994; 367:295–299.

15. Yu L, Loewenstein PM, Zhang Z, Green M. In vitro interaction of the human immunodeficiency virus type 1 Tat transactivator and the general transcription factor TFIIB with the cellular protein TAP. J Virol 1995; 69:3017–3023.

16. Wu-Baer F, Lane WS, Gaynor RB. Identification of a group of cellular cofactors that stimulate the binding of RNA polymerase II and TRP-185 to human immunodeficiency virus 1 TAR RNA. J Biol Chem 1996; 271:4201–4208.

17. Luban J, Bossolt KL, Franke EK, Kalpana GV, Goff SP. Human immunodeficiency virus type 1 Gag protein binds to cyclophilins A and B. Cell 1993; 73: 1067–1078.

18. Lori F, Malykh A, Cara A, et al. Hydroxyurea as an inhibitor of human immunodeficiency virus-type 1 replication. Science 1994; 266:801–805.

19. Feng Y, Broder CC, Kennedy PE, Berger EA. HIV-1 entry cofactor: functional cDNA cloning of a seven-transmembrane, G protein-coupled receptor. Science 1996; 272:872–877.

20. Alkhatib G, Combadiere C, Broder CC, et al. CC CKR5: a RANTES, MIP-1alpha, MIP-1beta receptor as a fusion cofactor for macrophage-tropic HIV-1. Science 1996; 272:1955–1958.

21. Paxton WA, Martin SR, Tse D, et al. Relative resistance to HIV-1 infection of CD4 lymphocytes from persons who remain uninfected despite multiple high-risk sexual exposure. Nat Med 1996; 2:412–417.

22. Liu R, Paxton WA, Choe S, et al. Homozygous defect in HIV-1 coreceptor accounts for resistance of some multiply-exposed individuals to HIV-1 infection. Cell 1996; 86:367–377.

23. Buseyne F, Janvier G, Teglas JP, et al. Impact of heterozygosity for the chemokine receptor CCR5 32-bp-deleted allele on plasma virus load and CD4 T lymphocytes in perinatally human immunodeficiency virus-infected children at 8 years of age. J Infect Dis 1998; 178:1019–1023.

24. Cairns JS, D'Souza MP. Chemokines and HIV-1 second receptors: the therapeutic connection. Nat Med 1998; 4:563–568.

25. Valdez H, Purvis SF, Lederman MM, Fillingame M, Zimmerman PA. Association of the CCR5delta32 mutation with improved response to antiretroviral therapy [letter]. JAMA 1999; 282:734.

26. Simmons G, Clapham PR, Picard L, et al. Potent inhibition of HIV-1 infectivity in macrophages and lymphocytes by a novel CCR5 antagonist. Science 1997; 276:276–279.

27. Rusconi S, La Seta-Catamancio S, Kurtagic S, et al. Aminooxypentane-RANTES, an inhibitor of R5 human immunodeficiency virus type 1, increases the interferon gamma to interleukin 10 ratio without impairing cellular proliferation. AIDS Res Hum Retroviruses 1999; 15:861–867.

28. Rusconi S, Merrill DP, La Seta-Catamancio S, Citterio P, Offord RE, Hirsch MS. Effective inhibition of HIV-1 isolated from patients with acute primary HIV-1 infection by aminooxypentane-RANTES [letter]. AIDS 1999; 13:1144–1145.

29. Mosier DE, Picchio GR, Gulizia RJ, et al. Highly potent RANTES analogues either prevent CCR5-using human immunodeficiency virus type 1 infection in vivo or rapidly select for CXCR4-using variants. J Virol 1999; 73:3544–3550.

30. He J, Chen Y, Farzan M, et al. CCR3 and CCR5 are co-receptors for HIV-1 infection of microglia. Nature 1997; 385:645–649.

31. Hughes MD, Johnson VA, Hirsch MS, et al. Monitoring plasma HIV-1 RNA levels in addition to CD4+ lymphocyte count improves assessment of antiretroviral therapeutic response. ACTG 241 Protocol Virology Substudy Team [see comments]. Ann Intern Med 1997; 126:929–938.

32. Arakaki R, Tamamura H, Premanathan M, et al. T134, a small-molecule CXCR4 inhibitor, has no cross-drug resistance with AMD3100, a CXCR4 antagonist with a different structure. J Virol 1999; 73:1719–1723.

33. Schols D, Este JA, Henson G, De Clercq E. Bicyclams, a class of potent anti-HIV agents, are targeted at the HIV coreceptor fusin/CXCR-4. Antiviral Res 1997; 35:147–156.

34. Gao WY, Cara A, Gallo RC, Lori F. Low levels of deoxynucleotides in peripheral blood lymphocytes: a strategy to inhibit human immunodeficiency virus type 1 replication. Proc Natl Acad Sci USA 1993; 90:8925–8928.

35. Lori F. Hydroxyurea and HIV: 5 years later–from antiviral to immune-modulating effects [editorial]. AIDS 1999; 13:1433–1442.

36. De Antoni A, Foli A, Lisziewicz J, Lori F. Mutations in the pol gene of human immunodeficiency virus type 1 in infected patients receiving didanosine and hydroxyurea combination therapy. J Infect Dis 1997; 176:899–903.

37. Lori F, Malykh AG, Foli A, et al. Combination of a drug targeting the cell with a drug targeting the virus controls human immunodeficiency virus type 1 resistance. AIDS Res Hum Retroviruses 1997; 13:1403–1409.

38. Buchkovich KJ, Greider CW. Telomerase regulation during entry into the cell cycle in normal human T cells. Mol Biol Cell 1996; 7:1443–1454.

39. Montaner JS, Zala C, Conway B, et al. A pilot study of hydroxyurea among patients with advanced human immunodeficiency virus (HIV) disease receiving chronic didanosine therapy: Canadian HIV trials network protocol 080. J Infect Dis 1997; 175:801–806.

40. Rutschmann OT, Opravil M, Iten A, et al. A placebo-controlled trial of didanosine plus stavudine, with and without hydroxyurea, for HIV infection. The Swiss HIV Cohort Study. AIDS 1998; 12:F71–F77.

41. Vila J, Biron F, Nugier F, Vallet T, Peyramond D. 1-Year follow-up of the use of hydroxycarbamide and didanosine in HIV infection [letter]. Lancet 1996; 348:203–204.

42. Vila J, Nugier F, Bargues G, et al. Absence of viral rebound after treatment of HIV-infected patients with didanosine and hydroxycarbamide [letter]. Lancet 1997; 350:635–636.

43. Lori F, Rosenberg E, Lieberman J, et al. Hydroxyurea and didanosine long-term treatment prevents HIV breakthrough and normalizes immune parameters. AIDS Res Hum Retroviruses 1999; 15:1333–1338.

44. Lori F, Jessen H, Lieberman J, Clerici M, Tinelli C, Lisziewicz J. Immune restoration by combination of a cytostatic drug (hydroxyurea) and anti-HIV drugs (didanosine and indinavir). AIDS Res Hum Retroviruses 1999; 15:619–624.

45. Ichimura H, Levy JA. Polymerase substrate depletion: a novel strategy for inhibiting the replication of the human immunodeficiency virus. Virology 1995; 211:554–560.

46. Allison AC, Kowalski WJ, Muller CD, Eugui EM. Mechanisms of action of mycophenolic acid. Ann NY Acad Sci 1993; 696:63–87.

47. Margolis D, Heredia A, Gaywee J, Oldach D, Drusano G, Redfield R. Abacavir and mycophenolic acid, an inhibitor of inosine monophosphate dehydrogenase, have profound and synergistic anti-HIV activity. J Acquir Immune Defic Syndr 1999; 21:362–370.

48. Mycophenolate mofetil in cadaveric renal transplantation. US Renal Transplant Mycophenolate Mofetil Study Group. Am J Kidney Dis 1999; 34:296–303.

49. Eberhard OK, Kliem V, Brunkhorst R. Five cases of Kaposi's sarcoma in kidney graft recipients: possible influence of the immunosuppressive therapy. Transplantation 1999; 67:180–184.

50. Biglino A, Sinicco A, Forno B, et al. Serum cytokine profiles in acute primary HIV-1 infection and in infectious mononucleosis. Clin Immunol Immunopathol 1996; 78:61–69.

51. Borzy MS. Interleukin 2 production and responsiveness in individuals with acquired immunodeficiency syndrome and the generalized lymphadenopathy syndrome. Cell Immunol 1987; 104:142–153.

52. Chehimi J, Starr SE, Frank I, et al. Impaired interleukin 12 production in human immunodeficiency virus-infected patients. J Exp Med 1994; 179:1361–1366.

53. Prince HE, Kermani-Arab V, Fahey JL. Depressed interleukin 2 receptor expression in acquired immune deficiency and lymphadenopathy syndromes. J Immunol 1984; 133:1313–1317.

54. Rook AH, Masur H, Lane HC, et al. Interleukin-2 enhances the depressed natural killer and cytomegalovirus- specific cytotoxic activities of lymphocytes from patients with the acquired immune deficiency syndrome. J Clin Invest 1983; 72:398–403.

55. Clerici M, Sarin A, Coffman RL, et al. Type 1/type 2 cytokine modulation of T-cell programmed cell death as a model for human immunodeficiency virus pathogenesis. Proc Natl Acad Sci USA 1994; 91:11811–11815.

56. Kinter AL, Bende SM, Hardy EC, Jackson R, Fauci AS. Interleukin 2 induces CD8+ T cell-mediated suppression of human immunodeficiency virus replication in CD4+ T cells and this effect overrides its ability to stimulate virus expression. Proc Natl Acad Sci USA 1995; 92:10985–10989.

57. Blanco J, Cabrera C, Jou A, Ruiz L, Clotet B, Este JA. Chemokine and chemokine receptor expression after combined anti-HIV-1 interleukin-2 therapy. AIDS 1999; 13:547–555.

58. Westby M, Marriott JB, Guckian M, Cookson S, Hay P, Dalgleish AG. Abnormal intracellular IL-2 and interferon-gamma (IFN-gamma) production as HIV-1-assocated markers of immune dysfunction. Clin Exp Immunol 1998; 111:257–263.

59. David D, Bani L, Moreau JL, et al. Regulatory dysfunction of the interleukin-2 receptor during HIV infection and the impact of triple combination therapy. Proc Natl Acad Sci USA 1998; 95:11348–11353.

60. Weiss L, Ancuta P, Girard PM, et al. Restoration of normal interleukin-2 production by CD4+ T cells of human immunodeficiency virus-infected patients after 9 months of highly active antiretroviral therapy. J Infect Dis 1999; 180: 1057–1063.

61. Teppler H, Kaplan G, Smith KA, Montana AL, Meyn P, Cohn ZA. Prolonged immunostimulatory effect of low-dose polyethylene glycol interleukin 2 in patients with human immunodeficiency virus type 1 infection. J Exp Med 1993; 177:483–492.

62. Teppler H, Kaplan G, Smith K, et al. Efficacy of low doses of the polyethylene glycol derivative of interleukin-2 in modulating the immune response of patients with human immunodeficiency virus type 1 infection. J Infect Dis 1993; 167: 291–298.

63. Jacobson EL, Pilaro F, Smith KA. Rational interleukin 2 therapy for HIV positive individuals: daily low doses enhance immune function without toxicity. Proc Natl Acad Sci USA 1996; 93:10405–10410.

64. Kovacs JA, Baseler M, Dewar RJ, et al. Increases in CD4 T lymphocytes with intermittent courses of interleukin-2 in patients with human immunodeficiency virus infection. A preliminary study [see comments]. N Engl J Med 1995; 332: 567–575.

65. Kovacs JA, Vogel S, Albert JM, et al. Controlled trial of interleukin-2 infusions in patients infected with the human immunodeficiency virus [see comments]. N Engl J Med 1996; 335:1350–1356.

66. Carr A, Emery S, Lloyd A, et al. Outpatient continuous intravenous interleukin-2 or subcutaneous, polyethylene glycol-modified interleukin-2 in human immunodeficiency virus-infected patients: a randomized, controlled, multicenter study. Australian IL-2 Study Group. J Infect Dis 1998; 178:992–999.

67. Davey RT, Jr., Chaitt DG, Piscitelli SC, et al. Subcutaneous administration of interleukin-2 in human immunodeficiency virus type 1-infected persons. J Infect Dis 1997; 175:781–789.

68. Levy Y, Capitant C, Houhou S, et al. Comparison of subcutaneous and intravenous interleukin-2 in asymptomatic HIV-1 infection: a randomised controlled trial. ANRS 048 study group. Lancet 1999; 353:1923–1929.

69. Kelleher AD, Roggensack M, Emery S, Carr A, French MA, Cooper DA. Effects of IL-2 therapy in asymptomatic HIV-infected individuals on proliferative responses to mitogens, recall antigens and HIV-related antigens. Clin Exp Immunol 1998; 113:85–91.

70. De Paoli P, Zanussi S, Simonelli C, et al. Effects of subcutaneous interleukin-2 therapy on CD4 subsets and in vitro cytokine production in HIV+ subjects. J Clin Invest 1997; 100:2737–2743.

71. Walker R, Hahn B, Kelly GG, Miller K, Piscitelli S, Figg WD, Davey RT, Falloon J, Kovacs JA, Polis MA, Masur H, Metcalf JA, Baseler M, Fyfe G, Thomas S, McCloskey RV, Lane HC. Effects of TNF-alpha antagonists thalidomide and monoclonal anti-TNF antibody (cA2) on reducing IL-2 associated toxicities: a randomized, controlled trial. 4th Conference on Retroviruses and Opportunistic Infections, Chicago, 1997, Abstract 36.

72. Krown SE, Gold JW, Niedzwiecki D, et al. Interferon-alpha with zidovudine: safety, tolerance, and clinical and virologic effects in patients with Kaposi sarcoma associated with the acquired immunodeficiency syndrome (AIDS). Ann Intern Med 1990; 112:812–821.

73. Arno A, Ruiz L, Juan M, et al. Efficacy of low-dose subcutaneous interleukin-2 to treat advanced human immunodeficiency virus type 1 in persons with ≤250/microL CD4 T-cells and undetectable plasma virus load. J Infect Dis 1999; 180:56–60.

74. Connors M, Kovacs JA, Krevat S, et al. HIV infection induces changes in CD4+ T-cell phenotype and depletions within the CD4+ T-cell repertoire that

are not immediately restored by antiviral or immune-based therapies. Nat Med 1997; 3:533–540.

75. Piketty C, Castiel P, Belec L, et al. Discrepant responses to triple combination antiretroviral therapy in advanced HIV disease. AIDS 1998; 12:745–750.

76. Chun TW, Engel D, Berrey MM, Shea T, Corey L, Fauci AS. Early establishment of a pool of latently infected, resting CD4(+) T cells during primary HIV-1 infection. Proc Natl Acad Sci USA 1998; 95:8869–8873.

77. Finzi D, Blankson J, Siliciano JD, et al. Latent infection of CD4+ T cells provides a mechanism for lifelong persistence of HIV-1, even in patients on effective combination therapy. Nat Med 1999; 5:512–517.

78. Natarajan V, Bosche M, Metcalf JA, Ward DJ, Lane HC, Kovacs JA. HIV-1 replication in patients with undetectable plasma virus receiving HAART. Highly active antiretroviral therapy [letter]. Lancet 1999; 353:119–120.

79. Zhang L, Ramratnam B, Tenner-Racz K, et al. Quantifying residual HIV-1 replication in patients receiving combination antiretroviral therapy [see comments]. N Engl J Med 1999; 340:1605–1613.

80. Chun TW, Engel D, Mizell SB, et al. Effect of interleukin-2 on the pool of latently infected, resting CD4+ T cells in HIV-1-infected patients receiving highly active anti-retroviral therapy. Nat Med 1999; 5:651–655.

81. Davey RT Jr, Bhat N, Yoder C, et al. HIV-1 and T cell dynamics after interruption of highly active antiretroviral therapy (HAART) in patients with a history of sustained viral suppression. Proc Natl Acad Sci USA 1999; 96: 15109–15114.

82. Barbaro G, Di Lorenzo G, Grisorio B, Soldini M, Barbarini G. Effect of recombinant human granulocyte-macrophage colony-stimulating factor on HIV-related leukopenia: a randomized, controlled clinical study. AIDS 1997; 11: 1453–1461.

83. Groopman JE, Mitsuyasu RT, DeLeo MJ, Oette DH, Golde DW. Effect of recombinant human granulocyte-macrophage colony-stimulating factor on myelopoiesis in the acquired immunodeficiency syndrome. N Engl J Med 1987; 317: 593–598.

84. Scadden DT, Bering HA, Levine JD, et al. GM-CSF as an alternative to dose modification of the combination zidovudine and interferon-alpha in the treatment of AIDS-associated Kaposi's sarcoma. Am J Clin Oncol 1991; 14(suppl 1):S40–S44.

85. Kaplan LD, Kahn JO, Crowe S, et al. Clinical and virologic effects of recombinant human granulocyte- macrophage colony-stimulating factor in patients receiving chemotherapy for human immunodeficiency virus-associated non-Hodgkin's lymphoma: results of a randomized trial. J Clin Oncol 1991; 9: 929–940.

86. Levine JD, Allan JD, Tessitore JH, et al. Recombinant human granulocyte-macrophage colony-stimulating factor ameliorates zidovudine-induced neutropenia in patients with acquired immunodeficiency syndrome (AIDS)/AIDS-related complex. Blood 1991; 78:3148–3154.

87. Deresinski SC. Granulocyte-macrophage colony-stimulating factor: potential therapeutic, immunological and antiretroviral effects in HIV infection [editorial]. AIDS 1999; 13:633–643.

88. San Miguel JF, Hernandez MD, Gonzalez M, et al. A randomized study comparing the effect of GM-CSF and G-CSF on immune reconstitution after autologous bone marrow transplantation. Br J Haematol 1996; 94:140–147.

89. Di Marzio P, Tse J, Landau NR. Chemokine receptor regulation and HIV type 1 tropism in monocyte-macrophages. AIDS Res Hum Retroviruses 1998; 14: 129–138.

90. Paxton WA, Kang S, Liu R, et al. HIV-1 infectability of CD4+ lymphocytes with relation to beta-chemokines and the CCR5 coreceptor. Immunol Lett 1999; 66:71–75.

91. Perno CF, Cooney DA, Gao WY, et al. Effects of bone marrow stimulatory cytokines on human immunodeficiency virus replication and the antiviral activity of dideoxynucleosides in cultures of monocyte/macrophages. Blood 1992; 80: 995–1003.

92. Matsuda S, Akagawa K, Honda M, Yokota Y, Takebe Y, Takemori T. Suppression of HIV replication in human monocyte-derived macrophages induced by granulocyte/macrophage colony-stimulating factor. AIDS Res Hum Retroviruses 1995; 11:1031–1038.

93. Koyanagi Y, O'Brien WA, Zhao JQ, Golde DW, Gasson JC, Chen IS. Cytokines alter production of HIV-1 from primary mononuclear phagocytes. Science 1988; 241:1673–1675.

94. Folks TM, Justement J, Kinter A, Dinarello CA, Fauci AS. Cytokine-induced expression of HIV-1 in a chronically infected promonocyte cell line. Science 1987; 238:800–802.

95. Perno CF, Yarchoan R, Cooney DA, et al. Replication of human immunodeficiency virus in monocytes. Granulocyte/macrophage colony-stimulating factor (GM-CSF) potentiates viral production yet enhances the antiviral effect mediated by 3'-azido-2'3'-dideoxythymidine (AZT) and other dideoxynucleoside congeners of thymidine. J Exp Med 1989; 169:933–951.

96. Hardy WD. Combined ganciclovir and recombinant human granulocyte-macrophage colony-stimulating factor in the treatment of cytomegalovirus retinitis in AIDS patients. J Acquir Immune Defic Syndr 1991; 4(suppl 1):S22–S28.

97. Scadden DT, Pickus O, Hammer SM, et al. Lack of in vivo effect of granulocyte-macrophage colony-stimulating factor on human immunodeficiency virus type 1. AIDS Res Hum Retroviruses 1996; 12:1151–1159.

98. ZP Bernstein SB, FA Hayes, M Gould, S Jacob, TB Tomasi. A pilot study in the use of GM-CSF in human immunodeficiency virus (HIV) infected individuals. Blood 1997; 90:133a.

99. Brites C, Badaro R, Pedral-Sampaio D, Bahia F, Pedroso C, Alcantara AP, Stellrecht K, Sasaki M, Matos J, Mongillo A, Whitmore J, Gilbert M. Granulocyte-macrophage-colony-stimulating factor (GM-CSF) reduces viral load and increases CD4 cell counts in individuals with AIDS. 38th Interscience Conference on Antimicrobial Agents and Chemotherapy, San Diego, 1998:I-243.

100. Skowron G, Stein D, Drusano G, et al. The safety and efficacy of granulocyte-macrophage colony-stimulating factor (sargramostim) added to indinavir- or ritonavir-based antiretroviral therapy: a randomized double-blind, placebo-controlled trial. J Infect Dis 1999; 180:1064–1071.

101. JB Angel, High K, Rhame F, Deresinski S, Brand D, Whitmore J, Agosti J, Gilbert M. Randomized, double-blind, placebo-controlled study of leukine (GM-CSF) in advanced HIV disease: significant improvements in overall infections, CD4 cell counts, and duration of viral suppression. 39th Interscience Conference on Antimicrobial Agents and Chemotherapy, San Francisco, 1999, 487, Abstract 693.

102. Kornbluth RS, Kee K, Richman DD. CD40 ligand (CD154) stimulation of macrophages to produce HIV-1-suppressive beta-chemokines. Proc Natl Acad Sci USA 1998; 95:5205–5210.

103. Cao Y, Qin L, Zhang L, Safrit J, Ho DD. Virologic and immunologic characterization of long-term survivors of human immunodeficiency virus type 1 infection. N Engl J Med 1995; 332:201–208.

104. Ogg GS, Jin X, Bonhoeffer S, et al. Quantitation of HIV-1-specific cytotoxic T lymphocytes and plasma load of viral RNA. Science 1998; 279:2103–2106.

105. Pantaleo G, Menzo S, Vaccarezza M, et al. Studies in subjects with long-term nonprogressive human immunodeficiency virus infection. N Engl J Med 1995; 332:209–216.

106. Rosenberg ES, Billingsley JM, Caliendo AM, et al. Vigorous HIV-1-specific CD4+ T cell responses associated with control of viremia. Science 1997; 278: 1447–1450.

107. Koup RA, Safrit JT, Cao Y, et al. Temporal association of cellular immune responses with the initial control of viremia in primary human immunodeficiency virus type 1 syndrome. J Virol 1994; 68:4650–4655.

108. Musey L, Hughes J, Schacker T, Shea T, Corey L, McElrath MJ. Cytotoxic-T-cell responses, viral load, and disease progression in early human immunodeficiency virus type 1 infection. N Engl J Med 1997; 337:1267–1274.

109. Brodie SJ, Lewinsohn DA, Patterson BK, et al. In vivo migration and function of transferred HIV-1-specific cytotoxic T cells. Nat Med 1999; 5:34–41.

110. Schmitz JE, Kuroda MJ, Santra S, et al. Control of viremia in simian immuno-deficiency virus infection by CD8+ lymphocytes. Science 1999; 283:857–860.

111. Krowka JF, Stites DP, Jain S, et al. Lymphocyte proliferative responses to human immunodeficiency virus antigens in vitro. J Clin Invest 1989; 83:1198–1203.

112. Pontesilli O, Carlesimo M, Varani AR, Ferrara R, D'Offizi G, Aiuti F. In vitro lymphocyte proliferative response to HIV-1 p24 is associated with a lack of CD4+ cell decline [letter]. AIDS Res Hum Retroviruses 1994; 10:113–114.

113. Schwartz D, Sharma U, Busch M, et al. Absence of recoverable infectious virus and unique immune responses in an asymptomatic HIV+ long-term survivor. AIDS Res Hum Retroviruses 1994; 10:1703–1711.

114. Kalams SA, Buchbinder SP, Rosenberg ES, et al. Association between virus-specific cytotoxic T-lymphocyte and helper responses in human immunodeficiency virus type 1 infection. J Virol 1999; 73:6715–6720.

115. Malhotra U, Berrey MM, Huang Y, et al. Effect of combination antiretroviral therapy on T-cell immunity in acute human immunodeficiency virus type 1 infection. J Infect Dis 2000; 181:121–131.

116. Pitcher CJ, Quittner C, Peterson DM, et al. HIV-1-specific CD4+ T cells are detectable in most individuals with active HIV-1 infection, but decline with prolonged viral suppression. Nat Med 1999; 5:518–525.

117. Matloubian M, Concepcion RJ, Ahmed R. CD4+ T cells are required to sustain CD8+ cytotoxic T-cell responses during chronic viral infection. J Virol 1994; 68:8056–8063.

118. Ogg GS, Jin X, Bonhoeffer S, et al. Decay kinetics of human immunodeficiency virus-specific effector cytotoxic T lymphocytes after combination antiretroviral therapy. J Virol 1999; 73:797–800.

119. Ranga U, Woffendin C, Verma S, et al. Enhanced T cell engraftment after retroviral delivery of an antiviral gene in HIV-infected individuals. Proc Natl Acad Sci USA 1998; 95:1201–1206.

120. Andersson J, Fehniger TE, Patterson BK, et al. Early reduction of immune activation in lymphoid tissue following highly active HIV therapy. AIDS 1998; 12:F123–F129.

121. Bucy RP, Hockett RD, Derdeyn CA, et al. Initial increase in blood CD4(+) lymphocytes after HIV antiretroviral therapy reflects redistribution from lymphoid tissues. J Clin Invest 1999; 103:1391–1398.

122. Badley AD, Dockrell DH, Algeciras A, et al. In vivo analysis of Fas/FasL interactions in HIV-infected patients. J Clin Invest 1998; 102:79–87.

123. Allison JP. CD28-B7 interactions in T-cell activation. Curr Opin Immunol 1994; 6:414–419.

124. Wong JK, Hezareh M, Gunthard HF, et al. Recovery of replication-competent HIV despite prolonged suppression of plasma viremia [see comments]. Science 1997; 278:1291–1295.

125. Jubault V, Burgard M, Le Corfec E, Costagliola D, Rouzioux C, Viard JP. High rebound of plasma and cellular HIV load after discontinuation of triple combination therapy [letter]. AIDS 1998; 12:2358–2359.

126. Staszewski S, Miller V, Sabin C, Berger A, Hill AM, Phillips AN. Rebound of HIV-1 viral load after suppression to very low levels [letter]. AIDS 1998; 12: 2360.

127. Neumann AU, Tubiana R, Calvez V, et al. HIV-1 rebound during interruption of highly active antiretroviral therapy has no deleterious effect on reinitiated treatment. Comet Study Group. AIDS 1999; 13:677–683.

128. Ortiz GM, Nixon DF, Trkola A, et al. HIV-1-specific immune responses in subjects who temporarily contain virus replication after discontinuation of highly active antiretroviral therapy. J Clin Invest 1999; 104:R13–R18.

129. Rosenberg E, Altfeld M, Poon S, Wilkes B, Philips M, Robbins G, Boswell S, Davis B, Sax E, Caliendo A, D'Aquila R, Walker B. Generation and maintenance of HIV-specific T-helper cell responses in persons treated during acute HIV-1 infection and augmentation of these responses following structured treatment interruption. Infectious Diseases Society of America, Philadelphia, Pennsylvania, 1999, Abstract 725.

130. Salk J. Prospects for the control of AIDS by immunizing seropositive individuals. Nature 1987; 327:473–476.

131. Sandstrom E, Wahren B. Therapeutic immunisation with recombinant gp160 in HIV-1 infection: a randomised double-blind placebo-controlled trial. Nordic VAC-04 Study Group. Lancet 1999; 353:1735–1742.

132. Goebel FD, Mannhalter JW, Belshe RB, et al. Recombinant gp160 as a therapeutic vaccine for HIV-infection: results of a large randomized, controlled trial. European Multinational IMMUNO AIDS Vaccine Study Group. AIDS 1999; 13:1461–1468.

133. Kundu SK, Katzenstein D, Valentine FT, Spino C, Efron B, Merigan TC. Effect of therapeutic immunization with recombinant gp160 HIV-1 vaccine on HIV-1 proviral DNA and plasma RNA: relationship to cellular immune responses. J Acquir Immune Defic Syndr Hum Retrovirol 1997; 15:269–274.

134. Leandersson AC, Bratt G, Hinkula J, et al. Induction of specific T-cell responses in HIV infection. AIDS 1998; 12:157–166.

135. Schooley RT, Spino C, Chiu S, DeGruttola V, Kuritzkes DR. Poor immunogenicity of HIV-1 envelope vaccines with alum or MF59 adjuvant in HIV-1 infected individuals: results of two randomized trials. 4th Conference on Retroviruses and Opportunistic Infections, Chicago, 1997, Abstract 756.

136. Levine AM, Groshen S, Allen J, et al. Initial studies on active immunization of HIV-infected subjects using a gp120-depleted HIV-1 Immunogen: long-term follow-up. J Acquir Immune Defic Syndr Hum Retrovirol 1996; 11:351–364.

137. Moss RB, Trauger RJ, Giermakowska WK, et al. Effect of immunization with an inactivated gp120-depleted HIV-1 immunogen on beta-chemokine and cytokine production in subjects with HIV-1 infection. J Acquir Immune Defic Syndr Hum Retrovirol 1997; 14:343–350.

138. Trauger RJ, Ferre F, Daigle AE, et al. Effect of immunization with inactivated gp120-depleted human immunodeficiency virus type 1 (HIV-1) immunogen on HIV-1 immunity, viral DNA, and percentage of CD4 cells. J Infect Dis 1994; 169:1256–1264.

139. Kahn J, Lagakos S, Mayer K, Murray H. A randomized, placebo controlled multicenter study of remune in subjects with 300-550 CD4 cells and unrestricted anti-retroviral treatments. 39th Interscience Conference on Antimicrobial Agents and Chemotherapy, San Francisco, California, 1999, Abstract LB-21.

140. Talesnik E, Vial PA, Labarca J, Mendez C, Soza X. Time course of antibody response to tetanus toxoid and pneumococcal capsular polysaccharides in patients infected with HIV. J Acquir Immune Defic Syndr Hum Retrovirol 1998; 19:471–477.

141. Valdez H, Smith K, Lederman M, Landay A, Kessler H, Connick E, Kuritzkes D, Spritzler J, Fox L, Roe J, Lederman H, Lederman MB, Evans T, ACTG 375 Team. Response to immunization with recall and neoantigens after 48 weeks of HAART. 6th Conference of Retroviruses and Opportunistic Infections, Chicago, IL, 1999.

142. Tubiana R, Gomard E, Fleury H, et al. Vaccine therapy in early HIV-1 infection using a recombinant canarypox virus expressing gp160MN (ALVAC-HIV): a double-blind controlled randomized study of safety and immunogenicity [letter]. AIDS 1997; 11:819–820.

143. Calarota S, Bratt G, Nordlund S, et al. Cellular cytotoxic response induced by DNA vaccination in HIV-1-infected patients. Lancet 1998; 351:1320–1325.

144. MacGregor RR, Boyer JD, Ugen KE, et al. First human trial of a DNA-based vaccine for treatment of human immunodeficiency virus type 1 infection: safety and host response. J Infect Dis 1998; 178:92–100.

145. Valentine F, De Gruttola V, the Remune 816 Study Team. Immunological and virological evaluations of the effects of HAART compared to HAART plus an inactivated HIV-1 immunogen after 32 weeks. 6th Conference on Retroviruses and Opportunistic Infections, Chicago, 1999, Abstract 346.

10

Human Immunodeficiency Virus and Hepatitis B and C Coinfection: Pathogenic Interactions, Natural History, and Therapy

Arthur Y. Kim and Raymond T. Chung
*Massachusetts General Hospital and Harvard Medical School,
Boston, Massachusetts*

Bruce Polsky
St. Luke's–Roosevelt Hospital Center, New York, New York

I. INTRODUCTION

In the wake of recent advances in antiretroviral therapy for human immunodeficiency virus (HIV) infection and the attendant reconstitution of the immune system, survival free from life-limiting opportunistic infections has improved significantly. In place of these opportunists, infections with hepatitis B (HBV) and C virus (HCV) will become increasingly important problems in HIV-positive individuals (1–3). Recent data from a European population showed that chronic viral liver disease represented the fifth most common cause of death for HIV-infected patients (4). In view of the shared routes of transmission between HIV and HBV and HCV infections, morbidity and mortality from hepatitis-related liver failure is expected to become an even more critical problem in the immediate future. This chapter considers our current understanding of the pathogenic interactions between HIV and HBV/HCV, the natural history of HIV and hepatitis B/C coinfection, and available treatment strategies for the coinfected individual.

II. HIV AND HBV

A. Epidemiology and Prevention

Recent data on the epidemiology of HBV infection estimate an overall prevalence of 4.9%, with black race, increasing numbers of lifetime sexual partners, and foreign birth as the strongest independent risk factors predicting infection (5). HBV infection is particularly common in homosexual men, resulting in an extremely high rate of coinfection with HIV (6).

The influence of HIV may have a significant impact on the epidemiology of HBV infection given increased rates of chronic carriage (7). Those infected with HIV are approximately three to six times more likely to become chronic carriers of HBV than those who are HIV negative (8, 9). Lower CD4 cell counts are positively associated with development of the chronic carrier state (9). This phenomenon appears to increase the reservoir of HBV infection in the population.

In HIV-infected persons before the era of highly active antiretroviral therapy (HAART), the hepatitis B vaccine appeared to be less effective than in immunocompetent persons (10–14). Although a complete course of vaccination is capable of preventing HBV infection in HIV-positive individuals, it is possible that administration of inactivated vaccine temporarily impairs the immune response to acute HBV infection in HIV-positive individuals during the period of administration (8). Persons with HIV-1 infection preceding HBV infection had a significantly higher risk of developing HBV carriage, viremia, prolonged alanine aminotransferase (ALT) elevation, and clinical illness (8). Although HBV vaccination is recommended for those with HIV, these data underscore the importance of reduction of high-risk sexual behavior for the prevention of HBV.

B. Pathogenesis of HBV and Effects of Immunosuppression with HIV

The preponderance of evidence suggests that the central event in HBV pathogenesis is the recognition of virus-infected hepatocytes by CD8+ cytotoxic T lymphocytes (CTL). In the great majority (>95%) of acute infections with HBV, the CTL responses leads to successful viral clearance (15). In rare instances, however, HBV may exert intrinsic cytopathic effects that are not immune mediated. These are generally found in states of either exogenous or endogenous immune suppression. The defect in cell-mediated immunity present in HIV infection (16–19), as with exogenous immunosuppression (20, 21), is known to stimulate HBV replication. The so-called fibrosing cholestatic variant of HBV, characterized by a paucity of cellular infiltrate and rapidly progressive cholestatic injury with very high levels of intracellular virus, has been described in organ transplant recipients and represents the most extreme example of HBV's cytopathic effects.

C. Natural History of HBV in HIV-Infected Individuals

On the basis of the observation that immunosuppression enhances HBV replication yet diminishes immunological hepatocyte damage, it is difficult to predict the effect of HIV coinfection on the course of HBV. Initial autopsy studies of coinfected patients who died of acquired immunodeficiency syndrome (AIDS) showed less severe liver injury in those with HBV than in those without HBV, implying that severe immunosuppression reduced histological injury in HBV (22). However, further data indicate a more complex interaction between the two viruses.

The course of HBV in HIV-positive persons has been best studied in cohorts of homosexual men. Most studies indicate that HIV infection is associated with an increased frequency of markers of replicative HBV infection (HBeAg, HBV DNA positivity), consistent with less immune suppression of viral replication (23–25), but a lower alanine aminotransferase activity, consistent with less immunopathogenic liver injury. In patients with evidence of ongoing HBV replication, coinfection with HIV apparently results in a much lower rate of spontaneous reduction in viral replication (26). A greater prevalence of HBeAg positivity in HIV-infected hosts has also been reported (27, 28) and may be a marker of HIV seroconversion in persons previously infected with HBV (29).

It has also been demonstrated that chronic replicative HBV can be seen in HIV-positive patients whose only marker is anti-HBcore antibody, with negative assays for HBsAg and anti-HBsAg antibody (30). This pattern of HBV serum markers may be more frequent in those who are also HCV positive, suggesting that occult infection with HBV may be an important contributor to liver disease in certain individuals (31).

1. Effects of HIV on Histological Markers

Although there is certainly some basis for the proposition that the net result of HIV's effect on HBV progression is accelerated liver disease, early studies did not find a significant acceleration of histological liver damage in HIV-coinfected individuals (32, 33). One study found a higher histological activity index in HIV-positive persons; however, it did not control for the presence of HCV and had a high rate of hepatitis delta virus (HDV) coinfection, which can aggravate the severity of preexisting HBV liver disease (37). A second study in a non-intravenous drug user (IVDU) cohort, which excluded coinfection with HCV or HDV, also found accelerated histological liver injury, in addition to finding a significant increase in HBV DNA and decrease in ALT activity. Although this study may have been confounded by duration of HBV infection, which was only crudely estimated (35), collectively these data suggest that the course of HBV liver disease may be more accelerated in HIV coinfection and that the weakening of the immune system leads to a net adverse consequence for the natural history of HBV.

Further, with reports of the fibrosing cholestatic variant of HBV in HIV-coinfected hosts, it appears that cytopathic liver injury can be seen in coinfection and may contribute to progression of liver disease (36). Taken together, the data suggest that the reactivation of hepatitis B viral replication frequently seen in HIV coinfection *may* lead to acceleration of liver disease progression. Further studies are necessary to elucidate the precise impact of HIV coinfection on the natural history of HBV disease.

2. Effects of HBV on HIV

Studies have shown disparate results with regard to the influence of HBV infection on the course of HIV. Most natural history studies have not detected any difference in HIV disease progression (37–39). One study did find that the presence of markers of HBV infection resulted in an adjusted relative risk of HIV disease progression of 3.6; however, this study did not account for all other factors that influence the rate of HIV disease progression and most subjects were HBsAg negative (40). One recent retrospective analysis revealed an association of HBV infection with elevated IgE levels, which in turn may be a marker of HIV disease progression (41). The clinical relevance of this finding is unclear. In sum, no conclusive data demonstrate an adverse effect of HBV infection on the natural history of HIV disease.

3. Effect of Immune Reconstitution on HBV

It is clear that removal of immunosuppression plays an important role in both the reactivation of HBV disease and its clearance. This phenomenon has been illustrated by cases of fulminant hepatitis attributable to reactivation of HBV after discontinuation of immunosuppressive drugs (42, 43). These have been conjectured to be a result of restored cellular immunity to hepatocytes expressing enhanced levels of viral antigens. It is thus not surprising that similar flares have been observed in HBV-positive individuals initiating HAART for HIV infection during immune reconstitution; these flares have been followed by successful resolution of HBV (44–46). This finding underscores the need to properly interpret liver function abnormalities in HIV/HBV-coinfected persons starting anti-HIV therapy and to consider baseline hepatitis virus status in all individuals about to embark on a course of HAART.

In summary, the net effect of HIV-related immunosuppression on the natural history of HBV infection appears to depend on the status of the immune system. Initial studies indicated a relative protection against ongoing inflammation with reactivation of HBV replication as AIDS progresses. The introduction of HAART and immune reconstitution can be accompanied by a flare of hepatitis, but it may be hypothesized that restoration of HBV-specific immunity may result in a beneficial virological outcome. Further studies are needed to confirm this hypothesis. Caution should be counseled for those patients with evidence of HBV-related cirrhosis, as the flare of hepatitis seen with reconstitution could theoretically lead to hepatic decompensation as was seen in early trials of interferon alfa.

D. Therapy

Interferon alfa therapy, discussed in further detail in the section on HCV, has been associated with sustained clearance of circulating HBsAg in immunocompetent individuals (47, 48) but may be less effective for hepatitis B infection in persons infected with HIV (49, 50). Indeed, elevations in HIV viral load may be correlated with a poorer response to interferon (51). Small studies indicate that cotreatment with both interferon alfa and zidovudine (ZDV) may be associated with successful clearance of hepatitis B in coinfected patients (52, 53), but this approach has short-term gain and problematic side effects (54).

Unlike HCV, however, antiretroviral drugs have been found that not only work against HIV but also have anti-HBV activity, particularly against HBV DNA polymerase, which possesses reverse transcriptase activity (55). Neither ZDV nor didanosine (ddI or dideoxyinosine) have apparent clinical activity against HBV (56–58). Although zalcitabine (2′,3′-dideoxycytidine) has *in vitro* activity against HBV (59), its use has been limited by the development of severe peripheral neuropathy. Much more promising are two other antiretroviral agents, lamivudine (3TC) and adefovir.

3TC, in doses typically used for HIV infection, has excellent activity against HBV, both in resolution of markers of viral replication (60) and in histologic activity (61). Attenuation of HBV in HIV-positive patients receiving 3TC as part of a dual nucleoside regimen (62) and as part of triple therapy (63) has been reported. Another report of reactivation of hepatitis B after 3TC withdrawal as part of multidrug therapy for HIV, followed by resolution of hepatitis after reintroduction, lends credence to its use against both infections

(64). Given reports that 3TC is effective in controlling hepatitis B in other states of immunosuppression, such as postorgan transplant or chemotherapy (65, 66), and is associated with restoration of specific immune responses against HBV (67), there is ample reason to believe that this drug will work successfully in patients coinfected with HIV.

Unfortunately, long-term treatment with 3TC alone results in development of resistant HBV in a significant portion of immunocompetent individuals (68), mediated by mutations in a specific active-site (YMDD) motif of the viral DNA polymerase (69). This resistance pattern has been reported in an HIV-coinfected individual (70). Other nucleoside/nucleotide analogues, such as adefovir or penciclovir, are potentially useful in treatment of 3TC-resistant mutants (71, 72). Adefovir has activity against HIV as well (73), even in the setting of resistance to 3TC via the HIV reverse transcriptase (RT) M184V mutation (74). Adefovir thus appears to be yet another promising agent for treatment of the coinfected individual, either in combination with 3TC or as salvage therapy when resistance arises.

A therapeutic strategy should decrease HBV viral load, attenuate disease progression, and prevent emergence of drug-resistant virus. Although specific trials in coinfected individuals are lacking, there is sufficient basis to believe that 3TC or adefovir, either in combination or in conjunction with interferon alfa, may be the treatment regimen of choice for active chronic hepatitis B in patients with HIV. The results of ongoing studies using combination 3TC/adefovir antiretroviral therapy will be of interest in those coinfected patients with replicative HBV disease.

III. HIV AND HCV

The remainder of this chapter considers the epidemiology and transmission of coinfection with hepatitis C, the basis of possible pathogenic interactions between the two viruses, the effect of HIV on the natural history of HCV, and therapeutic options for the coinfected patient.

A. Epidemiology of HCV/HIV Coinfection

The prevalence of HCV infection is estimated to be 1.8% in the United States, corresponding to 3.9 million persons. Of these, an estimated 2.7 million persons are estimated to harbor chronic infection (75). The sharing of common means of transmission of HIV and HCV—parenteral, sexual, or vertical—results in a prevalence of antibodies to HCV that varies widely depending on the specific risk factor from 5% to 85% of HIV-infected individuals (Table 1)

Table 1 Prevalence of HCV Infection in HIV-positive Individuals Stratified by Risk Factor

Population	Antibodies to HCV
Intravenous drug users	52–92% (77, 79, 80, 81)
Hemophiliacs	60–85% (82, 83)
Homosexual men	4–14% (84–86)
Infants born to HCV/HIV+ mothers	8–17% HCV alone 4% cotransmission (87, 88)

(76). Coinfection is by far most common in persons with blood exposures such as sharing of contaminated needles or receiving infected blood products. A sample cohort study of 272 HIV-infected patients revealed an overall prevalence of HCV antibodies of 41.3% (77). The rates of coinfection with HCV were highest among intravenous drug users (78.3%) and persons having received blood transfusions before 1990 (31.2%), as compared with heterosexual (18.3%) and homosexual (2.9%) individuals. The overall prevalence of HCV in HIV-infected persons is estimated at 8–41% (78, 79).

1. Pitfalls in the Diagnosis of HCV in the HIV-Positive Individual

Studies may be inaccurate in determining the actual prevalence of HCV in HIV-positive individuals. Due to a high frequency of false positives intrinsic to the first-generation anti-HCV enzyme-immunosorbent assays (EIA-1), the prevalence may have been overestimated in older studies (81). Next-generation assays (EIA-2, EIA-3) appear to have a comparatively increased sensitivity (89) and specificity (90) for detection of HCV in HIV-positive hosts.

On the other hand, a high rate of variation in antibody titers in immuno-suppressed patients may result in many false negatives using these assays (91). EIA-1 may underreport the incidence of HCV infection in 10–30% of HIV-positive persons (92), particularly if they have advanced HIV infection or AIDS (79). It is likely that HIV, via suppression of cell-mediated immunity, reduces the magnitude of antibody response to HCV (93–95).

It should therefore not be surprising that seroreversion, or complete loss of antibody response to HCV detectable by EIA-1, occurs in those with HIV at a rate 2.5 times higher than those without HIV (96). In one study of hemophiliacs, around 25% of coinfected persons positive by EIA-1 later reverted to negative, with the vast majority of seroreverters positive via EIA-2 and HCV

RNA by polymerase chain reaction (PCR) (97). This phenomenon has also been documented as occurring more frequently in other immunocompromised states (98). Even with newer generation assays, a single negative HCV antibody does not entirely exclude infection (99). In persons with appropriate risk factors and negative HCV antibodies, the possibility of seroreversion leading to a false-negative antibody result must be taken seriously and testing for HCV RNA performed to exclude the presence of HCV infection.

2. Cotransmission of HIV and HCV

Parenteral Transmission.   The strongest risk factor for the transmission of either virus is direct blood exposure, either by sharing of needles during intravenous drug users or infusion of virus via blood transfusion. Sharing of needles and syringes appears to be clearly associated with cotransmission of viruses (100, 101). Multiply-transfused individuals such as hemophiliacs have coinfection prevalence rates as high as 60–90% (78). Fortunately, due to advances in screening the blood supply, transmission of either virus via transfusion is now extremely rare, with an estimate of contamination with HIV of 1 in every 493,000 units of packed red blood cells, with HCV 1 in 103,000 units (102).

The primary vehicle for occupational transmission of either HIV or HCV is via needlestick exposure. The overall risk of infection with HIV if exposed in this fashion is estimated at 0.3%, compared with a rate of 2–8% for HCV (103, 104). Cases of simultaneous transmission of both viruses have been reported (105), one marked by an unusually rapid progression to hepatic failure and death (106). Conjunctival blood exposure, although generally a lower risk event than a needlestick, also resulted in coincident transmission of both HIV and HCV (107). Universal precautions remain a key component of prevention of occupational transmission, and although effective regimens exist for postexposure prophylaxis for HIV (108), it is unknown whether a similar approach for HCV is of benefit.

Sexual Transmission.   HCV is transmitted via heterosexual contact far less efficiently than HIV (109–113). Nevertheless, HCV exposure correlates with other markers of unprotected sex, and transmission via sexual means, although infrequent, is an important risk factor for both viruses (114, 115). In a study of prostitutes who denied intravenous drug use or blood transfusion, a positive test for HCV was significantly associated with HIV seropositivity, number of sex partners, and a history of genital ulcers (116). The presence of HIV coinfection in the index case resulted in a doubling of the likelihood that HCV would be transmitted to partners of HCV-positive sexually promiscuous individuals (117). It is likely that male-to-female transmission of HCV is more efficient than the converse (118).

In a study examining transmission of the two viruses to sexual partners of multitransfused men with hemophilia, 2.6% of female sexual partners were HCV positive, as opposed to 12.8% positive for HIV. Interestingly, in the same hemophiliac cohort, coinfected patients passed HCV more efficiently to their partners if HIV was also transmitted (119). A similar analysis of stable heterosexual partners of HCV-positive individuals also suggested that HIV may be a cofactor for the transmission of HCV (120).

Studies that address the sexual transmission of HCV in homosexuals have been limited. The much higher relative prevalence of HIV compared with HCV argues against a major role of sexual transmission of HCV in this population. Those reports suggesting homosexual transmission of HCV may have been confounded by the presence of intravenous drug use. Nonetheless, they collectively suggest that HCV seropositivity was associated with HIV infection, with HIV possibly serving as a risk factor for HCV transmission (121, 122).

Vertical Transmission.   Both HIV and HCV may be transmitted vertically *in utero* via the placenta at the time of delivery. HCV does not appear to be transmitted via breast milk (123). The efficiency of HIV-1 transmission by an untreated mother to her child is approximately 25% (124), whereas the vertical transmission rate of HCV alone is much lower (125). Large cohorts of coinfected pregnant women have revealed potential interactions between the two viruses, particularly with regard to mutual enhancement of viral transmission efficiency.

The efficiency of vertical transmission of HCV is enhanced by the presence of HIV. This efficiency appears to be dependent on the HCV viral load (126, 127), which is known to be significantly elevated in HIV-positive as compared with HIV-negative patients (128). An Italian cohort of 155 HCV-infected mothers revealed a fourfold enhancement of transmission of HCV in HIV-positive mothers (87). In a larger study of 511 HCV-infected mothers, if the maternal HCV RNA concentration was $<10^5$ copies/mL, no HCV infection could be detected in infants (88). The same study showed that HIV-1 enhanced transmission of HCV threefold, with an overall transmission rate in coinfected mothers of 15.1%. Another recent study of coinfected mothers found that of the infants who acquired HIV, 40% also acquired HCV, whereas in those who did not acquire HIV, only 7.5% became HCV infected (129).

Conversely, HCV may also enhance vertical transmission of HIV. One study found that the presence of HCV increased the risk of HIV transmission even when controlling for potential confounders such as maternal intravenous drug use (130).

The apparent reciprocal enhancement of vertical transmission has not been rigorously studied in the era of HAART. Nevertheless, these findings suggest important interactions between the two viruses. Efforts to prevent transmission of either virus from coinfected mothers to infants should involve reduction of maternal viral loads of both viruses (131), and elective cesarean delivery (132) might be considered for mothers who do not achieve virological control of both diseases.

In sum, the risk factors most strongly associated with coinfection of HIV and hepatitis C are parenteral. Although HCV is less efficiently transmitted via horizontal or vertical means, studies examining the dual transmission of these two infections imply that HIV is an important cofactor in the transmission of hepatitis C.

B. Pathogenic Interactions

There is little evidence to suggest a *direct* virological interaction between HCV and HIV in the liver. While HIV is lymphotropic, it does not infect hepatocytes directly. On the other hand, a number of studies have suggested but not proved that HCV may be lymphotropic, as viral sequences can be amplified from peripheral blood mononuclear cells of infected individuals.

The pace of scientific progress since the discovery of the viral genome (Fig. 1) has led to a clearer understanding of the HCV life cycle (Fig. 2). After infection of the hepatocyte and internalization by an as yet defined receptor, the 9.4-kb RNA genome is uncoated and undergoes two fates: it is translated by host cellular ribosomes into a long polyprotein, which is subsequently cleaved by both host (signal peptidase) and virus-derived pro-

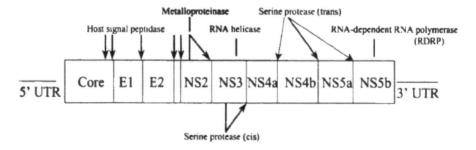

Figure 1 Structure of the hepatitis C virus polyprotein, including structural and nonstructural proteins and sites of host and viral protease actions.

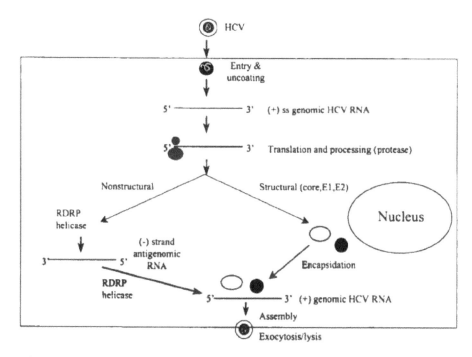

Figure 2   Schematic representation of the hepatitis C virus life cycle.

teases (NS2 metalloproteinase, NS3) to yield mature viral proteins. These proteins include structural components (core and the two envelope glycoproteins E1 and E2) that comprise the viral particle and the nonstructural proteins that are generally concerned with protein processing and genome replication. The virus-encoded RNA polymerase (NS5B) is unique in that it possesses RNA-dependent RNA polymerase activity and does not move through a DNA intermediate. Thus, this polymerase is insensitive to reverse transcriptase inhibitors. As with HBV, hepatocyte damage thought to occur as a result of the host cellular immune response to virus-infected hepatocytes. However, rare examples of a potential cytopathic HCV effect have also been described in the form of a fibrosing cholestatic picture similar to that described for HBV. These have also occurred in the setting of immunosuppression such as that found after solid organ transplant (133).

HCV's remarkable predilection for chronicity appears to lie in the inability of the host immune response to bring about viral clearance after acute infection. There is evidence that the breadth and depth of the cellular immune response to HCV is limited in individuals who fail to clear virus. Emerging data also suggest that HCV may subvert the host antiviral response by inhibit-

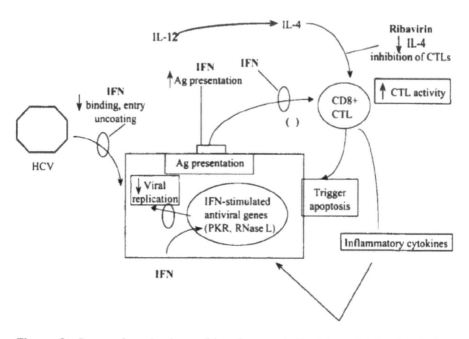

Figure 3 Proposed mechanisms of interferon and ribavirin action in chronic hepatitis C virus infection.

ing interferon-inducible protein kinases (Fig. 3). Both the E2 and the NS5A protein appear to inhibit PKR, which itself is responsible for inhibition of viral protein synthesis (134, 135). The observed alterations in cytokine production that attend HIV infection may ultimately lead to an aggravation of this already blunted endogenous interferon response. Observations of the balanced increase in both T_H1 and T_H2 cytokine expression in HIV coinfection suggests factors leading to increased tissue injury and fibrosis (increased T_H1 profile) but also a blunted antiviral effect (increased T_H2 profile) (136). The mechanisms underlying accelerated tissue injury and fibrosis remain unclear and require further study.

C. Natural History of HCV and HIV

In immunocompetent hosts, acute HCV infection is generally asymptomatic or minimally symptomatic. After exposure, the risk of progression to chronic hepatitis C infection is 50–80%, with an estimated overall 20% risk of cirrhosis (3, 137, 138). Once cirrhosis is present, hepatocellular carcinoma develops at a 1–4% annual incidence (129). In the United States, HCV is the leading cause of chronic liver disease and the most common reason for referral for liver transplantation (140). In view of the importance of the cellular immune response both in the control and the pathogenesis of HCV-induced liver disease, several studies have examined the impact of HIV/HCV coinfection on clinical outcomes.

1. Effect of HIV on HCV Viral Load

Mounting evidence indicates that HCV RNA levels are higher in individuals who are HIV positive than those who are HIV negative. Although two studies did not show this trend to be a statistically significant finding (141, 142), most others indicate that HIV results in at least a severalfold higher level of viremia as measurable by HCV RNA (94, 120, 143–148). Longitudinal data in injection drug users have compared HCV-positive patients before and after acquiring HIV infection. HCV RNA concentrations increased by 0.6 log after HIV seroconversion. This study also found that increased age and CD4 counts of <200 were correlated with significant increases in HCV viral load (92).

The best data regarding the natural history of HCV/HIV coinfection have been provided by hemophiliac cohorts, in whom the timing of infection can be estimated more precisely. In this population, it appears that circulating HCV RNA is present more frequently in HIV-positive than in HIV-negative individuals (143, 149). Ghany et al. (150) found higher HCV viral loads only if the CD4 count was less than 200, although this study was limited by small sample size. Another study observed that HCV RNA levels were many times higher in those coinfected with HIV than those who were not, with the additional finding that HCV RNA was inversely correlated with CD4 counts over time, implying a possible enhanced cytopathic effect of HCV in the presence of cell-mediated immunosuppression (151). In a matched cohort of hemophiliacs, a 1.0 log increase in HCV viral load was observed *immediately* after HIV seroconversion. In addition, HIV infection was associated with an accelerated *rate* of HCV RNA rise over the 2-year follow-up, resulting in a 20-fold HCV RNA elevation compared with those individuals who were HIV-negative (152). Thus, HIV coinfection, perhaps by impairing host immune surveillance of virally infected cells, appears to lead to an alteration in the "set point" of HCV infection.

2. Effect of HIV on Progression of HCV Liver Disease: Clinical Data

Does the association of increased HCV viral load in HIV-positive patients result in worsened clinical outcomes? In 1989, Martin et al. (153) published a case series of three HIV-positive patients who developed rapid onset of cirrhosis within 3 years after contracting non-A, non-B hepatitis. As described earlier, simultaneous transmission of the two viruses after a needlestick injury resulted in rapid development of liver failure (106). Although this is not the course in most coinfected patients, these cases raise the possibility that HIV promotes progression of HCV-associated liver disease.

In the Multicenter Hemophilia Cohort Study, a prospective analysis of 223 hemophiliacs found that all 11 subjects who developed progressive liver disease due to HCV were coinfected with HIV, with an overall risk of liver failure of 8.8% in coinfected hosts. Liver failure was observed when HCV was present for >10 years (83). Additional studies have verified the accelerated progression of liver disease when HIV-positive in separate hemophiliac populations (154–156). A similar hastening of HCV progression was seen in a population of intravenous drug users (157).

Studies suggest that a greater degree of immunosuppression as indicated by CD4 count correlates with worsening outcome due to hepatitis C. Rockstroh et al. (158) found that liver failure was observed only in coinfected patients whose CD4 count fell from 230 to 50 and not in any patients with stable CD4 counts.

Interestingly, the finding that indeterminate hepatitis C antibody responses in coinfected patients were associated with an increase in hepatic disease may lend credence to the theory that an insufficient humoral response related to immunosuppression is associated with acceleration of HCV progression (159). This would be consistent with the observation of an accelerated course of hepatitis C found in hypogammaglobulinemic states (160).

Extrahepatic manifestations of hepatitis C, including cryoglobulinemia, membranoproliferative glomerulonephritis, and porphyria cutanea tarda, have not been studied rigorously in HIV-positive patients. Porphyria cutanea tarda seems to occur with greater frequency in coinfected patients (161, 162). One recent series of patients with HCV-associated glomerular disease indicated that patients with HIV, particularly those with advanced AIDS, experienced a particularly rapid progression to renal failure requiring dialysis; pathological data excluded a potential confounder of HIV-related nephropathy (163).

3. Effect of HIV on Progression of HCV Liver Disease: Histology

Histological data are limited but also strongly suggest a hastening of HCV-related liver disease in HIV-positive individuals. A greater degree of piecemeal necrosis and fibrosis in liver biopsy specimens is found in coinfected individuals (164). In addition, when examining autopsy cases involving coinfected patients, inflammation, cholestasis, and fibrosis were also seen to a higher degree (165).

Although one study failed to show any differences in histological activity or cirrhosis in coinfected persons (166) and another appeared to find less portal inflammation in HIV-positive individuals (167), a subsequent study that controlled for the length of time from initial infection with HCV indicated a higher rate of cirrhosis in coinfected (25%) compared with HIV-negative (8.9%) individuals in the first 15 years after HCV infection (168). In another study, the mean interval from estimated time of HCV infection in parenterally acquired hepatitis C to the presence of cirrhosis was found to be 6.9 years in HIV-positive patients, compared with 23.2 years in HIV-negative individuals (169). In a study that controlled for alcohol use, HCV-related cirrhosis was found at a much higher rate (relative risk 2.6) in the HIV-coinfected compared with the HIV-uninfected host (170). Finally, the only series that compared sequential liver biopsy specimens found an accelerated progression of HCV-related cirrhosis in HIV-positive individuals, with the additional finding that a low CD4 count was associated with a faster rate of progression (171). Taken together, the bulk of evidence strongly supports the conclusion that HCV-related liver fibrosis progression is accelerated by HIV coinfection.

The mechanism by which HIV infection, which does not infect hepatocytes, accelerates the progression of HCV-related liver disease is unclear, but several possibilities merit consideration. The observed higher levels of HCV in coinfected hosts may suggest a cytopathic form of liver injury caused by direct toxic effects of viral proteins on hepatocytes. We have observed several cases of the fibrosing cholestatic variant (FCH) of HCV in HIV-infected persons, characterized by the rapid development of extensive parenchymal collapse, ballooning degeneration, periportal fibrosis, and a scant inflammatory infiltrate. As with HBV, the paucity of inflammation suggests that the rapid progression may be attributable to the cytopathic effects of HCV. However, HCV RNA levels have not been markedly elevated in these and several other cases of FCH described in organ transplant recipients (133, 172, 173), suggesting that additional or other cooperative mechanisms may be contributing to the hepatocyte destruction.

What are potentially alternative explanations for the rapid progression of liver injury in the coinfected host? It is tempting to speculate that local alterations of cytokine profiles in HIV disease (e.g., endogenous interferon levels, transforming growth factor-β (TGF-β), tumor necrosis factor-α (TNF-α)) may lead to exaggerated activation of apoptotic pathways or to fibrogenesis. A recent report has suggested that occult HBV infection may be an unrecognized contributor to the acceleration of HCV-related liver disease (31); this finding warrants further investigation in a group of patients at risk for all three viral infections.

4. Effect of HCV on HIV Progression

Although the above data point toward a definite effect of HIV infection on HCV, it is conceivable, in view of the evidence for the lymphotropism of HCV, that a reciprocal interaction also occurs. In the era before routine HIV viral load testing, initial cross-sectional data appeared to indicate that the presence of hepatitis C infection did not influence surrogate markers of HIV infection (i.e., CD4 count, p24 antigen, etc.) (174) and that there was no apparent impact on the progression of HIV disease (79). This is consistent with the finding that hepatitis C does not independently affect CD4 counts (175). Longitudinal data over a 30-month period in 1990–1993 verified the lack of acceleration of clinical deterioration due to AIDS (176), and there also appeared to be no effect of HCV on mortality in HIV-infected patients (177, 178).

However, more recent data found that HCV infection was associated with clinical deterioration as defined by decrease in Karnofsky index, weight loss, AIDS-defining illness, or death (179). One retrospective study of hemophiliacs found that HCV genotype 1 infection was an independent risk factor in progression to AIDS (180); however, this finding has not been confirmed by other studies (181). In light of the fact that all of these studies were conducted before the introduction of HAART and may have been confounded by other factors that accelerated HIV disease, it is possible that the high mortality associated with AIDS and opportunistic infections during that era may have hidden any contributory effect of HCV to HIV progression. It will therefore be of interest to determine whether HCV infection prospectively influences HIV disease progression in the HAART era.

5. Effect of Antiretroviral Therapy and Immune Reconstitution on HCV

HAART has radically altered the natural history of HIV-1 infection. Accompanying the exceptional decreases in HIV viral load and rises in CD4 counts (182) has been marked attenuation of opportunistic infections (183). It could be expected that HCV-specific immune responses would also be restored in coinfected individuals, leading to the hypothesis that reconstitution of the immune system may in the short-term exacerbate disease but in the long-term assist control of HCV infection.

Before HAART, there appeared to be little interaction between antiretroviral therapy and HCV. Reduction in HCV-related disease was seen at the level of case reports (184, 185). More recently, it has been appreciated that a subset of patients during institution of HAART have developed clinically significant and even severe hepatitis (186). Although a certain amount may be secondary to drug hepatotoxicity, it is possible that activation of HCV causing direct cytopathic damage and the immune response to HCV may each be playing a role.

In one study of 19 coinfected patients, it was determined that HCV RNA and alanine aminotransferase levels increased in the first 2 months of treatment with protease inhibitors, but both returned to baseline within 6 to 9 months despite continuation of antiretroviral therapy, arguing against a major role of drug toxicity (187). Other studies have also found no alteration of HCV RNA levels on HAART (188, 189). It therefore appears unlikely that HAART in the short term has an anti-HCV effect, either directly or through reconstitution of the immune system. It remains to be seen whether long-term HIV suppression results in a reduction of the HCV set point. Interestingly, during institution of HAART in two patients who were HCV-antibody negative, severe hepatitis was found to be secondary to HCV as assessed by increases in plasma HCV RNA level and "seroreconversion" to a positive antibody (190). These data provide indirect evidence that HCV-specific immune responses are reactivated with the immune system during HAART.

Reactivation appears to be associated with an initial worsening of HCV-related liver disease. Histological samples of coinfected patients who began combination anti-HIV therapy revealed pronounced worsening in Knodell score, lobular necrosis, and inflammation as compared with pretreatment biopsies (191). A case report of progressive liver failure in a coinfected patient after institution of HAART with markedly increased HCV viremia was described, with histology showing marked worsening of necrotizing inflammation and cirrhosis presumed secondary to restoration of immune function. After discontinuation of HAART, liver indices improved as CD4 count fell (192), underscoring the importance of the immune system in the pathogenesis of HCV.

Although it appears that HAART transiently exacerbates HCV disease, it remains possible that immune reconstitution will favorably impact the progression of liver disease over the long term. Therefore, liver function test abnormalities in coinfected individuals initiating HAART may or may not reflect drug toxicity and may subside once the immune system is reconstituted. As with HBV, it is important to exclude the presence of advanced liver disease, given the potential risk for hepatic decompensation with an early flare. The flare of HCV-related inflammation appears to resemble the exacerbations of other opportunistic infections that occur during antiretroviral therapy. It is unknown whether pretreatment with anti-hepatitis C therapy such as interferon *before* initiation of HAART will attenuate the initial worsening of liver disease; prospective studies are needed to address this important issue.

D. Therapy

The current standard treatment for HCV in immunocompetent individuals is a combination of interferon alfa and ribavirin for a period of 6 to 12 months. Combination therapy has been found to achieve sustained clearance of HCV RNA, normalization of ALT, and improvement in liver histology in both naive individuals (193) and relapsers to interferon alfa therapy alone (194). Longer courses (12 months) of therapy are currently recommended for those individuals with genotype 1 HCV, whereas a shorter course (6 months) appears to be sufficient for genotype 2 and 3 infection. This section reviews the potential effects of interferon alfa and ribavirin on HIV disease, summarizes trials of antiviral therapy for HCV in HIV-positive patients, and considers future therapeutic options (195).

1. Interferon Alfa

An early interest in interferon alfa as a nonspecific antiviral agent with some anti-HIV activity in vitro (196) resulted in its introduction into trials for potential therapeutic use against HIV. Very high dose interferon, although accompanied by a high incidence of side effects, showed maintenance of CD4 count with fewer opportunistic infections compared with controls (197). When added to nucleoside inhibitors, interferon appears to result in transient decrease in HIV viral load, at the cost of more frequent side effects in the treatment group (198, 199). However, further trials with interferon have failed to demonstrate any long-term virologic benefit against HIV (200, 201), and in a subset of patients have apparently resulted in a decline of CD4+ count (202, 203).

Interferon alfa appears to exert its antiviral action against hepatitis C virus through several mechanisms. It appears to prevent binding, entry, and un-coating of virus into hepatocytes; stimulates endogenous ribonucleases that degrade viral RNA; increases viral peptide antigen display; and increases CTL activity (Fig. 3) (204). When used for the treatment of HCV, inter-feron alone does not appear to have the same efficacy against HCV disease in HIV-coinfected as compared with immunocompetent persons (205). Al-though initial end-of-treatment responses may be similar, long-term sustained responses appear to be achieved at a lower rate in coinfected individuals (206). The prospective trials (Table 2) thus far performed have not been randomized and have yielded inconsistent results, perhaps stemming from the differing regimens used.

Table 2 Trials of Interferon Alfa for Hepatitis C in HIV-infected Individuals

Study	No. of patients	IFN regimen	End of treatment response (%)	Sustained response (%)
Boyer et al. (1992) (207)	12	1,3,5 MIU TIW × 4–6 mo	33	n.a.
Nardiello et al. (1992) (208)	21	3 MIU TIW × 6 mo	45	27
Marriot et al. (1993) (209)	14	9 MIU q.d. × 3 mo then 9 MIU TIW × 3 mo then 6 MIU TIW × 3 mo then 3 MIU TIW × 3 mo	55	44
De Sanctis et al. (1993) (210)	20	3 MIU TIW × 18 mo	n.a.	25
Marcellin et al. (1994) (211)	20	3 MIU TIW × 6 wks	30	15
Arcias et al. (1994) (212)	10	3 MIU TIW × 6 mo	40	20
Pol et al. (1995) (213)	16	3 MIU TIW × 6 mo	23	0
Soriano et al. (1996) (214)	90	5 MIU TIW × 3 mo then 3 MIU TIW × 9 mo	32.5	23
Piliero et al. (1997) (215)	28	3 or 5 MIU TIW × 6 mo	25 or 11	0
Venkataramani et al. (1997) (216)	11	3 MIU TIW × 12 mo	18	n.a.
Causse (1997) (217)	76	3 MIU TIW × 6 mo	17.5	11
Mauss et al. (1998) (218)	17	5 MIU TIW × 6 mo	47	29

TIW, three times per week; n.a., not available.

2. Ribavirin

Interferon monotherapy is no longer standard treatment for chronic hepatitis C and should therefore not be used in coinfected individuals. As with regimens for HIV infection, combination therapy of interferon with ribavirin appears to be much more effective in achieving virologic endpoints and is the current standard of care in immunocompetent individuals.

Ribavirin is a synthetic guanosine analogue with activity against a broad spectrum of RNA viruses. Although its mechanism of action has yet to be fully clarified, ribavirin has been proposed to effect a change in the cytokine profile from a T_H2 to a more antiviral T_H1 response (Fig. 3) (219). Its primary toxicities are a dose-related hemolytic anemia, which can be treatment limiting, and teratogenicity. Clinical trials of ribavirin in HIV-infection performed before the era of HAART did not demonstrate promising anti-HIV activity (220–224). In vitro, ribavirin antagonizes the phosphorylation of certain antiretrovirals such as ZDV or stavudine (d4T), whereas it enhances the inhibitory effects of purine analogues such as ddI (225, 226). However, the clinical significance of any of these interactions is unknown (227). When used as monotherapy against HCV, ribavirin exhibited *no* effect on HCV RNA levels but led to reductions in ALT, suggesting that it may be working through cytokine modification rather than as a *direct* antiviral agent.

Data for efficacy of combination interferon alfa and ribavirin in coinfected individuals are sparse. Two small trials, each involving 10 patients, have suggested improved anti-HCV activity when compared with historical controls receiving interferon alone (228, 229). A recently reported trial of combination therapy in 21 coinfected individuals showed a significant decline in HCV RNA at 3 months; however, the average CD4+ cell count declined markedly (529 to 277 cells/mm^3) in the group that received ribavirin (230). Data are too limited to determine which genotypes are more likely to respond to combination therapy in coinfected patients.

3. Future Directions in HCV Therapy for Coinfected Individuals

The limited success with currently licensed antiviral therapy underscores the need to find anti-HCV therapies with improved efficacy and diminished toxicity for those coinfected with HIV. Pegylated interferon, which complexes interferon to the inert polyethylene glycol, leading to more sustained absorption and delivery of interferon, appears to be as effective as interferon and ribavirin in immunocompetent patients (231). Studies examining the efficacy of this once a week injection either alone or in combination with ribavirin are currently underway in coinfected patients. Ultimately, antivirals that specifically target HCV-specific enzymatic functions such as the HCV-encoded serine protease, helicase, or polymerase will prove useful in combination with preexisting therapies (232).

As understanding of the mechanisms underlying the clearance of HCV infection expands, immunological therapies may provide the basis for further therapy. The T_H2 response is associated with chronic infection with HCV (233). Immunomodulation promoting the T_H1 response, in the form of interleukin-2 and interleukin-12, may favor clearance of HCV infection. Already, a clinical benefit has been reported with recombinant interleukin-2 in combatting HIV infection (234); it appears to lower HCV viral load in coinfected patients (235). IL-2 may prove to be useful as an adjunct to currently strategies aimed at controlling HCV.

Finally, the treatment of last resort for end-stage liver disease related to HCV is liver transplantation. Although AIDS is an absolute contraindication to transplantation, in the era of increased longevity associated with HAART, this policy might be reconsidered for HIV-positive patients. One case of liver transplantation for a patient with HIV has been reported, specifically for HCV-related liver disease in a hemophiliac, with successful control of HIV on HAART 7 months posttransplant (236). The role for liver transplantation in the management of those patients who develop end-stage liver disease requires further clarification in view of the disparity between the rapidly growing candidate list and the limited availability of donor organs.

4.   Prevention of Hepatitis A Virus (HAV) Infection

Although data are limited, it would be prudent for the clinician to immunize coinfected patients against additional potential viral insults to the liver. Although HAV is a rare cause of fulminant hepatic failure in persons with no underlying liver disease, it has resulted in a higher incidence of fulminant disease in persons infected with HCV (237). In milder cases, the elevation in liver function tests and the self-limited illness may result in cessation of HAART, potentially precipitating treatment failure (238). The inactivated hepatitis A vaccine, given in two intramuscular doses spaced apart, appears to be safe in HIV-positive individuals (239).

Hepatitis C and HIV often travel together in the same host, and transmission is apparently enhanced when HCV viral load is higher. HIV appears to have a permissive effect on HCV replication and is correlated with a more rapid progression to cirrhosis. In the era of HAART, the evaluation of elevated liver function tests is complicated by the reactivation of chronic hepatitis. Current treatments for HCV in the setting of coinfection are under development. Prevention of further insults to the liver damage are of vital importance, including immunization against HAV and HBV and restriction of alcohol intake.

IV. CONCLUSION

It is clear that chronic viral hepatitis is both a common and crucial problem in HIV-infected patients. Considering the vital role of the immune system in the pathogenesis and control of both HBV and HCV, these viruses should be considered opportunistic infections that will contribute significantly to morbidity and mortality in coinfected hosts. Although restoration of the cellular immune system may play a role in the control and possible clearance of these infections, specific and effective therapies directed against these hepatitis viruses will be essential in the era of active antiretroviral therapy.

REFERENCES

1. Soriano V, Garcia-Samaniego J, Gutierrez M, Bravo R, Gonzalez-Lahoz J. High morbidity and mortality of chronic viral liver disease in HIV-infected individuals in Spain. J Infect 1994; 28:100–102.

2. Ockenga J, Tillmann HL, Trautwein C, Stoll M, Manns MP, Schmidt RE. Hepatitis B and C in HIV-infected patients. Prevalence and prognostic value. J Hepatol 1997; 27:18–24.

3. Darby SC, Ewart DW, Giangrande PL, Spooner RJ, Rizza CR, Dusheiko GM, Lee CA, Ludlam CA, Preston FE. Mortality from liver cancer and liver disease in haemophilic men and boys in UK given blood products contaminated with hepatitis C. Lancet 1997; 350:1425–1431.

4. Soriano V, Garcia-Samaniego J, Valencia E. Rodriguez-Rosado R. Munoz F. Gonzalez-Lahoz J. Impact of chronic liver disease due to hepatitis viruses as cause of hospital admission and death in HIV-infected drug users. Eur J Epidemiol 1999; 15:1–4.

5. McQuillan GM, Coleman PJ, Kurszon-Moran D, Moyer LA, Lambert SB, Margolis HS. Prevalence of hepatitis B virus infection in the United States: the National Health and Nutrition Examination Surveys, 1976 through 1994. Am J Public Health 1999; 89:14–18.

6. Twu SJ, Detels R, Nelson K, Visscher BR, Kaslow R, Palenicek J, Phair J. Relationship of hepatitis B virus infection to human immunodeficiency virus type 1 infection. J Infect Dis 1993; 167:299–304.

7. Ouattara SA, Meite M, Aron Y, Akran V, Gody M, Manlan LK, de-The G. Increase of the prevalence of hepatitis B virus surface antigen related to immunodeficiency inherent in acquired immune deficiency syndrome (AIDS). J Acquir Immune Defic Syndr 1990; 3:282–286.

8. Hadler SC, Judson FN, O'Malley PM, Altman NL, Penley K, Buchbinder S, Schable CA, Coleman PJ, Ostrow DN, Francis DP. Outcome of hepatitis B virus infection in homosexual men and its relation to prior human immunodeficiency virus infection. J Infect Dis 1991; 163:454–459.

9. Bodsworth NJ, Cooper DA, Donovan B. The influence of human immunodeficiency virus type 1 infection on the development of the hepatitis B virus carrier state. J Infect Dis 1991; 163:1138–1140.

10. Collier AC, Corey L, Murphy VL, Handsfield HH. Antibody to human immunodeficiency virus and suboptimal response to hepatitis B vaccination. Ann Intern Med 1988; 109;101–105.

11. Hadler SC, Francis DP, Maynard JE, Thompson SE, Judson FN, Echenberg DF, Ostrow DG, O'Malley PM, Penley KA, Altman NL. Long-term immunogenicity and efficacy of hepatitis B vaccine in homosexual men. N Engl J Med 1986; 315:209–214.

12. Loke RH, Murray-Lyon IM, Coleman JC, Evans BA, Zuckerman AJ. Diminished response to recombinant hepatitis B vaccine in homosexual men with HIV antibody: an indicator of poor prognosis. J Med Virol 1990; 31:109–111.

13. Rutstein RM, Rudy B, Codispoti C, Watson B. Response to hepatitis B immunization by infants exposed to HIV. AIDS 1994; 8:1281–1284.

14. Wong EK, Bodsworth NJ, Slade MA, Mulhall BP, Donovan B. Response to hepatitis vaccination in a primary care setting: influence of HIV infection, CD4+ lymphocyte count and vaccination schedule. Int J STD AIDS 1996; 7:490–494.

15. Rehermann B, Lau D, Hoofnagle JH, Chisari FV. Cytotoxic T lymphocyte responsiveness after resolution of chronic hepatitis B virus infection. J Clin Invest 1996; 97:1655–1665.

16. Lazizi Y, Grangeot-Keros, L, Delfraissy J-F, Boue F, Dubreuil P, Badur S, Pillot J. Reappearance of hepatitis B virus in immune patients infected with the human immunodeficiency virus type 1 [letter]. J Infect Dis 1988; 158:666–667.

17. Vento S, Di Perri G, Luzzati R, Cruciani M, Garofano T, Mengoli C, Concia E, Bassetti D. Clinical reactivation of hepatitis B in anti-HBs-positive patients with AIDS [letter]. Lancet 1989; 1:332–333.

18. Waite J, Gilson RJC, Weller IVD, Lacey CJ, Hambling MH, Hawkins A, Briggs M, Tedder RS. Hepatitis B virus reactivation or reinfection associated with HIV-1 infection. AIDS 1988; 2:443–448.

19. Vandercam B, Cornu C, Gala JL, Geubel A, Cahill M, Lamy ME. Reactivation of hepatitis B virus in a previously immune patients with human immunodeficiency virus infection [letter]. Eur J Clin Microbiol Infect Dis 1990; 9:701–702.

20. Lok ASF, Liang RHS, Chiu EKW, Wong K-L, Chan T-K. Reactivation of hepatitis B virus replication in patients receiving cytotoxic therapy. Report of a prospective study. Gastroenterology 1991; 100:182–188.

21. Kidd-Ljungren K. Reappearance of hepatitis B 10 years after kidney transplantation. N Engl J Med 1999; 341:127.

22. Rustki VK, Hoofnagle JH, Gerin JL, et al. Hepatitis B virus infection in the acquired immunodeficiency syndrome. Ann Intern Med 1984; 101:795–797.

23. Perrillo RP, Regenstein FG, Roodman ST. Chronic hepatitis B in asympatomatic homosexual men with antibody to human immunodeficiency virus. Ann Intern Med 1986; 105:382–383.

24. Bodsworth N, Donovan B, Nightingale BN. The effect of concurrent human immunodeficiency virus infection on chronic hepatitis B: a study of 150 homosexual men. J Infect Dis 1989; 160:577–582.

25. Fang JWS, Lau JYN, Davis GL. HIV-induced HBV breakthrough during interferon-alpha therapy [letter]. Am J Gastroenterol 1993; 88:1293–1294.

26. Krogsgaard K, Lindhardt BO, Nielson JO, Andersson P, Kryger P, Aldershvile J, Gerstoft J, Pedersen C. The influence of HTLV-III infection on the natural history of hepatitis B virus infection in male homosexual HBsAg carriers. Hepatology 1987; 7:37–41.

27. McDonald JA, Harris S, Waters JA, Thomas HC. Effect of human immunodeficiency virus (HIV) infection on chronic hepatitis B hepatis viral antigen display. J Hepatol 1987; 4:337-342.

28. Mai AL, Yim C, O'Rourke K, Heathcote EJ. The interaction of human immunodeficiency virus and hepatitis B infection in infected homosexual men. J Clin Gastroenterol 1996; 22:299–304.

29. Gilson RJC, Hawkins AE, Beecham MR, Ross E, Waite J, Briggs M, McNally T, Kelly GE, Tedder RS, Weller IVD. Interactions between HIV and hepatitis B virus in homosexual men: effects on the natural history of infection. AIDS 1997; 11:597–606.

30. Hofer M, Joller-Jemelka HI, Grob PJ, Luthy R, Opravil M. Frequent chronic hepatitis B virus infection in HIV-infected patients positive for antibody for hepatitis B core antigen only. Eur J Clin Microbiol Infect Dis 1998; 17:6–13.

31. Cacciola I, Pollicino T, Squadrito G, Cerenzia G, Orlando ME, Raimondo G. Occult hepatitis B virus infection in patients with chronic hepatitis C liver disease. N Engl J Med 1999; 341:22–26.

32. Goldin RD, Fish DE, Hay A, Waters JA, McGarvey MJ, Main J, Thomas HC. Histological and immunohistochemical study of hepatitis B virus in human immunodeficiency virus infection. J Clin Pathol 1990; 43:203–205.

33. Bonacini M, Govindarajan S, Redeker AG. Human immunodeficiency virus infection does not alter serum transaminases and hepatitis B virus (HBV) DNA

in homosexual patients with chronic HBV infection. Am J Gastroenterol 1991; 86:570–573.

34. Housset C, Pol S, Carnot F, Dubois F, Nalpas B, Housset B, Berthelot P, Brechot C. Interactions between human immunodeficiency virus-1, hepatitis delta virus and hepatitis B virus infections in 260 chronic carriers of hepatitis B virus. Hepatology 1992; 15:578–583.

35. Colin J-F, Cazals-Hatem D, Loriot MA, Martinot-Peignoux M, Pham BN, Auperin A, Degott C, Benhamou JP, Erlinger S, Valla D, Marcellin P. Influence of human immunodeficiency virus infection on chronic hepatitis B in homosexual men. Hepatology 1999; 29:1306–1310.

36. Fang JWS, Wright TL, Lau JYN. Fibrosing cholestatic hepatitis in a patient with human immunodeficiency virus and hepatitis B virus coinfection. Lancet 1993; 342:1175.

37. Schechter MT, Craib KJP, Le TN, Willoughby B, Douglas B, Sestak P, Montaner JS, Weaver MS, Elmslie KD, O'Shaughnessy MV. Progression to AIDS and predictors of AIDS in seroprevalent and seroincident cohorts of homosexual men. AIDS 1989; 3:347–353.

38. Solomon RE, Van Raden M, Kaslow RA, Lyter D, Visscher B, Farzadegan H, Phair J. Association of hepatitis B surface antigen and core antibody with acquisition and manifestation of human immunodeficiency virus type 1 (HIV-1) infection. Am J Public Health 1990; 80:1475–1478.

39. Scharschmidt BF, Held MJ, Hollander HH, Read AE, Lavine JE, Veereman G, McGuire RF, Thaler MM. Hepatitis B in patients with HIV infection: relationship to AIDS and patient survival. Ann Intern Med 1992; 117:837–838.

40. Eskild A, Magnus P, Petersen G, Sohlberg C, Jensen F, Kittelsen P, Skaug K. Hepatitis B antibodies in HIV-infected homosexual men are associated with more rapid progression to AIDS. AIDS 1992; 6:571–574.

41. de Asis ML, Rosenstreich DL, Chang CJ, Gourevitch MN, Small CB. Effect of prior hepatitis B infection on serum IgE levels in patients with human immunodeficiency virus infection. Ann Allergy Asthma Immunol 1998; 80:35–38.

42. Hanson CA, Sutherland DE, Snover DC. Fulminant hepatic failure in an HBsAg carrier renal transplant patient following cessation of immunosuppressive therapy. Transplantation 1985; 39:311–312.

43. Flowers MA, Heathcote J, Wanless IR, Sherman M, Reynolds WJ, Cameron RG, Levy GA, Inman RD. Fulminant hepatitis as a consequence of reactivation of hepatitis B virus infection after discontinuation of low-dose methotrexate therapy. Ann Intern Med 1990; 112:381–382.

44. Carr A, Cooper DA. Restoration of immunity to chronic hepatitis B infection in an HIV-infected patient on protease inhibitor. Lancet 1997; 349:995–996.

45. Mastroianni CM, Trinchieri V, Santopadre P, Lichtner M, Forcina G, D'Agostino
     C, Corpolongo A, Vullo V. Acute clinical hepatitis in an HIV-seropositive hep-
     atitis B carrier receiving protease inhibitor therapy. AIDS 1998; 12:1939–1940.

46. Velasco M, Moran A, Tellez MJ. Resolution of chronic hepatitis B after riton-
     avir treatment in an HIV-infected patient. N Engl J Med 1999; 340:1765–1766.

47. Di Martino V, Lunel F, Cadranel JF, Hoang C, Parlier Y, Le Charpentier Y,
     Opolon P. Long-term effects of interferon-alpha in five HIV-positive patients
     with chronic hepatitis B. J Viral Hepat 1996; 3:253–260.

48. Wong DKH, Yim C, Naylor CD, Chen E, Sherman M, Vas S, Wanless IR,
     Read S, Li H, Heathcote EJ. Interferon alfa treatment of chronic hepatitis B:
     randomized trial in a predominantly homosexual male population. Gastroen-
     terology 1995; 108:165–171.

49. McDonald JA, Caruso L, Karayiannis P, Scully LJ, Harris JR, Forster GE,
     Thomas HC. Diminished responsiveness of male homosexual chronic hepati-
     tis B virus carriers with HTLV-III antibodies to recombinant alpha-interferon.
     Hepatology 1987; 7:719–723.

50. Brook MG, McDonald JA, Karayiannis P, Caruso L, Forster G, Harris JR.
     Randomized controlled trial of interferon alfa 2A for the treatment of chronic
     hepatitis B virus (HBV) infection; factors that influence response. Gut 1989;
     30:1116–1122.

51. Chen DK, Yim C, O'Rourke K, Krajden M, Wong DK, Heathcote EJ. Long-
     term follow-up of a randomized trial of interferon therapy for chronic hepatitis
     B in a predominantly homosexual male population. J Hepatol 1999; 30:556–
     563.

52. Marcellin P, Boyer N, Colin JF, Martinot-Peignoux M, Lefort V, Matheron S,
     Erlinger S, Benhamou JP. Recombinant alpha interferon for chronic hepatitis
     B in anti-HIV positive patients receiving zidovudine. Gut 1993; 32S:S106.

53. Visco G, Alba L, Grisetti S, Guarascio P, Narciso P, Sette P, Struglia C, Tossini
     G, Tozzi V. Zidovudine plus interferon alfa-2b treatment in patients with HIV
     and chronic active viral hepatitis. Gut 1993; 34S:S107–S108.

54. Janssen HL, Berk L, Heijtink RA, ten Fate FJ, Schalm SW. Interferon-alpha and
     zidovudine combination therapy for chronic hepatitis B: results of a randomized
     placebo-controlled trial. Hepatology 1993; 17:383–388.

55. Locarnini S, Birch C. Antiviral chemotherapy for chronic hepatitis B infection:
     lessons learned from treating HIV-infected patients. J Hepatol 1999; 30:536–
     550.

56. Gilson RJ, Hawkins AE, Kelly GK, Gill SK, Weller IV. The effect of zidovudine
     on hepatitis B viral replication in homosexual men with symptomatic HIV-1
     infection. AIDS 1991; 5:217–220.

57. Fried MW, Korenman JC, Di Bisceglie AM, Park Y, Waggoner JG, Mitsuya H, Hartman NR, Yarchoan R, Broder S, Hoofnagle JH. A pilot study of 2',3'-dideoxyinosine for the treatment of chronic hepatitis B. Hepatology 1992; 16:861–864.

58. Catterall AP, Moyle GJ, Hopes EA, Harrison TJ, Gazzard BG, Murray-Lyon IM. Dideoxyinosine for chronic hepatitis B infection. J Med Virol 1992; 37:307–309.

59. Yokota T, Mochizuki S, Konno K, Mori S, Shigeta S, De Clercq E. Inhibitory effects of selected antiviral compounds on human hepatitis B virus DNA synthesis. Antimicrob Agents Chemother 1991; 35:394–397.

60. Dienstag JL, Perrillo RP, Schiff ER, Bartholomew M, Vicary C, Rubin M. A preliminary trial of lamivudine for chronic hepatitis B infection. N Engl J Med 1995; 333:1657–1661.

61. Lai C-L, Chien R-N, Leung NWY, Chang T-T, Guan R, Tai DI, Ng KY, Wu PC, Dent JC, Barber J, Stephenson SL, Gray DF. A one-year trial of lamivudine for chronic hepatitis B. N Engl J Med 1998; 339:61–68.

62. Schnittman SM, Pierce PF. Potential role of lamivudine (3TC) in the clearance of chronic hepatitis B virus infection in a patient coinfected with human immunodeficiency virus type 1. Clin Infect Dis 1996; 23:638–639.

63. Nagai K, Hosaka H, Kubo S, Nakamura N, Shinohara M, Nonaka H. Highly active antiretroviral therapy used to treat concurrent hepatitis B and human immunodeficiency virus infections. J Gastroenterol 1999; 34:275–281.

64. Altfeld M, Rockstroh JK, Addo M, Kupfer B, Irmgard P, Will H, Spengler U. Reactivation of hepatitis B in a long-term anti-HBs-positive patients with AIDS following lamivudine withdrawal. J Hepatol 1998; 29:306–309.

65. Herrero JI, Quiroga J, Sangro B, Sola I, Riezu-Boj JI, Pardo F, Prieto J. Effectiveness of lamivudine in treatment of acute recurrent hepatitis B after liver transplantation. Dig Dis Sci 1998; 43:1186–1189.

66. Ahmed A, Keeffe EB. Lamivudine therapy for chemotherapy-induced reactivation of hepatitis B virus infection. Am J Gastroenterol 1999; 94:249–251.

67. Boni C, Bertoletti A, Penna A, Cavalli A, Pilli M, Urbani S, Scognamiglio P, Boehme R, Panebianco R, Fiaccadori F, Ferrari C. Lamivudine treatment can restore T cell responsiveness in chronic hepatitis B. J Clin Invest 1998; 102:968–975.

68. Honkoop P, Niesters HGM, de Man RAM, Osterhaus AD, Schalm SW. Lamivudine resistance in immunocompetent chronic hepatitis B. J Hepatol 1997; 26:1393–1395.

69. Bartholomew MM, Jansen RW, Jeffers LJ, Reddy KR, Johnson LC, Bunzendahl H, Condreay LD, Tzakis AG, Schiff ER, Brown NA. Hepatitis-B-virus

resistance to lamivudine given for recurrent infection after orthotopic liver transplantation. Lancet 1997; 349:20–22.

70. Wolters LM, Niesters HG, de Man RA, Schalm SW. Antiviral treatment for human immunodeficiency virus patients co-infected with hepatitis B virus: combined effect for both infections, an obtainable goal? Antiviral Res 1999; 42:71–76.

71. Xiong X, Flores C, Yang H, Toole JJ, Gibbs CS. Mutations in hepatitis B DNA polymerase associated with resistance to lamivudine do not confer resistance to adefovir in vitro. Hepatology 1998; 28:1669–1673.

72. Ono-Nita SK, Kato N, Shiratori Y, Lan KH, Yoshida H, Carrilho FJ, Omata M. Susceptibility of lamivudine-resistant hepatitis B virus to other reverse transcriptase inhibitors. J Clin Invest 1999; 103:1635–1640.

73. Deeks SG, Collier A, Lalezari J, Pavia A, Rodrigue D, Drew WL, Toole J, Jaffe HS, Mulato AS, Lamy PD, Li W, Cherrington JM, Hellmann N, Kahn J. The safety and efficacy of adefovir dipivoxil, a novel anti-human immunodeficiency virus (HIV) therapy, in HIV-infected adults: a randomized, double-blind, placebo-controlled trial. J Infect Dis 1997; 176:1517–1523.

74. Miller MD, Anton KE, Mulato AS, Lamy PD, Cherrington JM. Human immunodeficiency virus type 1 expressing the lamivudine-associated M184V mutation in reverse transcriptase shows increased susceptibility to adefovir and decreased replication capability in vitro. J Infect Dis 1999; 179:92–100.

75. Alter MJ, Kruszon-Moran D, Nainan OV, McQuillan GM, Gao F, Moyer LA, Kaslow RA, Margolis HS. The prevalence of hepatitis C virus infection in the United States, 1988 through 1994. N Engl J Med 1999; 341:556–562.

76. Conry-Cantilena C, VanRaden M, Gibble J, Melpolder J, Shakil AO, Viladomiu L, Cheung L, DiBisceglie A, Hoofnagle J, Shih JW. Routes of infection, viremia, and liver disease in blood donors found to have hepatitis C virus infection. N Engl J Med 1996; 334:1691–1696.

77. Quaranta JF, Delaney SR, Alleman S, Cassuto JP, Dellamonica P, Allain JP. Prevalence of antibody to hepatitis C virus (HCV) in HIV-1 infected patients. J Med Virol 1994; 42:29–32.

78. Sherman KE, Freeman S, Harrison S, Andron L. Prevalence of antibody to hepatitis C virus in patients infected with the human immunodeficiency virus. J Infect Dis 1991; 163:414–415.

79. Quan CM, Krajden M, Grigoriew GA, Salit IE. Hepatitis C virus infection in patients infected with the human immunodeficiency virus. Clin Infect Dis 1993; 17:117–119.

80. Polywka S, Laufs R. Hepatitis C virus antibodies among different groups at risk and patients with suspected non-A, non-B hepatitis. Infection 1991; 19:81–84.

81. Hayashi PH, Flynn N, McCrudy SA, Kuramoto IK, Holland PV, Zeldis JB. Prevalence of hepatitis C virus antibodies among patients infected with human immunodeficiency virus. J Med Virol 1991; 33:177–180.

82. Rumi MG, Colombo M, Grigeri A, Mannucci PM. High prevalence of antibody to hepatitis C virus in multitransfused hemophiliacs with normal transaminase levels. Ann Intern Med 1990; 112:379–380.

83. Eyster MW, Diamondstone LS, Lien JM, Ehmann WC, Quan S, Goedert JJ, for the Multicenter Hemophilia Cohort Study. Natural history of hepatitis C virus infection in multitransfused hemophiliacs: effect of coinfection with human immunodeficiency virus. J Acquir Immune Defic Syndr 1993; 6:602–610.

84. Esteban JI, Esteban R, Viladomiu L, Lopez-Talavera JC, Gonzalez A, Hernandez JM, Roget M, Vargas V, Genesca J, Buti M. Hepatitis C virus antibodies among risk groups in Spain. Lancet 1989; 2:294–297.

85. Sonnerborg A, Abebe A, Strannegard O. Hepatitis C virus infection in individuals with or without human immunodeficiency virus type 1 infection. Infection 1990; 18:347–351.

86. Fainboim H, Gonzalez J, Fassio E, Martinez A, Otegui L, et al. Prevalence of hepatitis viruses in an anti-human immunodeficiency virus-positive population from Argentina, a multicentre study. J Viral Hepat 1999; 6:53–57.

87. Tovo PA, Palomba E, Ferraris G, Principi N, Ruga E, Dallacasa P, Maccabruni A. Increased risk of maternal-infant hepatitis C virus transmission for women coinfected with human immunodeficiency virus type 1. Italian Study Group for HCV Infection in Children. Clin Infect Dis 1997; 25:1121–1124.

88. Thomas DL, Villano SA, Riester KA, Hershow R, Mofenson LM, Landesman SH, Hollinger FB, Davenny K, Riley L, Diaz C, Tang HB, Quinn TC. Perinatal transmission of hepatitis C virus from human immunodeficiency virus type-1 infected mothers. Women and Infants Transmission Study. J Infect Dis 1998; 177:1480–1488.

89. Marcellin P, Colin JF, Martinot-Peignoux M, Pham BN, Lefort V, Picault AB, Degott C, Erlinger S, Benhamou JP. Hepatitis C virus infection in anti-HIV positive and negative French homosexual men with chronic hepatitis: comparison of second- and third-generation anti-HCV testing. Liver 1993; 13:319–322.

90. Flomenberg P, Balliet K, Bernstein B, Gutierrez E, Carrigan D. High specificity of hepatitis C second-generation enzyme immunoassay in HIV-infected patients. J Acquir Immune Defic Syndr 1995; 9:97–98.

91. Collier J, Heathcote J. Hepatitis C viral infection in the immunosuppressed patient. Hepatology 1998; 27:2–6.

92. Thomas DL, Shih JW, Alter HJ, Vlahov D, Cohn S, Hoover DR, Cheung L, Nelson KE. Effect of human immunodeficiency virus on hepatitis C virus infection among injecting drug users. J Infect Dis 1996; 174:690–695.

93. Marcellin P, Martinot-Peignoux M, Elias A, Branger M, Courtois F, Level R, Erlinger S, Benhamou JP. Hepatitis C virus (HCV) viremia in human immunod-eficiency virus-seronegative and -seropositive patients with indeterminate HCV recombinant immunoblot assay. J Infect Dis 1994; 170:433–435.

94. Cribier B, Rey D, Schmitt C, Lang JM, Kirn A, Stoll-Keller F. High hepatitis C viraemia and impaired antibody response in patients coinfected with HIV. AIDS 1995; 9:1131–1136.

95. Sorbi D, Shen D, Lake-Bakarr G. Influence of HIV disease on serum anti-HCV antibody titers: a study of intravenous drug users [letter]. J Acquir Immune Defic Syndr 1996; 13:295–296.

96. Chamot E, Hirschel B, Wintsch J, Robert CF, Gabriel V, Deglon JJ, Yerly S, Perrin L. Loss of antibodies against hepatitis C virus in HIV-seropositive intravenous drug users. AIDS 1990; 4:1275–1277.

97. Ragni MV, Ndimbie OK, Rice EO, Bontempo FA, Nedjar S. The presence of hepatitis C virus (HCV) antibody in human virus-positive hemophilic men undergoing HCV "seroreversion." Blood 1993; 82:1010–1015.

98. Lok AS, Chien D, Choo QL, Chan TM, Chiu EK, Cheng IK, Houghton M, Kuo G. Antibody response to core, envelope and nonstructural hepatitis C virus antigens; comparison of immunocompetent and immunosuppressed patients. Hepatology 1993; 18:497–502.

99. Lefrere JJ, Guiramand S, Lefrere F, Mariotti M, Aumont P, Lerable J, Petit JC, Girot R, Morand-Joubert L. Full or partial seroreversion in patients infected by hepatitis C virus. J Infect Dis 1997; 175:316–322.

100. Schoenbaum EE, Hartel D, Selwyn PA, Klein RS, Davenny K, Rogers M, Feiner C, Friedland G. Risk factors for human immunodeficiency virus infection in intravenous drug users. N Engl J Med 1989; 321:874–879.

101. Stark K, Muller R, Bienzle U, Guggenmoos-Holzmann I. Frontloading: a risk factor for HIV and hepatitis C virus infection among injecting drug users in Berlin. AIDS 1996; 10:311–317.

102. Schreiber GB, Busch MP, Kleinman SH, Korelitz JJ. The risk of transfusion-transmitted viral infection. N Engl J Med 1996; 334:1685–1690.

103. Cardo DM, Culver DH, Ciesielski CA, Srivastava PU, Marcus R, Abiteboul D, Heptonstall J, Ippolito G, Lot F, McKibben PS, Bell DM. Case control study of a HIV-seroconversion in health care workers after percutaneous exposure. N Engl J Med 1997; 337:1485–1490.

104. Puro V, Petrosillo N, Ippolito G. Risk of hepatitis C seroconversion after occu-pational exposures in health care workers. Am J Infect Control 1995; 23:273–277.

105. Garces JM, Yazbeck H, Pi-Sunyer T, Gutierrez-Cebollada J, Lopez-Colomes JL. Simulteanous human immunodeficiency virus and hepatitis C infection following a needlestick injury. Eur J Clin Microbiol Infect Dis 1996; 15:92–94.

106. Ridzon R, Gallagher K, Ciesielski C, Mast EE, Ginsberg MB, Robertson BJ, Luo C-C, DeMaria A. Simultaneous transmission of human immunodeficiency virus and hepatitis C virus from a needle-stick injury. N Engl J Med 1997; 336:919–922.

107. Ippolito G, Puro V, Petrosillo N, De Carli G, Micheloni G, Magliano E. Simultaneous infection with HIV and hepatitis C virus following occupational conjunctival blood exposure [letter]. JAMA 1998; 280:28.

108. Update: provisional Public Health Service recommendations for chemoprophylaxis after occupational exposure to HIV. MMWR Morb Mortal Wkly Rep 1996; 45:468–472.

109. Brettler DB, Mannucci PM, Gringeri A, Rasko JE, Forsberg AD, Rumi MG, Garsia RJ, Rickard KA, Colombo M. The low risk of hepatitis C virus transmission among sexual partners of hepatitis C-infected hemophilic males: an international multicenter study. Blood 1992; 80:540–543.

110. Hallam NF, Fletcher ML, Read SJ, Majid AM, Kurtz JB, Rizza CR. Low risk of sexual transmission of hepatitis C virus. J Med Virol 1993; 40:251–253.

111. Thomas DL, Zenilman JM, Alter MJ, Shih JW, Galai N, Carella AV, Quinn TC. Sexual transmission of hepatitis C virus among patients attending Baltimore sexually transmitted disease clinics—an analysis of 309 sex partnerships. J Infect Dis 1995; 171:768–775.

112. Sawanpanyalert P, Boonmar S, Maeda T, Matsura Y, Miyamura T. Risk factors for hepatitis C virus infection among blood donors in an HIV-epidemic area in Thailand. J Epidemiol Community Health 1996; 50:174–177.

113. Wyld R, Robertson JR, Brettle RP, Mellor J, Prescott L, Simmonds P. Absence of hepatitis C virus transmission but frequent transmission of HIV-1 from sexual contact with doubly-infected individuals. J Infect 1997; 35:163–166.

114. Salvaggio A, Conti M, Albano A, Pianetti A, Muggiasca ML, Re M, Salvaggio L. Sexual transmission of hepatitis C virus and HIV-1 infection in female intravenous drug users. Eur J Epidemiol 1993; 9:279–284.

115. Daikos GL, Lai S, Fischl MA. Hepatitis C virus infection in a sexually active inner city population. The potential for heterosexual transmission. Infection 1994; 22:72–76.

116. Pineda JA, Rivero A, Rey C, Hernandez-Quero J, Vergara A, Munoz J, Aguado I, Santos J, Torronteras R, Gullardo JA. Association between hepatitis C virus seroreactivity and HIV infection in non-intravenous drug abusing prostitutes. Eur J Clin Microbiol Infect Dis 1995; 14:460–464.

117. Lissen E, Alter HJ, Abad MA, Torres Y, Perez-Romero M, Leal M, Pineda JA, Torronteras R, Sanchez-Quijano A. Hepatitis C virus infection among sexually promiscuous groups and the heterosexual partners of hepatitis C virus infected index cases. Eur J Clin Microbiol Infect Dis 1993; 12:827–831.

118. Thomas DL, Cannon RO, Shapiro CN, Hook EW III, Alter MJ, Quinn TC. Hepatitis C, hepatitis B, and human immunodeficiency virus infections among non-intravenous drug-using patients attending clinics for sexually transmitted diseases. J Infect Dis 1994; 169:990–995.

119. Eyster ME, Alter HJ, Aledort LM, Quam S, Hatzakin A, Goedert JJ. Heterosexual co-transmission of hepatitis C virus (HCV) and human immunodeficiency virus (HIV). Ann Intern Med 1991; 115:764–768.

120. Soto B, Rodrigo L, Garcia-Bengoechea M, Sanchez-Quijano A, Riestra S, Arenas JI, Andreu J, Rodriguez M, Emperanza JI, Torres Y. Heterosexual transmission of hepatitis C virus and the possible role of coexistent human immunodeficiency virus infection in the index case. A multicentre study of 423 pairings. J Intern Med 1994; 236:515–519.

121. Ndimbie OK, Kingsley LA, Nedjar S, Rinaldo CR. Hepatitis C virus infection in a male homosexual cohort: risk factor analysis. Genitourin Med 1996; 72:213–216.

122. Bodsworth NJ, Cunningham P, Kaldor J, Donovan B. Hepatitis C virus infection in a large cohort of homosexually active men: independent association with HIV-1 infection and injecting drug use but not sexual behavior. Genitourin Med 1996; 72:118–122.

123. Manzini P, Saracco G, Cerchier A, Riva C, Musso A, Ricotti E, Palomba E, Scolfaro C, Verme G, Bonino F. Human immunodeficiency virus infection as risk factor for mother-to-child hepatitis C virus transmission; persistence of anti-hepatitis C virus in children is associated with the mother's anti-hepatitis C virus immunoblotting pattern. Hepatology 1995; 21:328–332.

124. Connor EM, Sperling RS, Gelber R, Kiselev P, Scott G, O'Sullivan MJ, VanDyke R, Bey M, Shearer W, Jacobsen RL, Jimenez E, O'Neill E, Bazin B, Delfraissey JF, Culnane M, Coombs R, Elkins M, Moye J, Stratton P, Balsley J. Reduction of maternal-infant transmission of human immunodeficiency virus type 1 with zidovudine treatment. N Engl J Med 1994; 331:1173–1180.

125. Lam JPH, McOmish F, Burns SM, Yap PL, Mok JYQ, Simmonds P. Infrequent vertical transmission of hepatitis C virus. J Infect Dis 1993; 167:572–576.

126. Ohto H, Terazawa S, Sasaki N, Sasaki N, Hino K, Ishiwata C, Kako M, Vjiie N, Erdo C, Matsui A, Okamoto H, Mishiro S. Transmission of hepatitis C virus from mother to infants. N Engl J Med 1994; 330:744–750.

127. Lin HH, Kao JH, Hsu HY, Ni YH, Yeh SH, Hwang LH, Chang MH, Hwang SC, Chen PJ, Chen DS. Possible role of high-titer maternal viremia in perinatal transmission of hepatitis C virus. J Infect Dis 1994; 169:638–641.

128. Giovannini M, Tagger A, Ribero ML, Zuccotti G, Pogliani L, Grossi A, Ferroni P, Fiocchi A. Maternal-infant transmission of hepatitis C virus and HIV infections: a possible interaction [letter]. Lancet 1990; 335:1166.

129. Papaevangelou V, Pollack H, Rochford G, Kokka R, Hou Z, Chernoff D, Hanna B, Krasinski K, Borkowsky W. Increased transmission of vertical hepatitis C virus (HCV) infection to human immunodeficiency virus (HIV)-infected infants of HIV- and HCV-coinfected women. J Infect Dis 1998; 178:1047–1052.

130. Hershow RC, Riester KA, Lew J, Quinn TC, Mofenson LM, Davenny K, Landesman S, Cotton D, Hanson IC, Hillyer GV, Tang HB, Thomas DL. Increased vertical transmission of human immunodeficiency virus from hepatitis C virus-coinfected mothers. Women and Infants Transmission Study. J Infect Dis 1997; 176:414–420.

131. Mofenson LM, Lambert JS, Stiehm ER, Bethel J, Meyer WA 3rd, Whitehouse J, Moye J Jr, Reichelderfer P, Harris DR, Fowler MG, Mathieson BJ, Nemo GJ. Risk factors for perinatal transmission of human immunodeficiency virus type 1 in women treated with zidovudine. N Engl J Med 1999; 341:385–393.

132. The International Perinatal HIV Group. The mode of delivery and the risk of vertical transmission of human immunodeficiency virus type 1—a meta-analysis of 15 prospective cohort studies. N Engl J Med 1999; 340:977–987.

133. Toth CM, Pascual M, Chung RT, Graeme-Cook F, Dienstag JL, Bhan AK, Cosimi AB. HCV-associated fibrosing cholestatic hepatitis after renal transplantation: response to interferon alfa therapy. Transplantation 1998; 66:1254–1258.

134. Gale MJ, Blakely CM, Kwieciszewski B, Tan SL, Dossett M, Tang NM, Korth MJ, Polyak SJ, Gretch DR, Katze MG. Control of PKR protein kinase by the hepatitis C virus nonstructural 5A protein: molecular mechanisms of kinase recognition. Mol Cell Biol 1998; 18:5208–5218.

135. Taylor DR, Shi ST, Romano PR, Barber GN, Lai MMC. Inhibition of the interferon-inducible protein kinase PKR by HCV E2 protein. Science 1999; 285:107–110.

136. Spengler U, Rockstroh JK. Hepatitis C in the patient with human immunodeficiency virus infection. J Hepatol 1998; 29:1023–1030.

137. Seeff LB, Buskell-Bales Z, Wright EC, Durako SJ, Alter HJ, Iber FL, Hollinger FB, Gitnick G, Knodell RG, Perillo RP, Stevens CE, Hollingsworth CG, National HLBISG. Long term mortality after transfusion-associated non-A, non-B hepatitis. N Engl J Med 1992; 327:1906–1911.

138. Tong MJ, El-Farra NS, Reikes AR, Co RL. Clinical outcomes after transfusion-associated hepatitis C. N Engl J Med 1995; 332:1463–1466.

139. Seeff LB. Natural history of hepatitis C. Hepatology 1997; 26(suppl 1):21S–28S.

140. Detre KM, Belle SH, Lombardero M. Liver transplantation for chronic viral hepatitis. Viral Hepat Rev 1996; 2:219–228.

141. Pol S, Rothschild C, Poussin K. HIV coinfection does not modify HCV infection profile in hemophiliacs [abstract]. J Hepatol 1994; 21:S122.

142. Berger A, Depka Prondzinski M, Doerr HW, Rabenau H, Weber B. Hepatitis C plasma viral load is associated with HCV genotype but not with HIV coinfection. J Med Virol 1996; 48:339-343.

143. Allain JP, Dailey SH, Laurian Y, Vallari DS, Rafowicz A, Desai SM, Devare SG. Evidence for persistent hepatitis C virus (HCV) infection in hemophiliacs. J Clin Invest 1991; 88:1672–1679.

144. Sherman KE, O'Brien J, Gutierrez AG, Harrison S, Uredea M, Neuwald P, Wilber J. Quantitative evaluation of hepatitis C virus RNA in patients with concurrent human immunodeficiency virus infections. J Clin Microbiol 1993; 31:2679–2682.

145. Telfer P, Brown D, Devereux H, Lee CA, Dusheiko GM. HCV RNA levels and HIV infection; evidence for a viral interaction in haemophilic patients. Br J Haematol 1994; 88:397–399.

146. Cribier B, Schmitt C, Rey D, Uhl G, Lang JM, Vetter D, Kirn A, Stoll-Keller F. HIV increases hepatitis C viraemia irrespective of hepatitis C virus genotype. Res Virol 1997; 148:267–271.

147. Beld M, Penning M, Lukashov V, McMorrow M, Roos M, Pakker N, van den Hoek A, Goudsmit J. Evidence that both HIV- and HIV-induced immunodeficiency enhance HCV replication among HCV seroconverters. Virology 1998; 244:504–512.

148. Bonanici M, Govindarajan S, Blatt LM, Schmid P, Conrad A, Lindsay KL. Patients coinfected with human immunodeficiency virus and hepatitis C virus demonstrate higher levels of hepatic HCV RNA. J Viral Hepat 1999; 6:203–208.

149. Chambost H, Gerolami V, Halfon P, Thuret I, Michel G, Sicardi F, Rousseau S, Perrimond H, Cartouzou G. Persistent hepatitis C virus RNA replication in haemophiliacs: role of co-infection with human immunodeficiency virus. Br J Haematol 1995; 91:703–707.

150. Ghany MG, Leissinger C, Lagier R, Sanchez-Pescador R, Lok AS. Effect of human immunodeficiency virus infection on hepatitis C virus infection in hemophiliacs. Dig Dis Sci 1996; 41:1265–1272.

151. Matsuda J, Tsukamoto M, Gohchi K, Saitoh N, Gotoh M. Hepatitis C virus (HCV) RNA and human immunodeficiency virus (HIV) p24 antigen in the cryoglobulin of hemophiliacs with HIV and/or HCV infection. Clin Infect Dis 1994; 18:832–833.

152. Eyster ME, Fried MW, Di Bisceglie AM, Goedert JJ. Increasing hepatitis C virus RNA levels in haemophiliacs; relationship to human immunodeficiency virus infection in a haemophiliac population. Blood 1994; 84:1020–1023.

153. Martin P, Di Bisceglie AM, Kassianides C, Lisker-Melman M, Hoofnagle JH. Rapidly progressive non-A, non-B hepatitis in patients with human immunodeficiency virus infection. Gastroenterology 1989; 97:1559–1561.

154. Telfer P, Sabin C, Devereux H, Scott F, Dusheiko GM, Lee C. The progression of HCV-associated liver disease in a cohort of haemophilic patients. Br J Haematol 1994; 87:555–561.

155. Makris M, Preston FE, Rosendaal, FR, Underwood JCE, Rice KM, Triger DR. The natural history of chronic hepatitis C in haemophiliacs. Br J Haematol 1996; 94:746–752.

156. Lesens O, Deschenes M, Steben M, Belanger G, Tsoukas CM. Hepatitis C virus is related to progressive liver disease in human immunodeficiency virus-positive hemophiliacs and should be treated as an opportunistic infection. J Infect Dis 1999; 179:1254–1258.

157. Pol S, Lamorthe B, Thi NT, Thiers V, Carnot F, Zylberberg H, Berthelot P, Brechot C, Nalpas B. Retrospective analysis of the impact of HIV infection and alcohol use on chronic hepatitis C in a large cohort of drug users. J Hepatol 1998; 28:945–950.

158. Rockstroh JK, Spengler U, Sudhop T, Ewig S, Theisen A, Hammerstein U, Bierhoff E, Fischer HP, Oldenburg J, Brackmann HH, Sauerbruch T. Immunosuppression may lead to progression of hepatitis C virus associated liver disease in hemophiliacs coinfected with HIV. Am J Gastroenterol 1996; 91:2563–2568.

159. Diamondstone LS, Blakley SA, Rice JC, Clark RA, Goedert JJ. Prognostic factors for all-cause mortality among hemophiliacs infected with human immunodeficiency virus. Am J Epidemiol 1995; 142:304–313.

160. Bjoro K, Froland SS, Yun Z, Samdal HH, Haaland T. Hepatitis C infection in patients with primary hypogammaglobulinemia after treatment with contaminated immune globulin N Engl J Med 1994; 331:1607–1611.

161. Castanet J, Lacour JP, Bodokh J, Bekri S, Ortonne JP. Porphyria cutanea tarda in association with human immunodeficiency virus infection: is it related to hepatitis C virus infection? Arch Dermatol 1994 130:774–775.

162. O'Connor WJ, Murphy GM, Darby C, Fogarty J, Mulcahy F, O'Moore R, Barnes L. Porphyrin abnormalities in acquired immunodeficiency syndrome. Arch Dermatol 1996; 132:1443–1447.

163. Cheng J-T, Anderson HL, Markowitz GS, Appel GB, Pogue VA, D'Agati VD. Hepatitis C virus-associated glomerular disease in patients with human immunodeficiency virus coinfection. J Am Soc Nephrol 1999; 10:1566–1574.

164. Garcia-Samaniego J, Soriano V, Castilla J, Bravo R, Moreno A, Carbo J, Iniguez A, Gonzalez J, Munoz F. Influence of hepatitis C virus genotypes and HIV infection on histological severity of chronic hepatitis C. Am J Gastroenterol 1997; 92:1130–1134.

165. Bierhoff E, Fischer HP, Willsch E, Rockstroh J, Spengler U, Brackmann HH, Oldenburg J. Liver histopathology in patients with concurrent chronic hepatitis C and HIV infection. Virchows Arch 1997; 430:271–277.

166. Castro A, Pereiro C, Pedreira JD, Agulla JA, Amal F. Influence of HIV infection on chronic hepatitis C in intravenous drug addicts. J Hepatol 1992; 16(suppl 1):84.

167. Guido M, Rugge M, Fattovich G, Rocchetto P, Cassaro M, Chemello L, Noventa F, Giustina G, Alberti A. Human immunodeficiency virus infection and hepatitis C pathology. Liver 1994; 14:314–319.

168. Sanchez-Quijano A, Andreu J, Gavilan F, Luque F, Abad MA, Soto B, Munoz J, Aznar JM, Leal M, Lissen E. Influence of human immunodeficiency virus type 1 infection on the natural course of chronic parenterally acquired hepatitis C. Eur J Clin Microbiol Infect Dis 1995; 14:949–953.

169. Soto B, Sanchez-Quijaro A, Rodrigo L, del Olmo JA, Garcia-Bengoechea M, Hernandez-Quero J, Rey C, Abad MA, Rodriguez M, Sales Gilabert M, Gonzalez F, Miron P, Caruz A, Relimpio F, Torronteras R, Leal M, Lissen E. Human immunodeficiency virus infection modifies the natural history of chronic parenterally-acquired hepatitis C with an unusually rapid progression to cirrhosis. J Hepatol 1997; 26:1–5.

170. Pol S, Fontaine H, Carnot F, Zylberberg H, Berthelot P, Brechot C, Nalpas B. Predictive factors for development of cirrhosis in parenterally acquired chronic hepatitis C: a comparison between immunocompetent and immunocompromised patients. J Hepatol 1998; 29:12–19.

171. Benhamou Y, Bochet M, Di Martino V, Charlotte F, Azria F, Coutellier A, Vidaud M, Bricaire F, Opolon P, Katlama C, Poynard T. Liver fibrosis progression in human immunodeficiency virus and hepatitis C virus coinfected patients. Hepatology 1999; 30:1054–1058.

172. Zylberberg H, Carnot F, Mamzer MF, Blancho G, Legendre C, Pol S. Hepatitis C virus-related fibrosing cholestatic hepatitis after renal transplantation. Transplantation 1997; 63:158–160.

173. Rosenberg PM, Farrell JJ, Abraczinskas DR, Graeme-Cook, FM, Dienstag JL, Chung RT. Rapidly progressive fibrosing cholestatic hepatitis C virus: a fatal variant in HIV-coinfected individuals. Am J Gastroenterol. In press, 2000.

174. Llibre JM, Garcia E, Aloy A, Valls J. Hepatitis C virus infection and progression of infection due to human immunodeficiency virus [letter]. Clin Infect Dis 1993; 16:182.

175. Prince HE, Fang CT. Unaltered lymphocyte subsets in hepatitis C virus-seropositive blood donors. Transfusion 1992; 32:166–168.

176. Dorrucci M, Pezzotti P, Phillips AN, Lepri AC, Rezza G. Coinfection of hepatitis C virus with human immunodeficiency virus and progression to AIDS. J Infect Dis 1995; 172:1503–1508.

177. Macias J, Pineda JA, Leal M, Abad MA, Garcia-Pesquera F, Delgado J, Gallardo JA, Sanchez-Quijano A, Lissen E. Influence of hepatitis C virus infection on the mortality of antiretroviral-treated patients with HIV disease. Eur J Clin Microbiol Infect Dis 1998; 17:167–170.

178. Wright TL, Hollander H, Pu X, Held MJ, Lipson P, Quan S, Polito A, Thaler MM, Bacchetti P, Scharschmidt BF. Hepatitis C in HIV-infected patients with and without AIDS: prevalence and relationship to survival. Hepatology 1994; 20:1152–1155.

179. Piroth L, Duong M, Quantin C, Abrahamowicz M, Michardiere R, Aho LS, Grappin M, Buisson M, Waldner A, Portier H, Chavanet P. Does hepatitis C virus co-infection accelerate clinical and immunological evolution of HIV-infected patients? AIDS 1998; 12:381–388.

180. Sabin CA, Telfer P, Philips AN, Bhagani S, Lee CA. The association between hepatitis C virus genotype and human immunodeficiency virus disease progression in a cohort of hemophilic men. J Infect Dis 1997; 175:164–168.

181. Piroth L, Bourgeois C, Dantin S, Waldner A, Grappin M, Portier H, Chavanet P. Hepatitis C virus (HCV) genotype does not appear to be a significant prognostic factor in HIV-HCV-coinfected patients. AIDS 1999; 13:523–524.

182. Hammer SM, Squires KE, Hughes MD, Grimes JM, Demeter LM, Currier JS, Eron JJ JR, Feinberg JE, Balfour HH Jr, Deyton LR, Chodakewitz JA, Fischl MA. A controlled trial of two nucleoside analogues plus indinavir in persons with human immunodeficiency virus infection and CD4 cell counts of 200 per cubic millimeter or less. N Engl J Med 1997; 337:725–733.

183. Jacobson MA, French M. Altered natural history of AIDS-related opportunistic infections in the era of potent combination antiretroviral therapy. AIDS 1997; 12(suppl A):S157–S163.

184. Garofano T, Vento S, Di Perri G, Concia E, Bassetti D. AZT induces remission of chronic active C virus hepatitis in subjects with HIV-1 infection. G Ital Chemother 1991; 38:193–194.

185. Vento S, Garofano T, Di Perri G, Cruciani M, Concia E, Bassetti D. Zidovudine therapy associated with remission of chronic hepatitis C in HIV-1 carriers. AIDS 1991; 5:776.

186. Karras A, Rabian C, Zylberberg H, Hermine O, Duchatella V, Durand F, Valla D, Viard JP. Severe anoxic hepatic necrosis in an HIV-1-hepatitis C-co-infected patient starting antiretroviral triple combination therapy [letter]. AIDS 1998; 12:827–829.

187. Rutschmann OT, Negro F, Hirschel B, Hadengue A, Anwar D, Perrin LH. Impact of treatment with human immunodeficiency virus (HIV) protease inhibitors on hepatitis C viremia in patients coinfected with HIV. J Infect Dis 1998; 177:783–785.

188. Zylberberg H, Chaix ML, Rabian C, Rouzioux C, Aulong B, Brechot C, Viard JP, Pol S. Tritherapy for human immunodeficiency virus infection does not modify replication of hepatitis C virus in coinfected subjects. Clin Infect Dis 1998; 26:1104–1106.

189. Rockstroh JK, Theisen A, Kaiser R, Sauerbruch T, Spengler U. Antiretroviral triple therapy decreases HIV viral load but does not alter hepatitis C virus (HCV) serum levels in HIV-HCV-co-infected haemophiliacs [letter]. AIDS 1998; 12:829–830.

190. John M, Flexman J, French MA. Hepatitis C virus-associated hepatitis following treatment of HIV-infected patients with HIV protease inhibitors: an immune restoration disease? AIDS 1998; 12:2289–2293.

191. Vento S, Garofano T, Renzini C, Casali F, Ferraro T, Concia E. Enhancement of hepatitis C virus replication and liver damage in HIV-coinfected patients on antiretroviral combination therapy. AIDS 1998; 12:116–117.

192. Zylberberg H, Pialoux G, Carnot F, Landau A, Brechot C, Pol S. Rapidly evolving hepatitis C virus-related cirrhosis in a human immunodeficiency virus-infected patient receiving triple antiretroviral therapy. Clin Infect Dis 1998; 27:1255–1258.

193. McHutchison JG, Gordon SC, Schiff ER, Shiffman ML, Lee WM, Rustgi VK, Goodman ZD, Ling MH, Cort S, Albrecht J. Interferon alfa-2b alone or in combination with ribavirin as initial treatment for chronic hepatitis C. Hepatitis Interventional Therapy Group. N Engl J Med 1998; 339:1485–1492.

194. Davis GL, Esteban-Mur R, Rustgi V. Interferon alfa-2b alone or in combination with ribavirin for the treatment of relapse of chronic hepatitis C. International Hepatitis Interventional Therapy Group. N Engl J Med 1998; 339:1493–1499.

195. Soriano V, Rodriguez-Rosado R, Garcia-Samaniego J. Management of chronic hepatitic C in HIV-infected patients. AIDS 1999; 13:539–546.

196. Hartshorn KL, Vogt MW, Chou TC, Blumberg RS, Byington R, Schooley RT, Hirsch MS. Synergistic inhibition of human immunodeficiency virus in vitro by azidothymidine and recombinant alfa interferon. Antimicrobiol Agents Chemother 1987; 31:168–172.

197. Lane HC, Davey V, Kovacs JA, Feinberg J, Metcalf JA, Herpin B, Walker R, Deyton L, Davey RT Jr, Falloon J. Interferon-alpha in patients with asymptomatic human immunodeficiency virus (HIV) infection. A randomized, placebo-controlled trial. Ann Intern Med 1990; 112:805–811.

198. Fischl MA, Richman DD, Saag M, Meng TC, Squires KE, Holden-Wiltse J, Meehan PM. Safety and antiviral activity of combination therapy with zidovu-

dine, zalcitabine, and two doses of interferon-alpha-2a in patients with HIV:
AIDS Clinical Trials Group Study 197. J Acquir Immune Defic Syndr 1997;
16:247–253.

199. Kovacs JA, Bechtel C, Davey RT Jr, Falloon J, Polis MA, Walker RE, Metcalf
      JA, Davey V, Piscitelli SC, Baseler M, Dewar R, Salzman NP, Masur H, Lane
      HC. Combination therapy with didanosine and interferon-alpha in human im-
      munodeficiency virus-infected patients: results of a phase I/II trial. J Infect Dis
      1996; 173:840–848.

200. Fernandez-Cruz E, Lang J-M, Frissen J, Furner V, Chateauvert M, Boucher
      CA, Dowd P, Stevens J. Zidovudine plus interferon versus zidovudine alone in
      HIV-infected symptomatic or asymptomatic persons with CD4+ cell counts >
      150 × 106/L: results of the Zidon trial. AIDS 1995; 9:1025–1036.

201. Soriano V, Garcia-Lerma G, Bravo R, Garcia-Samaniego J, Gonzalez J, Castro
      A, Gonzalez-Lahoz J. Lack of antiretroviral effect of alpha-interferon in HIV-
      infected patients treated for chronic hepatitis C [letter]. J Infect 1997; 35:319–
      320.

202. Vento S, Di Perri G, Cruciani M, Garofano T, Cancia E, Basseti D. Rapid
      decline of CD4+ cells after IFN alpha treatment in HIV-1 infection [letter].
      Lancet 1993; 341:958–959.

203. Soriano V, Bravo R, Samaniego JG, Gonzalez J, Odriozola PM, Arroyo E,
      Vicano JL, Castro A, Colmenero M, Carballo E. CD4+ T-lymphocytopenia
      in HIV-infected patients receiving interferon therapy for chronic hepatitis C.
      AIDS 1994; 8:1621–1622.

204. Peters M, Davis GL, Dooley JS, Hoofnagle JH. The interferon system in acute
      and chronic viral hepatitis. In: Popper H, Schaffner F, eds. Progress in Liver
      Diseases. New York: Grune and Stratton, 1986:453–467.

205. Marcellin P, Boyer N, Behamou J-P, Erlinger S. Interferon-alfa therapy for
      chronic hepatitis C in special patient populations. Dig Dis Sci 1996; 12(suppl):
      126S–30S

206. Dieterich DT, Purow JM, Rajapaksa R. Activity of combination therapy with
      interferon alfa-2b plus ribavirin in chronic hepatitis C patients co-infected with
      HIV. Sem Liver Dis 1999; 19(suppl 1):87–94.

207. Boyer N, Marcellin P, Degott C, Saimot AG, Erlinger S, Benhamou JP. Recom-
      binant interferon-alfa for chronic hepatitis C in patients positive for antibody
      to human immunodeficiency virus. J Infect Dis 1992; 165:723–726.

208. Nardiello S, Gargiulo M, Pizzella T. Interferon treatment for chronic HCV and
      NANB hepatitis in HIV seropositive patients [abstract]. In: Program and Ab-
      stracts of the 8th International Conference on AIDS (Amsterdam). Amsterdam,
      The Netherlands: CONGREX Holland BV, 1992:B149. Abstract 3373.

209. Marriott E, Navas S, Del Romero J, Garcia S, Castillo I, Quiroga JA, Carreno V. Treatment with recombinant alpha-interferon of chronic hepatitis C in anti-HIV-positive patients. J Med Virol 1993; 40:107–111.

210. De Sanctis GM, Errera G, Barbacini G, Leonetti G, Bergami N, Chireu LV. Long term outcome of chronic hepatitis infection in HIV + subjects treated with interferon [abstract]. In: Program and Abstracts of the 9th International Conference on AIDS (Berlin). Berlin, Germany: Insititute for Clinical and Experimental Virology of the Free University of Berlin, 1993:B10. Abstract 1822.

211. Marcellin P, Boyer N, Areias J. Comparison of efficacy of alfa-interferon in former intravenous drug addicts with chronic hepatitis with or without HIV-infection. Gastroenterology 1994; 107:A9.

212. Arcias J, Pedroto I, Barrias S, Maros P, Freitas T, Saraiva AM. Pilot study of interferon alpha 2b treatment of chronic hepatitis C in patients coinfected with the human immunodeficiency virus [abstract 264]. Hepatology 1994; 20:162A.

213. Pol S, Trinh T, Thiers V, Jaffredo F, Carnot F. Chronic hepatitis of drug users: influence of HIV infection [abstract 933]. Hepatology 1995; 22:340A.

214. Soriano V, Garcia-Samaniego J, Bravo R, Gonzalez J, Castro A, Castilla J, Martinez-Odriozola P, Colmenero M, Carballo E, Suarez D, Rodriguez-Pinero FJ, Moreno A, del Romero J, Pedreira J, Gonzalez-Lahoz J. Interferon alfa for the treatment of chronic hepatitis C in patients infected with human immun-odeficiency virus. Clin Infect Dis 1996; 23:585–591.

215. Piliero PJ, Szebeny IS, Bartholome WC, et al. Recombinant interferon therapy for chronic hepatitis C in patients with HIV. Abstracts of the 4th Conference on Retroviruses and Opportunistic Infections, Washington, 1997:672.

216. Venkataramani A, Roud R, Beaumont C, Lyche K. Interferon therapy in patients coinfected with hepatitis C (HCV) and human immunodeficiency virus (HIV) [Abstract 738]. Hepatology 1997; 26:313A.

217. Causse X. Chronic hepatitis C should be treated even among HIV patients. A prospective, multicenter study conducted in France [Abstract 734]. Hepatology 1997; 26:312A.

218. Mauss S, Klinker H, Ulmer A, Willers R, Weissbrich B, Albrecht H, Haussinger D, Jablonowski H. Response to treatment of chronic hepatitis C with interferon alpha in patients infected with HIV-1 is associated with higher CD4+ cell count. Infection 1998; 26:16–19.

219. Ning Q, Brown D, Parodo J, Cattral M, Gorczynski R, Cole E, Fung L, Ding JW, Liu MF, Rotstein O, Phillips MJ, Levy G. Ribavirin inhibits viral-induced macrophage production of TNF, IL-1, the procoagulant fgl2 prothrombinase and preserves Th1 cytokine production but inhibits Th2 cytokine response. J Immunol 1998; 160:3487–3493.

220. Crumpacker C, Heagy W, Bubley G, Monroe JE, Finberg R, Hussey S, Schnipper L, Lucey D, Lee TH, McLane MF, Essex M, Mulder C. Ribavirin treatment of the acquired immunodeficiency syndrome (AIDS) and the acquired-immunodeficiency-syndrome-related complex (ARC). A phase 1 study shows transient clinical improvement associated with suppression of the human immunodeficiency virus and enhanced lymphocyte proliferation. Ann Intern Med 1987; 107:664–674.

221. Schulof RS, Parenti DM, Simon GL, Paxton H, Meyer WA 3rd, Schlesselman SB, Courtless J, LeLacheur S, Sztein MB. Clinical, virologic, and immunologic effects of combination therapy with ribavirin and isoprinosine in HIV-infected homosexual men. J Acquir Immune Defic Syndr 1990; 3:485–492.

222. Roberts RB, Hollinger FB, Parks WP, Rasheed S, Laurence J, Heseltine PNR, Makuch RW, Lubina JA, Johnson KM. A multicenter clinical trial of oral ribavirin in HIV-infected people with lymphadenopathy: virologic observations. Ribavirin-LAS Collaborative Group. AIDS 1990; 4:67–72.

223. Roberts RB, Dickinson GM, Heseltine PNR, Leedom JM, Mansell PWA, Rodriguez S, Johnson KM, Lubina JA, Makuch RW. A multicenter clinical trial of oral ribavirin in HIV-infected patients with lymphadenopathy. J Acquir Immune Defic Syndr 1990; 3:884–892.

224. The Ribavirin ARC Study Group. Multicenter clinical trial of oral ribavirin in symptomatic HIV-infected patients. J Acquir Immune Def Syndr 1993; 6:32–41.

225. Baba M, Pauwels R, Balzarini J, Herdewijn P, DeClercq E, Desmyter J. Ribarvirin antagonizes the inhibitory effects of pyrimidine 2′-3′-dideoxynucleosides but enhances inhibitory effects of purine 2′,3′-dideoxynucleosides on replication of human immunodeficiency virus in vitro. Antimicrob Agents Chemother 1987; 31:1613–1617.

226. Balzarini J, Lee CK, Herdewijn P, De Clercq E. Mechanism of the potentiating effect of ribavirin on the activity of 2′,3′-dideoxyinosine against human immunodeficiency virus. J Biol Chem 1991; 266:21509–21514.

227. Balzarini J, Naesens L, Robins MJ, De Clercq E. Potentiating effect of ribavirin on the in vitro and in vivo antiretrovirus activities of 2′,3′-dideoxyinosine and 2′,3′-dideoxy-2,6-diaminopurine riboside. J Acquir Immune Defic Syndr 1990; 3:1140–1147.

228. Zylberberg H, Landau A, Chaix M-L, Fontaine H, Pialoux G, Brechot C, Pol S. Ribavirin does not modify HIV replication in HCV-HIV coinfected subjects under antiretroviral regimen [Abstract 1267]. Hepatology 1998; 28:479A.

229. Landau A, Batisse D, Duong JP. Efficacy of combination therapy with interferon-alpha 2b and ribavirin for chronic hepatitis C in HIV-infected patients. Program and abstracts of the 39th ICAAC; September 26–29, 1999, San Francisco, CA. Abstract 113.

230. Dieterich D, Weisz K, Goldman D. Interferon (IFN) and ribavirin (RBV) therapy for hepatitis C (HCV) in HIV-coinfected patients. Program and abstracts of the 39th ICAAC; September 26–29, 1999, San Francisco, CA. Abstract 102.

231. Shiffman M, Pockros PJ, Reddy R. A controlled, randomized, multicenter descending dose phase II trial of pegylated interferon alfa-2a (PEG) vs standard interferon alfa-2a (IFN) for treatment of chronic hepaitis C. Gastroenterology 1999; 116:A1275.

232. Davis GL, Nelson DR, Reyes GR. Future options for the management of hepatitis C. Semin Liver Dis 1999; 19(suppl 1):103–112.

233. Tsai SL, Liaw YF, Chen MH, Huang CY, Kuo GC. Detection of type 2-like T-helper cells in hepatitis C virus infection: implications for hepatitis C virus chronicity. Hepatology 1997; 25:440–458.

234. Davey RT, Chaitt DG, Piscitelli SC, Wells M, Kovacs JA, Walker RE, Falloon J, Polis MA, Metcalf JA, Masur H, Fyfe G, Lane HC. Subcutaneous administration of interleukin-2 in human immunodeficiency virus type 1 infected persons. J Infect Dis 1997; 175:783–789.

235. Uberti-Foppa C, De Bona A, Morsica G, Guffanti M, Gianotti N, Boeri E, Lazzarin A. Recombinant interleukin-2 for treatment of HIV reduces hepatitis C viral load in coinfected patients. AIDS 1999; 13:140–141.

236. Ragni MV, Dodson SF, Hunt SC, Bontempo FA, Fung JJ. Liver transplantation in a hemophilia patient with acquired immunodeficiency syndrome. Blood 1999; 93:1113–1114.

237. Vento S, Garofano T, Renzini C, Cainelli F, Casali F, Ghironzi G, Ferraro T, Concia E. Fulminant hepatitis associated with hepatitis A virus superinfection in patients with chronic hepatitis C. N Engl J Med 1998; 338:286–290.

238. Berggren RE, Burman W, Keiser P. Impact of acute hepatitis A on 35 HIV-1-infected patients. Program and abstracts of the 39th ICAAC; September 26–29, 1999, San Francisco, CA. Abstract 97.

239. Bodsworth NJ, Neilsen GA, Donovan B. The effect of immunization with inactivated hepatitis A vaccine on the clinical course of HIV-1 infection: 1-year follow-up. AIDS 1997; 11:747–749.

240. Lechner F, Wong DKH, Dunbar PR, Chapman R, Chung RT, Dohrenwend P, Robbins G, Phillips R, Klenerman P, Walker BD. Analysis of successful immune responses in persons infected with hepatitis C virus. J Exp Med 2000; 191:1499–1512.

Index

About the Editors

PAUL A. VOLBERDING is Professor of Medicine at the University of California, San Francisco, and Director of the UCSF Positive Health Program at San Francisco General Hospital. A leading figure in AIDS research, Dr. Volberding has authored or coauthored more than 100 technical articles and abstracts and has coauthored or contributed chapters to more than 25 books and monographs. He served as Co-Chairperson to the VI International Conference on AIDS, held in June 1990, in San Francisco, California, as well as President of the International AIDS Society (1990–1992). The Founder and Board Chair of the International AIDS Society-USA Inc., he is a member of the Institute of Medicine of the National Academy of Sciences, the HIV Research Agenda Committee of the AIDS Clinical Trials Group of the ACTG, and the Scientific Advisory Committee for the RAND Study of AIDS care, utilization, and outcome. Dr. Volberding received the B.A. degree (1971) from the University of Chicago, Illinois, and the M.D. degree (1975) from the University of Minnesota, Minneapolis.

MARK A. JACOBSON is Professor of Medicine in Residence, Positive Health Program, Infectious Diseases, and Clinical Pharmacology, Department of Medicine, University of California at San Francisco, and the Medical Service, San Francisco General Hospital, where he is also Director of the AIDS Clinical Trials Unit. An authority on AIDS research, Dr. Jacobson has authored many book chapters, articles, and abstracts in leading medical journals. He has recently served as Chair of the HIV complications Research Agenda Committee of the National Institute of Allergy and Infectious Diseases Adult AIDS Clinical Trials Group. He received the B.A. degree (1971) from the University of California, Berkeley, and the M.D. degree (1981) from the University of California, San Francisco.

Milton Keynes UK
Ingram Content Group UK Ltd.
UKHW031128141024
449569UK00006B/366